Manual of Veterinary Dietetics

Manual of Veterinary Dietetics

C.A. Tony Buffington, DVM, PhD, DACVN

Cheryl Holloway, RVT

Sarah K. Abood, DVM, PhD

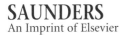

SAUNDERS
An Imprint of Elsevier

SAUNDERS
An Imprint of Elsevier

11830 Westline Industrial Drive
St. Louis, Missouri 63146

MANUAL OF VETERINARY DIETETICS   0-7216-0123-5

NOTICE

Veterinary medicine is an ever-changing field. Standard safety precautions must be followed, but as new
research and clinical experience broaden our knowledge, changes in treatment and drug therapy may
become necessary or appropriate. Readers are advised to check the most current product information
provided by the manufacturer of each drug or therapeutic diet to be administered to verify the
recommended dose, the method and duration of administration, and contraindications. It is the
responsibility of the licensed prescriber, relying on experience and knowledge of the patient, to
determine dosages and the best treatment for each individual patient. Neither the publisher nor the
author assumes any liability for any injury and/or damage to persons or property arising from this
publication.

International Standard Book Number 0-7216-0123-5

Publishing Director: Linda Duncan
Senior Editor: Liz Fathman
Developmental Editor: Shelly Dixon
Publishing Services Manager: Patricia Tannian
Project Manager: Sarah Wunderly
Senior Book Designer: Amy Buxton

Printed in United States
Last digit is the print number: 9   8   7   6   5   4   3   2   1

We wrote this handbook of clinical dietetics for veterinarians, veterinary students, and technicians in companion animal practice. We intend it primarily as a guide to diet and feeding recommendations for healthy and sick patients. We base recommendations on physical and nutritional assessment of the patients and the wishes and abilities of clients. We have tried to focus on indications, possible adverse reactions, contraindications, and ongoing evaluation of the efficacy of the interventions suggested. We also have provided suggestions for implementing the recommendations, and for client communication and education. These recommendations reflect our background in academic clinical practice in Columbus, Ohio, and East Lansing, Michigan, where we communicate with and advise veterinarians, technicians, and students on these issues on a daily basis.

A sound scientific basis for therapeutic recommendations depends on well-designed and controlled clinical trials in the patient population of interest. Few of these trials have been conducted for the myriad of therapeutic diets currently marketed by pet food manufacturers. We have tried to make recommendations based on relevant evidence whenever possible and have tried to point out areas of limited knowledge that would benefit from more clinical research. We hope to stimulate discussion and more research to fill in the many gaps in our understanding of the effects of diets and nutrients on our patients.

Introduction

We have chosen to present the information in this handbook somewhat differently from most pet nutrition books, because we intend it to help practitioners—clinicians, technicians, and students—help owners with concerns about their pets, rather than to teach nutrition. The client's concern for the quality of various commercial foods, the validity of advertising claims, and requests for recipes for "homemade" foods all may lead owners to seek nutritional advice. We initiate discussions of diet and nutrition with new clients and teach owners how to identify normal body condition, choose a satisfactory diet for their pet, the

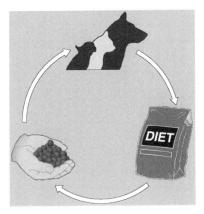

basics of feeding management, and ways to introduce new foods to "finicky" eaters. We also provide information on diets and feeding management of breeding animals, discuss diet and nutrient needs for different life stages when the physiologic status of a patient changes, and make diet and feeding recommendations for sick animals. In these circumstances nutrition may be part of the problem, or it may be part of the solution.

To determine the role of nutrition in any given situation, we recommend the method depicted in the illustration. This method, developed by the curriculum committee of the American College of Veterinary Nutrition (ACVN), helps ensure that all the important nutritional factors related to each clinical situation are considered. As veterinarians and animal technicians, we usually begin by assessing the following relevant factors.

- Animal factors—signalment, physiologic status, food intake, and environment.
- Diet factors—quality, completeness, balance, nutrient availability, and palatability.
- Feeding factors—diet availability and the method of feeding.
- Owner factors—owner attitudes, wishes, needs, and abilities.
- Client communications—veterinarian's and technician's ability to communicate information, instructions, and advice.

Finally, all the information collected is synthesized into an opinion of the role these factors play in the given situation.

Our goal is to sustain the nutritional health of the pets we care for without adversely affecting the quality of the bond between our clients and their pets. An associated issue in our practice is that many urban clients do not have extensive experience as pet owners, and appreciate advice that may seem elementary to animal care professionals. The depth of the nutritional assessment will depend on our initial evaluation of the patient. The veterinarian, technician, or both may participate in the intervention, depending on the complexity of the case and amount of time required for data collection and client education.

Animal Factors

We begin by considering the age, physiologic state, and amount of activity of the patient. If we are lucky, we can begin our relationship with the client when the pet is a puppy or kitten so we can get the owner off to a good start. This is the time we recommend a diet we trust, and discuss any information, or misinformation, the client may have received about feeding the new pet. We become concerned when clients reveal that they are feeding a "fad" or home-prepared diet, they are giving a variety of supplements, or they are providing an overly rigid diet or feeding regimen a well-meaning breeder has recommended. Listening to clients' concerns and explaining that commercial pet food quality has improved so much that home-prepared diets and supplementation no longer are necessary (and could be hazardous) usually will convince them of the wisdom of feeding a prepared pet food. If not, we recommend that they have their pet examined frequently to ensure that all continues to go well.

The initial visit also is the time to explain that urban pets, like urban people, are at risk of obesity because of the ready availability of highly palatable foods and the lack of opportunities for calorie-burning activities. To prevent future problems with obesity and begging for food, many clients need help learning to feed their pet to a moderate body condition and to establish a tradition of non–food-related interactions with their pet. We teach owners to feed whatever amount of food is necessary to maintain a moderate (3/5 or

5/9) body condition (see Fig. 1-1 in Chapter 1). If they have limited experience with animals, we show them the elements of moderate body condition by having them palpate the ribs and waist of their pet under our supervision, so that we can advise them if the animal needs more, less, or the same amount of food. Another advantage of teaching owners to feed according to body condition is that most people use (or should use) the same method themselves. Few people know how many cups or calories of food they need to eat to maintain moderate body condition. People usually decrease intake when their clothes become a little snug, and we can teach our clients to do essentially the same thing with their pets.

We can also help clients maintain their pet's body condition by recommending non–food-related interactions. Teaching the pet tricks, playing with it, and walking it regularly instead of feeding it when it wants attention all help maintain a bond that does not depend on food. Owners sometimes confuse begging for attention with begging for food. They can differentiate the two by throwing a favorite toy for the pet to fetch when it looks longingly at them. If it fetches the toy, it was more interested in attention than food.

Diet Factors

One of the most common nutrition-related client questions is, "what should I feed my pet?" The practitioner can learn to answer this question confidently by obtaining diet histories on all patients and creating a list of diets that seem to perform well for these animals. The list of satisfactory foods will vary with geography and socioeconomic status of clients in the practice but will always be based on clinical experience and personal judgment rather than on marketing claims that may be irrelevant to individual circumstances. As practitioners, we have a daily opportunity to evaluate the quality of diets. We can then recommend those diets with which we have had positive experiences and recommend against diets when a pattern of inadequacy is discerned. Moreover, the absence of a product from the list does not mean that it is unacceptable, only that we have insufficient experience with it to make a recommendation. This method of choosing diets is analogous to the decision-making process for many pharmaceutical preparations we use and recommend each day.

Feeding Factors

Owners can adjust the frequency and timing of feeding of their pets to their convenience to maintain moderate body condition and to facilitate toilet habits. Although both the amount and timing of feeding may be important during some physiologic states, the majority of urban pets are inactive, neutered adults. These pets do not need many calories to maintain themselves in a moderate body condition, so they may consume only small volumes of food, sometimes much less than label suggestions. Manufacturer's feeding directions are only initial guidelines, often established based on the intake of quite active animals. We explain to owners that individual animals might need to eat twice, or half, as much as label recommendations to maintain moderate body condition, depending on their temperament and activity.

The number of feedings necessary to maintain the desired condition ranges from continuous availability of food to one small meal per day. We generally recommend that owners feed dogs shortly before their walk, usually after work. A small meal in the morning before they leave for work is all right; feeding the majority of the food when the owner is at home reduces begging if the owner feeds only small amounts to maintain moderate body condition.

Owner Factors

Owners who spend large amounts of time at home with the pet seem especially likely to want to provide their pet with treats. We can help them do this without sacrificing the pet's body condition by teaching them the difference between replacing calories and supplementing them. If they want to feed treats, they need to understand that these should replace some of the pet's regular food, not be added to it. Some clients are willing to set part of the daily ration of dry food apart to provide as treats, or to reduce the daily ration so that they can provide treats. As long as the treats do not account for more than about 25% of the daily calories, this practice is not dangerous to the pet and may bring great enjoyment to the owner.

The ACVN approach also permits the practitioner to divide nutrition-related diseases into those that are nutrient sensitive, diet induced, and feeding related. In addition, it provides an organized approach to evaluation of manufacturers' claims for new diets by stressing the importance of assessing the appropriateness of the animals tested, the diet changes made, and the feeding protocols used in studies. Results obtained in young, healthy animals with induced disease fed a diet on a free-choice basis and consuming relatively large quantities per day may not predict the response of aged animals that have naturally occurring disease and eat small amounts of food. Consideration of all these aspects helps us make better informed diet therapy decisions.

We attempt to provide a basis for dietary decision-making in this book. Because manufacturers regularly introduce new foods to fill veterinary and client needs, we emphasize desirable nutrient profiles rather than specific foods. Selecting an appropriate food helps ensure our patients' general health and performance, because pets often cannot obtain adequate nutrition by eating a variety of foods as humans do.

Client Communication

Our ability to communicate with clients determines our success. Effective nutritional support depends on obtaining an accurate diet history and successful compliance with recommendations by the pet owner. Effective communication requires us to do the following:
- Determine the emotional state of the owner.
- Evaluate the owner's knowledge and understanding of the situation.
- Ask open-ended questions.
- Actively listen to client responses.
- Accurately interpret verbal cues such as silence.
- Recognize nonverbal cues from the client's body language.
- Provide clear, unambiguous instructions.

We try to determine the emotional state of owners first because it determines their ability to provide information and understand instructions. Clients who are frightened, worried, or angry may not be able to think clearly, and first may need to be calmed and comforted. This often happens when the owner brings an animal in for emergency treatment.

We need to learn to identify who actually feeds the pet, because that person can provide the most accurate information on what is being fed, how much, and how often. We can obtain only partial or incomplete information when the primary caretaker of the pet is not present; when this happens, we recommend sending home a comprehensive diet history form that the primary caretaker can complete and telephone us about, or mail or fax back as soon as possible.

Once we decide the client is ready and able to provide a history, we try to ask open-ended questions. Open-ended questions are those that do not result in a black or white, yes or no, answer. They invite the client to describe what happens to their individual pet in their unique environment. Using open-ended questions may require more time; we allow the client to provide information by "painting a picture" we might not otherwise be able to see. Asking open-ended questions also avoids the temptation for clients to provide answers they think we may want to hear.

Actively listening to what our clients say involves using our own body language to indicate that we are really hearing what they have to say. Body language that tells clients we are open and ready to listen includes facing them squarely, smiling and making eye contact, nodding the head while listening, standing or sitting with arms unfolded and palms open, and leaning forward toward the client. Actively listening also means responding in a way that tells clients we have heard what they said. Active responses include clarifying (asking another question if the client's response was unclear), paraphrasing (putting the client's information into our own words to make sure we have gotten the right perspective or angle), reflecting (repeating what was said to show support), and summarizing (bringing disjointed events and information into focus or bringing closure to an interview). Active listening skills require some measure of patience and tolerance, as well as practice. There are numerous books, websites, and workshops available for training in this area. Two examples we like are: *Listening: The Forgotten Skill (A Self-Teaching Guide)* by Madelyn Burley-Allen and *Nutrition Counseling Skills for Medical Nutrition Therapy* by Linda G. Snetselaar.

What should we do when clients remain silent in the examination room? How do we interpret silence as a [verbal] clue? In an effort to prevent long periods of silence, some practitioners continue talking, thinking that the client has not quite grasped the explanation or intention, whereas others abruptly cut the interview short and make a hasty exit. Silence on the part of the client could mean one of three things: they understand what the practitioner is saying and are waiting for him or her to continue; they do not understand what the practitioner has said and are hesitant to ask questions; or they simply require a bit of time to process the information the practitioner has just shared and to formulate their question. It is imperative that clients be allowed the necessary time to think before reacting to information on which their next decision will be based. Along the same line, how should we interpret short responses, such as "okay," "I see," or "I get it"? These types of verbal cues may or may not indicate that the client is following what the practitioner is saying and is in agreement. For some clients these phrases represent a noncommitment and are said just to keep up their end of the interview, but most practitioners and technicians would interpret these responses to mean the client understands and will comply.

Suggestions for handling the minimally responsive or quiet clients include the following:
- If you tend to talk quickly, slow your speaking pace
- Ask the client to help determine if the communication was clear by restating what was just told to them or ask if something did not make sense
- If the direct approach is preferred, ask the client, "Does your silence mean I confused you? If so, what was the last thing that made sense?"

Another important verbal cue is the word "But. . .", usually followed by some telling piece of information to which the practitioner should pay close attention for shaping or designing dietary recommendations. Many clients will not directly say what they cannot or will not do in regard to the practitioner's recommendations; however, they may exclaim, "But she really loves those bacon strips I fry up every morning." This verbal cue indicates a behavior that the client is reluctant to change, despite the best arguments, and the practitioner will need to determine if there is a way the owner can moderate the behavior to minimize any dietary and health risks to their pet.

Recognizing and interpreting nonverbal cues are just as important as trying to interpret what the client is (or is not) saying. Most practitioners can spot an "engaged" client; one who is making direct eye contact, is nodding the head with the body leaning forward, all poised and ready to take in information. But what does it mean when the client is standing with crossed arms, frowning, making little to no eye contact, has clenched hands, or is sitting with the body completely turned away and one leg crossed over the other? Rather than ignoring this closed, unresponsive, or negative communication signal, the practitioner should acknowledge it up front by telling the client, "I get the impression this is hard for you," and then wait for the client to respond.

Providing clear, unambiguous instructions is often more difficult than it sounds. If most people who garage their car are asked how they get to work, most will forget to mention that they open the garage door before leaving the garage! The same concept can be applied to giving go-home feeding instructions to clients. Clients better remember information given during the first third of any communication, so organize what information is to be given and how it will be given. For common questions (or the most common dietary recommendations), consider preparing a written handout with clear, concise instructions that the client can read and follow once they get home. Having the owner write down the instructions given and review them with the practitioner also works well. Other guidelines for sharing or conveying information include the following points.
- Limit the amount of information given at any one time.
- Give specific, concrete, and simple instructions.
- Use oral and written material together (draw stick figures or use pictures from wall charts, books, or brochures).
- Check the client's comprehension by asking the client to restate the key features of the instructions.
- Do not assume the client can read, write, or do simple math.
- Do not assume that clinical terms, such as vomiting and diarrhea, mean the same thing to practitioners and clients—clarify exactly what is meant and what the client should look for.
- Ask for and discuss the client's feelings (and biases) about the information provided.
- Repeat important information.

- Whenever possible, involve all members of the household, or significant others, in the therapeutic process.

Successful client communication skills are interwoven throughout the iterative process of animal, diet, and feeding management. Although it helps to have some natural talent at interviewing or expressing empathy, the best practitioners and technicians mindfully practice these skills on a daily basis. Regardless of the point at which the iterative process is entered, a few key questions to consider when approaching or developing the best strategy for effectively communicating with individual clients about their pets are: Why is the client here? Is the dietary problem the client describes all or only part of the problem? What are the nutrition behaviors and related concerns that can be addressed?

C.A. Tony Buffington
  The Ohio State University
Sarah Abood
  Michigan State University
Cheryl Holloway
  The Ohio State University

CONTENTS

1   Nutritional Assessment,   1

History,   1
Physical Examination,   2
Laboratory Evaluation,   6
Summary of Nutritional Assessment,   6

2   Normal Dogs,   9

Feeding During Gestation and Lactation,   9
Puppy Care and Feeding,   11
  Growing puppies,   *13*
Adult Dogs,   15
  Nutrition and behavior,   *16*
Performance Dogs,   18
Geriatric Dogs,   20
  Nutrient needs of healthy old dogs,   *22*
  Choosing foods for geriatric dogs,   *23*
  Feeding management,   *23*
Summary,   23
  Pregnancy and lactation,   *23*
  Neonates,   *24*
  Growing puppies,   *25*
  Adult dogs,   *25*
  Performance dogs,   *25*
  Geriatric dogs,   *25*

3   Normal Cats,   27

Gestation and Lactation,   27
Growing Cats,   28
Adult Cats,   30
Geriatric Cats,   31
  Healthy geriatric cats,   *31*
  Feeding considerations,   *33*
Nutrient Needs Specific to Cats,   34
Summary,   36
  Gestating and lactating cats,   *36*
  Growing cats,   *37*
  Adult cats,   *37*
  Geriatric cats,   *37*

4   Diet and Feeding Factors,   39

Commercial Diets,   39
  Characteristics of a satisfactory diet,   39
  Pet foods,   39
  Pet food labeling,   43
Feeding Factors,   47
  Changing the diet of "finicky" eaters,   47
Summary,   48
  Characteristics of a satisfactory diet,   48
  Pet food labeling,   48
  Feeding factors,   48

5   Clinical Dietetics,   49

Cancer,   50
Critical Care,   54
  Nutrition and sick or injured animals,   54
  Nutritional assessment,   59
  Routes of nutrient delivery,   60
  Diet selection,   67
  Feeding,   67
  Parenteral nutrition,   69
  Returning to normal food intake,   71
Dental Disease,   72
  Natural diets,   72
  Soft versus hard foods,   73
  Textured food,   73
  Treats and biscuits,   73
  Nonnutritional dental aids,   74
  Feeding,   74
  Conclusion,   74
Endocrine Disease,   75
  Diabetes mellitus,   75
  Hyperlipidemia,   79
Gastrointestinal Disease,   82
  Acute gastroenteritis and vomiting or small bowel diarrhea,   82
  Gastric dilatation-volvulus,   83
  Borborygmus and flatulence,   84
  Hairballs in cats,   84
  Chronic small bowel diarrhea,   84
  Chronic large bowel diarrhea,   85
  Constipation,   87
  Inflammatory bowel disease,   88
  Megacolon in cats,   89
  Lymphangiectasia and exocrine pancreatic insufficiency,   90

Pancreatitis, 91
Chronic liver disease, 92
Idiopathic hepatic lipidosis in cats, 93
Heart Disease, 94
Congestive heart failure, 94
Dilated cardiomyopathy in dogs, 96
Dilated cardiomyopathy in cats, 97
Kidney Disease, 100
Obesity, 109
Obesity and disease, 109
Prevention, 111
Obesity therapy program, 111
Summary, 116
Skin Disease, 117
Diagnosis, 117
Urinary Tract Disease, 125
Stones, 125
Idiopathic cystitis in cats, 133
Sick Geriatric Cats, 134
Oral disease, 135
Chronic renal failure, 135
Cardiovascular disease, 136
Hyperthyroidism, 136
Cancer, 136
Diabetes mellitus, 137
Conclusions, 137
Sick Geriatric Dogs, 137
Diet-Induced Problems, 138
Vitamin A, 138
Vitamin E and thiamin deficiencies, 139
Nutritional secondary hyperparathyroidism, 140

6   Contemporary Issues in Clinical Nutrition, 143
Contemporary and Alternative Veterinary Medicine, 143
Evaluating Information on the World Wide Web, 147
Evidence-Based Medicine, 151
The Transtheoretical Model of Behavioral Change and Its Role in Obesity
   Therapy, 156

7   Nutrition for Exotic Pets, 163

Appendices,
A. Nutrient Comparison Tables for Commercial Dog Foods, 171
B. Nutrient Comparison Tables for Commercial Cat Foods, 181

C. Diet History Sheet,   187

D. Food Transition Sheet,   191

E. Detailed Feeding Directions for Prevention of Nutrition-Related Developmental Orthopedic Disease,   193

F. Protein Calculation Sheet,   195

G. Enrichment Recommendations for Indoor Cats,   197

H. Veterinary Diets for Dogs,   201

I. Veterinary Diets for Cats,   215

J. Basic Homemade Diet for Cats and Dogs,   231

K. Gastrostomy Tubes,   233

L. Exchange Lists,   235

Nutritional Assessment

The $nutritional$ $assessment$ begins with a determination of the patient's signalment, a review of the history (including dietary and feeding history), and the physical examination. Based on the presenting signs and the findings of this initial evaluation, the examiner chooses whether to conduct a cursory, intermediate, or detailed evaluation of the animal, its diet, and the owner's feeding practices (Table 1-1).

For animals at relatively low risk for nutritional problems, such as an adult with a moderate body condition score and normal findings on physical examination, a cursory evaluation usually suffices. If the owner is feeding a satisfactory diet and food intake seems reasonable, further investigation is not usually necessary. A satisfactory diet is one that is made by a reputable manufacturer and that has passed feeding trials for all life stages; more detailed information on dietary evaluation is presented in Chapter 4. An intermediate evaluation may be useful if the physical examination findings are normal and the animal is in a higher-risk group; is gestating, lactating, growing, or geriatric; is living in a multiple-pet household; or is an endurance athlete. The intermediate evaluation examines the quality and availability of the diet (especially in multiple-pet households) and calculates protein intake, in addition to the information sought in the cursory evaluation (described in the section on geriatric pets). A more detailed nutritional assessment is indicated when the animal is in a higher-risk group, when any abnormality is identified on the physical examination, or when the animal is receiving an uncommon (unknown or homemade) diet. Detailed evaluation includes all of the above plus further investigation of the pet's diet and nutrition-related features of the environment. Additional information concerning the detailed nutrition assessment is included in the clinical sections.

HISTORY

For an accurate dietary history to be obtained, the person who feeds the animal should be interviewed, and leading questions should be avoided as much as possible. The goal is to identify the presence and significance of factors that could put the patient at risk for malnutrition.

Obtaining an accurate dietary history is also important for establishing possible nutritional causes of identified problems or their manifestations. These problems may be the result of nutrient deficiencies, toxicities, or imbalances. If this is suspected to be the case,

Table 1-1
Determining the Depth of Nutritional Assessment

Signalment	Presentation Examination	Diet	Feeding	Assessment
Low risk	Normal	Satisfactory	Satisfactory	Cursory—satisfactory diet, adequate food intake
High risk	Normal	Satisfactory	Questionable	Intermediate—cursory assessment plus determination of information regarding environment and protein intake
High risk	Abnormal	Questionable	Questionable	Detailed—intermediate assessment plus determination of further details as appropriate

the diet should be changed to one known to be satisfactory and one in which the examiner has confidence based on clinical experience.

Some of the symptoms or problems that may be present in patients fed an inadequate diet are presented in Table 1-2.

PHYSICAL EXAMINATION

The physical examination permits assessment of the animal's condition and comparison of physical findings with impressions formed when the history is taken. An important part of the physical examination is the assignment of a body score (BCS) and a muscle condition score (Figures 1-1 and 1-2). Body and muscle condition scoring provide another indicator of the nutritional adequacy of the diet and the level of food intake of an animal.

The animal should be weighed and the weight recorded in the medical record. For the purpose of comparison it is helpful to use the same scale and to weigh patients at the same time of day each time they are weighed, to minimize variation in gut and bladder fill.

Nutritional assessment questions to be answered during the taking of the history and the physical examination include the following.
1. Are the animal's weight, body condition, and muscle mass acceptable?
2. If the animal is overweight, is too much food being offered? Is too little exercise being provided?
3. If the animal is underweight, is enough food being offered?

Table 1-3 presents some physical signs suggestive of malnutrition, along with the potential causes.

Table 1-2
History and Clinical Signs Associated with Inappropriate Diet or Food Intake

Historical Feature or Clinical Sign	Potential Deficiency	Possible Cause
Isolation, environment associated with poverty, dental disease, unconventional diet	Various nutrients	Inadequate intake of a balanced diet
Decreased production or performance	Various nutrients	Imbalanced diet or inadequate intake of a balanced diet
Weight loss	Various nutrients	Imbalanced diet or inadequate intake of a balanced diet
Drug ingestion (antacids, anticonvulsants, laxatives, antibiotics, chemotherapeutic agents)	Varies depending on drug	Inadequate nutrient absorption; decreased nutrient utilization
Malabsorption (diarrhea, weight loss, steatorrhea)	Carbohydrate, protein, fat, calcium, magnesium, zinc; vitamins A, D, E, K	Inadequate nutrient absorption
Parasite infestation	Iron	Inadequate nutrient absorption
Gastrointestinal surgery	Energy, protein, fat, calcium, magnesium, zinc; vitamins A, D, E, K	Inadequate nutrient absorption
Heritable defects	Varies depending on defect	Inadequate nutrient absorption
Blood loss	Iron	Increased nutrient losses
Centesis	Protein	Increased nutrient losses
Dialysis	Protein, water-soluble vitamins, zinc	Increased nutrient losses
Diarrhea	Protein, electrolytes, zinc	Increased nutrient losses
Draining wounds	Protein	Increased nutrient losses
Nephrotic syndrome	Protein	Increased nutrient losses
Fever	Energy	Increased requirements
Hyperthyroidism	Energy	Increased requirements
Physiologic demands	Various nutrients	Increased requirements
Surgery, trauma, burns, infection	Various nutrients	Increased requirements

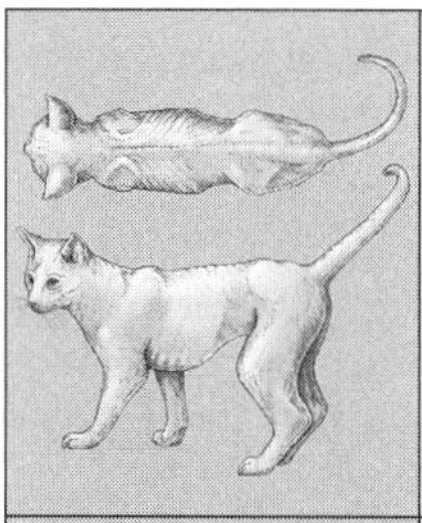

BCS 1   Emaciated

What you see   Obvious ribs, pelvic bones, and spine (backbone), no body fat or muscle mass
What you feel   Bones with little covering muscle

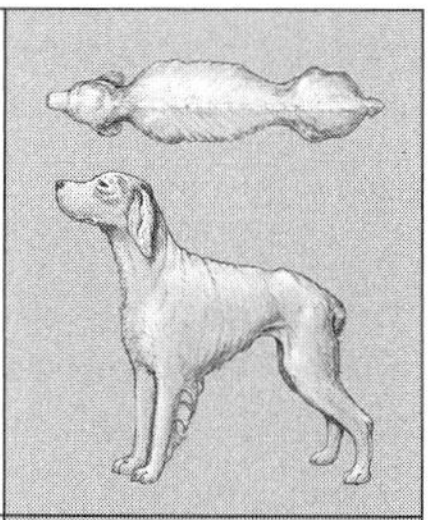

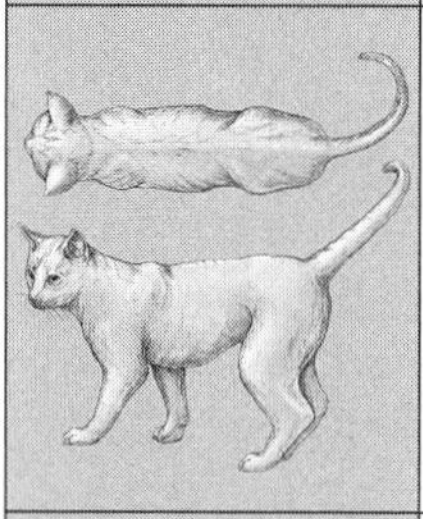

BCS 2   Thin

What you see   Ribs and pelvic bones, but less prominent; tips of spine; an "hourglass" waist (looking from above) and a tucked-up abdomen (looking from the side)
What you feel   Ribs (and other bones) with no palpable fat, but muscle present

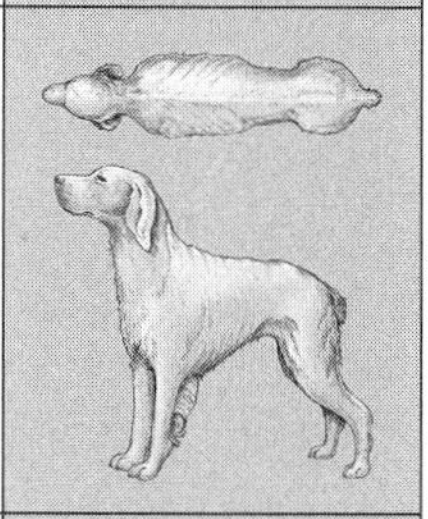

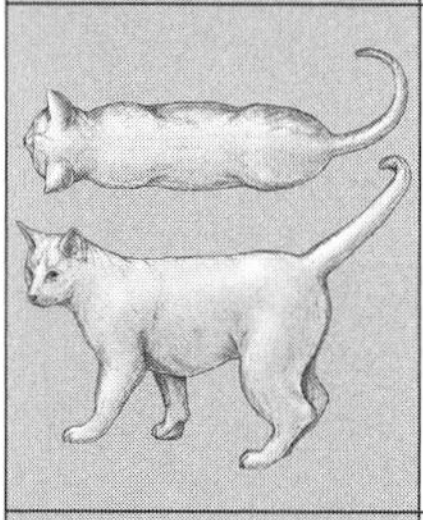

BCS 3   Moderate

What you see   Less prominent hourglass and abdominal tuck
What you feel   Ribs, without excess fat covering

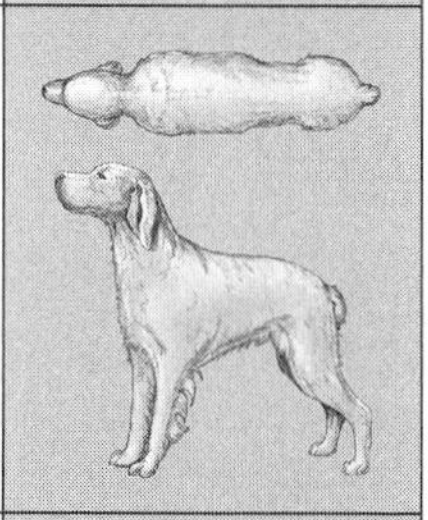

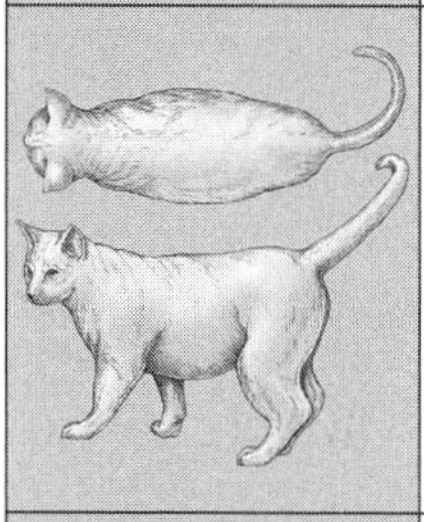

BCS 4   Stout

What you see   General fleshy appearance; hourglass and abdominal tuck hard to see
What you feel   Ribs, with difficulty

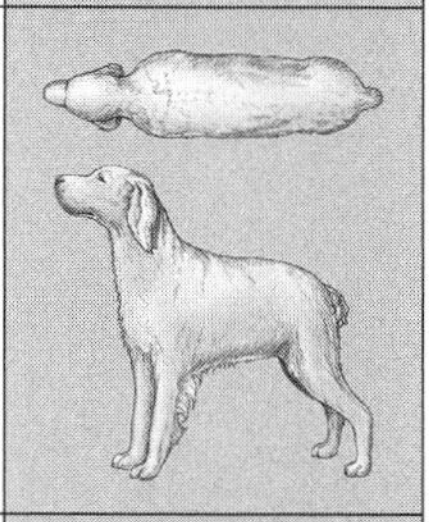

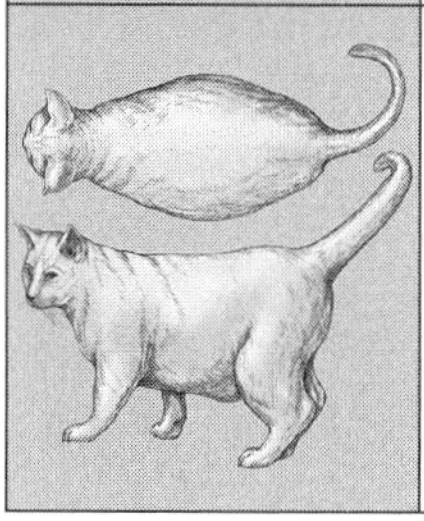

BCS 5   Obese

What you see   Sagging abdomen, large deposits of fat over chest, abdomen, and pelvis
What you feel   Nothing (except general flesh)

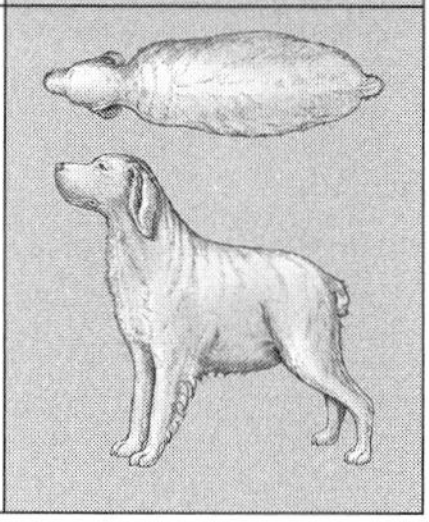

Figure 1-1 Body condition scoring.

3 Normal muscle mass
Muscle easily palpated over the temporal bones, ribs, lumbar vertebrae, and pelvic bones

No visible bony prominences when viewed from a distance

2 Moderate muscle wasting
Thin layer of muscle covering the temporal bones, ribs, lumbar vertebrae, and pelvic bones on palpation

Bony prominences slightly visible from a distance

1 Marked or
severe muscle wasting
No muscle covering the temporal bones, ribs, lumbar vertebrae, and pelvic bones on palpation

Bony prominences highly visible from a distance

"Overcoat syndrome"
Clinically, body condition score (BCS) and muscle condition score (MCS) are not directly related, because of the "overcoat syndrome" (OS), which occurs when an animal has less muscle and more fat, making an MCS of 1 or 2 look relatively normal. We suspect OS when the history and physical do not match. Palpation is required for a diagnosis of OS. Although some areas of the body may feel relatively normal (as shown at right), marked wasting is felt over bony prominences.

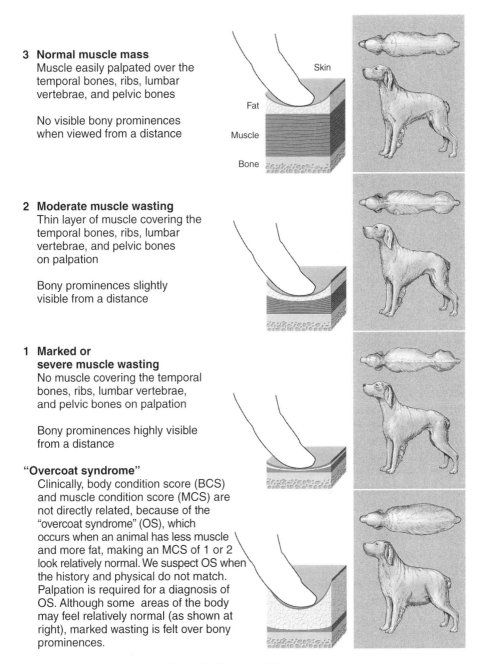

Figure 1-2 Muscle condition scoring.

Table 1-3
Physical Signs that Suggest Malnutrition

Sign	Nutritional Causes	Nonnutritional Causes	Cautions
Cachexia: fat loss, muscle wasting	Inadequate food availability	Inadequate food intake	Nonspecific finding
Haircoat: dry, coarse, lusterless, easily pluckable	Inadequate energy, protein, essential fatty acid, copper, zinc, vitamin B$_6$, folate intake	Fever, chronic disease	Nonspecific finding
Skin: dry, thin flaky, pressure sores, poor wound healing			Nonspecific finding
Hyperkeratosis	Vitamin A, zinc deficiency		
Eyes: xerophthalmia (dry eye), blindness	Vitamin A deficiency		
Retinal degeneration	Taurine deficiency		
Skeleton: bowed legs, "rubber jaw," beaded ribs, pathologic fractures	Vitamin D, calcium, phosphorus deficiency	Hyperparathyroidism (primary or secondary to renal failure)	
Bone pain	Vitamin A toxicity	Tumor, fracture, developmental orthopedic disease	Nonspecific finding

LABORATORY EVALUATION

Laboratory evaluation plays a limited role in diagnosing nutrition-related problems. Table 1-4 lists some common laboratory tests, potential nutritional and nonnutritional causes of abnormal values, and factors of which to be aware when evaluating the results of these tests. In most cases laboratory parameters lack sufficient predictive value to be diagnostic for nutrition-related problems.

SUMMARY OF NUTRITIONAL ASSESSMENT

For the nutritional status of the patient to be adequately assessed, it is important to first establish the patient's risk level by evaluating the signalment and physical condition of the patient and the dietary history. Evaluation of the physical condition must include the assignment of a body condition score. This score, along with the body weight and physiologic status of the patient, is used to determine the nutritional adequacy of the patient's current feeding regimen. In addition to the physical examination, a dietary history is obtained by asking the person who cares for the animal questions regarding current

Table 1-4
Laboratory Evaluation Results

Test	Nutritional Causes	Nonnutritional Causes	Cautions	Action
Albumin	Decreased: inadequate protein intake	Increased: infection, burns, trauma, congestive heart failure, fluid overload, recumbence, severe liver disease	False-normal values may occur in dehydrated patients or after infusion of albumin, plasma, or blood	Increase protein intake
Total iron-binding capacity	Decreased: inadequate protein intake	Decreased: similar to albumin	False-normal values may occur in iron-deficient patients	
BUN	When creatinine levels are normal, decreased BUN signifies inadequate protein intake; increased BUN signifies excessive protein intake, recent meal	Decreased: severe liver disease, anabolic state Increased: kidney disease, congestive heart failure, gastrointestinal hemorrhage, steroid therapy, dehydration, shock		
Creatinine	Decreased: inadequate energy intake Increased: cooked meat diet (small increase)	Decreased: decreased muscle mass Increased: kidney disease, severe muscle trauma		
Prothrombin time	Increased: vitamin K deficiency	Increased: anticoagulant ingestion, severe liver disease		
Total lymphocyte count	Decreased: inadequate food intake	Decreased: stress, steroid therapy, renal failure, cancer	Significant day-to-day fluctuation can occur	
Red blood cell parameters	Decreased hemoglobin and hematocrit: nutritional anemia (decreased MCV may signify iron, copper, cobalt deficiency; no change in MCV may signify inadequate food intake; increased MCV may signify folate deficiency)	Decreased hemoglobin and hematocrit: anemia caused by blood loss, hemolysis, chronic disease		

BUN, Blood urea nitrogen; *MCV*, mean corpuscular volume.

dietary and feeding behavior. Once the patient's risk level is established, it is possible to determine the depth of the overall assessment. It may be necessary to look further into the current diet, life-style, and environment of the patient. A laboratory evaluation can be completed to further assist in the nutritional assessment. Only after all these factors are considered can an adequate evaluation be made of the nutritional status of the patient, and any needed changes or adjustments be recommended.

Normal Dogs

Healthy dams of good breeding produce healthy offspring. The probability of producing healthy, vigorous puppies can be improved by breeding animals from lines known to be free of genetic problems, by avoiding inbreeding, and by breeding bitches between 2 and 6 years of age. When these criteria have been met, success depends primarily on the diet and feeding management of mother and offspring.

FEEDING DURING GESTATION AND LACTATION

Before a bitch is bred, she should receive a physical examination, her vaccinations should be updated, and worming should be performed if necessary. The dog should be of normal body weight and moderate body condition; excess weight may predispose to dystocia, whereas underweight bitches may have difficulty conceiving. Moderate body condition should be attained *before* breeding if problems are to be avoided later. Owners should be asked to measure the dam's usual food intake at this time; it will be important to remind them of this information when the puppies are weaned.

The dam should be fed an excellent-quality commercial diet during gestation. During the first 6 weeks of pregnancy she should maintain her normal weight and feeding schedule. A decrease in food intake commonly occurs during the third to fifth week after breeding, and this is a good indicator of pregnancy. During the final 3 weeks of gestation, the dam's weight should increase to approximately 25% more than at breeding, depending on the size of the litter. She may be gradually switched to a puppy growth diet during this period to meet the increased nutrient needs of late pregnancy and lactation, to avoid an abrupt dietary change at parturition, and to ensure that the pups have the food available to them when they start eating on their own. It may be necessary to increase feeding frequency during this period to ensure adequate intake if a large litter is present. Carbohydrate-free, meat-only diets should not be fed during this period to avoid the risk of hypoglycemia and decreased puppy survival at birth. Figure 2-1 shows the changes in body weight versus time during pregnancy.

Lactation is the time of greatest nutritional stress in the life of the dam (unless she also is a racing sled dog). In addition to meeting her own nutrient needs, she must supply all the necessary nutrients to a litter of pups that will double in body weight in 10 days. Her nutrient needs increase to approximately three times maintenance by the third week of lactation, depending on the size of the litter. Because the dam is "eating for many," she needs to be fed the best food available to her owner on a free-choice (ad libitum) basis.

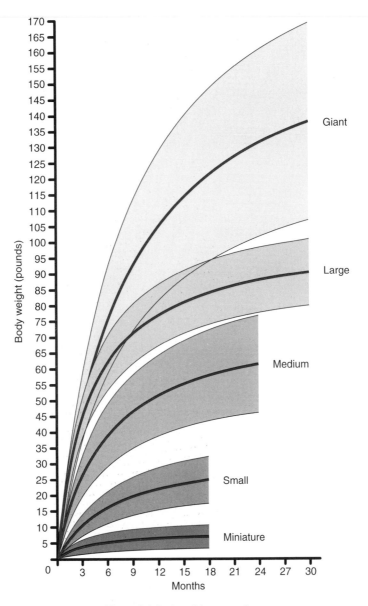

Figure 2-1 Body weight versus time.

Pups should be encouraged to begin eating by 3 weeks of age. This reduces the lactation demand on the dam and prepares the pups for weaning. Allowing the pups to "play" in a thick gruel of the dam's food mixed with water will soon give them the idea. Hot tap water should be added to the food approximately 20 minutes before feeding to improve digestibility and palatability and increase water intake.

Puppies should be weaned when they are 6 to 8 weeks old. On the day before they are to be removed from the dam, she should be separated from the pups for the day. The pups should be fed, and food (but not water) should be withheld from the dam. The puppies should be reunited with the dam overnight, and food (but not water) should be withheld from both dam and puppies. The puppies are removed from the mother and weaned the next day. This technique helps the dam "dry off" without problems. After the pups are weaned, return the dam to the diet she was consuming prior to breeding at *half* the amount the owner measured, increasing her food intake to this previously measured amount over the next 2 to 3 days. See Appendix A for comparisons of nutrients in foods designed for gestating and lactating dogs.

PUPPY CARE AND FEEDING

The first week of the puppies' lives is the most critical to their survival. Newborn animals are physiologically immature; body fat percentage is low—1% to 2% compared with 12% to 35% in adults—and they do not develop adequate glycogen reserves until after the first few days of nursing. Puppies have rapid respiratory rates (15 to 35 breaths per minute from 24 hours to 5 weeks of age) and heart rates (200 to 220 beats per minute from 24 hours to 5 weeks of age). The first nutritional concern with puppies is that they receive colostrum immediately after birth; all pups should be held up to a nipple to ensure they get colostrum within 24 hours of birth. The next priority is that they stay warm. Neonatal pups cannot regulate their body temperature (which is 94° to 97° F for the first 14 days). They need to be kept in an environment that is 85° to 90° F during the first week, and 80° to 85° F during the second week of life. Hypothermia makes pups unable to eat, which may result in their rejection by the dam.

A good way to ensure that pups are eating and developing normally is to weigh them daily. Pups should gain 1 to 2 g per day per pound of anticipated adult body weight. For example, if the anticipated adult body weight is 50 pounds, the pups should gain 50 to 100 g ($1^1/_2$ to 3 oz) per day.

Surveys indicate that a high percentage of deaths before weaning are due to a relatively small number of causes: infectious diseases, congenital defects, and malnutrition. The malnutrition usually results from the death of or neglect by the mother, lactation failure, or a litter that is too large for the milk supply. In these circumstances milk substitutes must be used to feed the puppies. As shown in Table 2-1 the composition of cow's milk is quite different from that of dog's and cat's milk, and cow's milk should not be fed by itself.

Table 2-1
Composition of Animal Milk*

	Volume (ml)	Protein (g)	Fat (g)	Lactose (g)	Calcium (mg)	Phosphorus (mg)
Cat	70	6.7	4.9	7.1	25	50
Dog	85	5.9	6.9	3.2	190	130
Cow	140	4.7	5.3	6.9	190	140

* Values indicated are per 100 kcal.

Several companies have developed milk replacers for dogs and cats; until a commercial product can be purchased, the combination of 1 quart (950 ml) whole cow's milk, 4 egg yolks, and 1 tablespoon (15 ml) corn oil may be fed. This homemade formula can be used for a day or so.

Orphaned puppies can be fed four times daily if the temperature of the environment is maintained at an appropriate level. Feeding every 6 hours is optimal, but feeding at approximately 8:00 AM, 12:00 noon, 4:00 PM, and 9:00 PM (do not wake pups to feed them) is adequate if the pups are kept at the proper temperature.

Most milk replacers supply about 1 kcal/ml. Puppies need approximately 15 to 20 kcal (milliliters) per 100 g ($3^{1}/_{2}$ oz) of body weight per day. The milk and equipment used for feeding must be as clean as possible. Larger puppies can be fed from a small baby bottle nipple; for smaller puppies, a doll bottle nipple or one made for puppies can be used. Feed milk, at least initially, at body temperature. If diarrhea develops, maintain the amount of fluid given, but reduce the solids by diluting the formula 25% to 50%. As with puppies raised by their mothers, orphan pups should be encouraged to eat from a pan by 3 weeks of age and should complete the transition to a growth diet by 6 to 8 weeks. See Appendix A for nutrient comparison tables for puppy milk replacers.

To ensure that orphaned or inadequately mothered puppies are maintained in an appropriate environment, an incubator can be constructed for them (Figure 2-2). This can be made from a cardboard box, a dry heating pad, a thermometer, cloth towels, newspaper, a cup, and a sponge. The heating pad cover should be pinned to the towel so that the heating element is secured under the towel and covers approximately half the floor area of the box, allowing the orphan to choose a comfortable temperature relative to the heat source. The cup should be taped in a corner of the box, and a moistened sponge kept in it to humidify the air. The thermometer should be hung in the box near the floor, and the top of the box should be covered to help retain the heat.

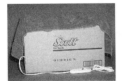

Side view

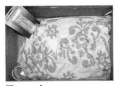

Top view

How to build an incubator
1. Obtain a large cardboard box
2. Place a dry heating pad in the bottom so that it covers approximately half the floor area of the box
3. Cover bottom (and heating pad) with towel
4. Pin towel to heating pad so the heating pad remains covered by the towel
5. Tape a plastic cup to one corner of the box
6. Place a moist sponge (keep it moist) in the cup to help maintain humidity of the box
7. Tape a thermometer in a corner of the box so temperature can be monitored
8. Cover the top of the box and place the box on newspapers to help with insulation

Figure 2-2 Incubator, with instructions for use.

CLIENT COMMUNICATION TIPS: Gestation and Lactation

- Plan to discuss with the owner the importance of body condition scoring (BCS) and what kind of conditioning you recommend for the bitch during the different stages of gestation and lactation.
- Plan to discuss how and when to make adjustments in energy intake, the need to increase intake in late gestation, and the need to decrease intake at the time of weaning to the prebreeding level.
- Advise clients that dams should not be fed the least expensive dog food on the market during gestation and lactation, nor should they be fed a product with which the veterinarian (or the owner) is unfamiliar ("go with what you know").
- Recommended diets should be from manufacturers that have both a growth and an adult product with which the clinician is familiar and that meet the clinician's criteria for adequately supporting late gestation and peak lactation.
- Provide the client with the practice's top list of manufacturers for adult and growth products.
- Discuss with the staff the criteria for determining which diets everyone in the practice recommends, as well as diets to avoid recommending. Which foods are on the practice's "A list," and why. Which are on the practice's "B list," and why. Help staff identify clients who are receptive to learning more about dietary recommendations.

TECH TIPS: Gestation and Lactation

Pregnancy is one of the most nutritionally stressful times in a dog's life. Client education is a very important part to the successful outcome of producing a litter. The following guidelines are recommended.

- Obtain a complete dietary history (see Appendix C), being careful to note the types and amounts of food eaten before pregnancy.
- Carefully evaluate BCS, muscle condition score (MCS), skin, and haircoat, then teach owners how to do the same (see Figures 1-1 and 1-2).
- If recommendations for a food change are given, instruct the owner on the proper way to transition the pet onto a new food (see Appendix D).
- Instruct the owner always to provide plenty of water and to add water to food if necessary to help keep up with milk production.

Growing Puppies

The first 6 months of life is the period of most rapid growth and greatest nutrient needs for most dogs. However, it is possible to feed a puppy too much. This can create problems, particularly in large-breed dogs. Overfed, rapidly growing large- and giant-breed dogs may develop a variety of orthopedic problems, including hyperflexion or extension of the carpus, osteochondrosis, hip dysplasia, fractures of the coronoid processes, radius curvus, wobbler syndrome, and enostosis. Owners of large-breed dogs should receive some dietary and feeding-management advice to help them avoid diet-related orthopedic problems in their pets.

Diet

Because the early growth period may be the most critical nutritional period in a dog's life, only high-quality diets tested in feeding trials should be fed. The diet recommended should be one the veterinarian trusts, based on positive experiences with it. Some owners prefer to feed large- and giant-breed dogs "adult" rather than "puppy" foods to try to avoid problems. These diets may be adequate, but it is important to determine exactly which diet the owner intends to feed to ensure that it is adequate for growth based on feeding trials. Once an adequate diet has been chosen, vitamin or mineral supplements are an unnecessary expense and are much more likely to cause than to prevent problems. See Appendix A for nutrient comparison tables for large-breed puppy or growth foods.

Feeding

Proper feeding management is usually much more important than dietary choice in preventing orthopedic problems, because most of these problems are caused by overfeeding.

Experimental studies of nutritional and developmental orthopedic diseases (DODs) have shown that restriction of food intake so that the pup maintains a lean body condition during the period of growth is the best insurance against nutrition-related problems. Owners need to be taught how to recognize the desired body condition and be reminded not to trust feeding recommendations on food packaging, as they may not be accurate for a particular dog in a specific environment.

Young growing animals should be maintained in a lean body condition. This means that the ribs should be easily felt and barely seen in smooth-coated dogs. Feeding to this condition will minimize the risk of orthopedic problems and still permit the animal to reach its genetic potential for adult size. The dog should be fed the amount of food necessary to maintain this body condition, and the range is large. Some dogs can have food available continuously, whereas others may need to be restricted to brief access to food once or twice a day. If owners understand this from the start, it becomes much easier for them to adjust the amount of food they offer their pets. Recommendations on dog food labels can be used as an initial estimate but should not be used as a substitute for the "eye of the master" with regard to adjusting intake as the animal grows.

Feeding to achieve a body condition rather than feeding a number of cups or cans of food per day is the best insurance against orthopedic problems in growing dogs; however, clients should be advised that genetic peculiarities and trauma can also cause DOD, and that these problems cannot be prevented by diet.

Detailed feeding directions to avoid developmental orthopedic disease.

1. Determine the diet fed (brand name, product name, form [canned, dry, semimoist]) and the daily amount consumed by the dog.
2. Assign a BCS using a scale of 1 to 5, in which 1 is cachexic, 2 is lean, 3 is moderate, 4 is stout, and 5 is obese.
3. If BCS is greater than 3/5, reduce daily food intake by approximately 10%, and feed this amount until the dog has reached a BCS of 2/5 or 3/5.
4. Once the desired body condition of 2/5 is attained, increase food intake only enough to sustain this body condition until the patient is completely grown. If the amount fed declines to an amount that concerns the owner, a food of lower energy density that is complete and balanced for growth (or all life stages), based on feeding trials conducted according to protocols approved by the Association of American Feed Control Officials (AAFCO), may be substituted on an equal-energy basis.

5. Manufacturer's feeding recommendations may be used as a starting point if the animal already has a BCS of 2/5 but the amount fed should be reduced as described in direction 3 if necessary. Because of the variability in growth rates and activity among dogs, they should be fed whatever amount is necessary to maintain a BCS of 2/5 during the growth period. Once their adult stature is achieved, their condition may be allowed to rise to 3/5 if desired by the owner.
6. Suggest a feeding frequency that is appropriate for conditions and that accommodates the circumstances of the owner—from once daily to free choice.
7. Keep fresh, clean, liquid water available at all times.
8. The puppy may be switched to a recommended adult food at 6 months of age (or earlier depending on the nutritional claim), or at suture removal for neutering procedures that occur after 3 months of age.
9. Following these recommendations should minimize the risk of nutrition-related DOD, and make supplementation of any kind unnecessary.

CLIENT COMMUNICATION TIPS: Growing Puppies

- Plan to review the importance of BCS at each well-puppy visit.
- Provide client with the practice's top list of manufacturers for puppy growth products and adult maintenance products.
- Provide client with two or three options for commercial treats, and talk about replacing calories in the food bowl instead of adding to them.
- Explain the value of regular exercise and obedience training at each well-puppy visit; provide client with a list of two or three obedience trainers in your area.
- If your client insists on feeding a homemade diet, recommend that they use the service provided at www.petdiets.com.
- Talk to clients about decreased energy needs as a result of neutering and spaying, when to switch from growth to adult food, and how you see that process occurring during the first 12 months of the puppy's life.
- For owners with large- or giant-breed pups, identify concerns about DOD, and discuss the key nutrients of concern; the rapid-growth phase (i.e., the "window of opportunity" for DOD); the variety of appropriate commercial diets available; and the relative risk of genetics, trauma, and nutrition in the pathogenesis of DOD.
- Discuss with the staff the criteria for determining which diets everyone in the practice recommends, as well as diets to avoid recommending. Which foods are on the practice's "A list," and why. Which are on the practice's "B list," and why. Help staff identify clients who are receptive to learning more about dietary recommendations.

ADULT DOGS

Healthy adult dogs have relatively small nutrient requirements compared with those in the reproductive stages of life. They may be maintained for years on a wide range of commercial or homemade diets with apparently little consequence. This adaptability may be an explanation for the fervent belief of some owners that a seemingly peculiar diet is beneficial for their pets. The probability of a diet-related problem, however, should be lower for animals fed properly formulated commercial diets, because these diets have been more

TECH TIPS: Dog Growth

When clients ask how much to feed a new puppy, the best thing to do is to teach them how to assign a BCS to their pet (see Figure 1-1). They will then be able to adjust the amount of food offered as necessary during the puppy's growth period. It is also a good idea to provide clients with a body condition scoring sheet, which provides a ready reference at home, as well as a pet food measuring cup. These are available through most pet food manufacturers on request.
- A handout of feeding directions for owners of large-breed puppies is provided in Appendix E.
- Schedule at least one follow-up appointment during the growing stage to assure that weight and body condition match the guidelines.
- Explain any feeding changes that may need to be made after spaying or neutering. A dog's energy needs may go down by as much as 25% after this procedure, so adjusting food intake at this stage is crucial to preventing future weight problems.

thoroughly tested, and have been fed to millions of animals successfully for generations. Because no adverse consequences are observed in a single animal does not mean that a diet provides superior nutrition.

Adult dogs may be fed on a free-choice basis or they may be fed at certain times, with the owner determining the size of each meal. Self-feeding is more convenient, and ensures that timid animals are not denied access to food in group-feeding situations. Self-feeding has the disadvantage of reducing owner contact with the pet and decreasing opportunities to evaluate the animal's body condition and general health. Pets that tend to overeat should be fed once or twice daily in amounts sufficient to maintain moderate body condition. See Appendix A for nutrient comparison tables for foods for adult dogs.

Nutrition and Behavior

Some pet owners and veterinarians have speculated that diet may play some role in the pathophysiology of and therapy for aggression in dogs. Some have reported that a high-protein diet has a calming effect, whereas others believe that the behavior of aggressive or hyperactive dogs might be improved by changing from a high-protein (28% to 32% dry

CLIENT COMMUNICATION TIPS: Adult Dogs

- Review the importance of BCS at each healthy-pet visit.
- Remember to mention the health benefits of regular exercise.
- If the client feeds commercial treats, provide two or three options for low-calorie products and emphasize the importance of replacing calories in the food bowl instead of adding to them.
- If the client would like to feed a homemade diet, recommend that the service provided at www.petdiets.com be used, and ask that the client include the clinician's e-mail address so that they can receive a report or updates.
- Discuss with the staff the criteria for determining which diets everyone in the practice recommends, as well as diets to avoid recommending. Which foods are on the practice's "A list," and why. Which are on the practice's "B list," and why. Help staff identify clients who are receptive to learning more about dietary recommendations.

TECH TIPS: Adult Dogs

> At this stage, clients should be aware of their pets' eating habits. Type of diet and amount of food should be noted for future reference; if an animal's eating habits change because of a health problem, the owner may be able to catch it early. If owners have not been educated about the BCS, the technique should be discussed at this time (see Figure 1-1).
>
> The following materials should also be provided:
> - Body condition scoring sheet
> - A pet food measuring cup
>
> These are available through most of the major pet food companies on request.

matter basis [DMB]) to a low-protein diet (12% to 20% DMB). One reason for this speculation is the knowledge that catecholamines and serotonin are synthesized from amino acids—tyrosine in the case of the catecholamines, and tryptophan in the case of serotonin.

The effect of dietary protein and tryptophan on the behavior of dogs in two studies has been reported. In 1996 Dodman and colleagues investigated the effect of diets containing 17%, 25%, and 32% protein on the behavior of 12 dogs with dominance aggression, 12 with hyperactivity, 12 with territorial aggression, and 14 without behavioral problems. All dogs were fed each of the diets for 2 weeks, and owners were instructed to score their dogs' behavior daily. No change was found in the behavior of the dogs with dominance aggression or hyperactivity or the healthy dogs. In seven of the dogs with fear-related territorial aggression, aggression scores were statistically significantly reduced when dogs were fed the low-protein (reduced approximately 38%) or medium-protein (reduced approximately 23%) diet, compared with territorial aggression when fed the high-protein diet. According to the authors these results suggested that a reduction in protein intake is not generally useful in the treatment of behavioral problems in dogs but may be appropriate in dogs with fear-related territorial aggression. Protein intake in this group when fed the 17%-protein diet was estimated to be about 1 g per pound of body weight per day.

In a subsequent study the effect of high- and low-protein diets with or without tryptophan supplementation on the behavior of 11 dogs with dominance aggression, 11 with territorial aggression, and 11 with hyperactivity was studied. The four diets were fed for 1 week each in random order with a transitional period of more than 3 days between each diet. Two diets contained approximately 18% protein, and the other two contained approximately 30%. Two of the diets (one low-protein and one high-protein) were supplemented with 1.45 g of tryptophan per kilogram of food. Owners scored the dogs' behavior daily, and mean weekly values of five behavioral measures and serum concentrations of serotonin and tryptophan were determined at the end of each dietary period. The behavioral scores in dogs with dominance aggression were generally low (less than 2 on a 10-point scale in all groups), being highest when these dogs were fed the unsupplemented high-protein diet. Consumption of the tryptophan-supplemented low-protein diet was associated with statistically significantly lower behavioral scores (an approximate 14% reduction, from 3.7 to 3.2 on a 10-point scale) than consumption of the low-protein diet without supplemental tryptophan in dogs with territorial aggression. No changes in serum concentrations of serotonin or tryptophan were identified. The authors concluded that adding tryptophan to high-protein diets or changing to a low-protein diet may reduce dominance aggression, and that tryptophan supplementation of a low-protein diet may be helpful in reducing territorial aggression.

The small number of animals studied, the short duration of the studies, and the small effect found suggest that protein or amino acids do not have large effects on the behavior of dogs. In certain subsets of dogs, however, such as those with fear aggression, further studies may be worthwhile. In these patients protein intakes should be measured before therapy to determine the potential for a significant reduction without compromising the patient's nutritional status. This issue is explained in greater depth in the section on geriatric nutrition later in this chapter. With regard to an independent effect of tryptophan, without a more thorough evaluation of the balance of neurotransmitters that interact with and modulate the effects of serotonin, it may be difficult to document specific, particularly therapeutic, effects.

The uncertainty regarding whether or to what extent protein affects behavior in dogs and the limited number of clinical trials in relevant patient populations is echoed in human medicine. As Dr. John Fernstrom, a long-time researcher of the effects of protein and amino acids on behavior, recently commented, "[S]everal lines of investigation have shown that the chemistry and function of both the developing and the mature brain are influenced by diet. Examples are . . . the effects of tryptophan or tyrosine intake (alone or as a constituent of dietary protein) on the production of the brain neurotransmitters derived from them (serotonin and the catecholamines, respectively). Sometimes the functional effects are clear and the underlying biochemical mechanisms are not; in other cases (such as the amino acids tyrosine and tryptophan), the biochemical effects are well understood, whereas the effect on brain function is not. Despite the incomplete knowledge base on the effects of such nutrients, investigators, physicians, and regulatory bodies have promoted the use of these nutrients in the treatment of disease. Typically, these nutrients have been given in doses above those believed to be required for normal health; after they have been given in pure form, unanticipated adverse effects have occasionally occurred. If this pharmacologic practice is to continue, it is important from a public safety standpoint that each nutrient be examined for potential toxicities so that appropriate purity standards can be developed and the risks weighed against the benefits when considering their use."

PERFORMANCE DOGS

After reproduction, work places the greatest nutritional demand on dogs. Dogs engage in guard and police work, racing, and hunting. Hard work increases all nutrient needs. For most "weekend athlete" dogs, these increases are proportional to the increase in energy needs, so they can be met by eating more of the same diet. Studies of sled dogs in the field and beagles on treadmills, however, have suggested that diets designed to support hard work and maximize stamina should have high digestibility and low bulk and should provide 50% to 60% of dietary energy from fat, 30% to 40% from protein, and 10% to 20% from carbohydrate.

The digestibility of commercial dog foods ranges from approximately 70% to 85%. Food bulk—the fiber and mineral content—therefore represents 15% to 30% of the food. Increasing the fat content usually increases the digestibility of dry dog foods. Moreover, high-fat diets often are lower in mineral and plant fiber content. Reducing the bulk improves

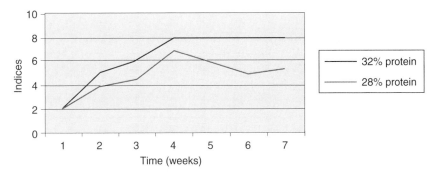

Figure 2-3 Red blood cell indices.

stamina by increasing nutrient density and reducing the volume of indigestible material in the colon.

In studies comparing the influence of fat and carbohydrate on stamina in racing sled dogs, red blood cell mass responded to training and racing and to dietary protein intake. Red blood cell indices increased during preseason training and were sustained during the racing season in dogs fed diets containing 32% or more of energy as protein, but not in dogs fed diets containing 28% or less of energy as protein (Figure 2-3).

If a dog is maintained on dry food when not in training, its diet should be changed to one that contains more fat and protein over a period of 1 to 2 weeks before training commences. This should ensure that tissue protein reserves are replete prior to the stress of training and should help to avoid the risks of abruptly switching to a high-fat diet. High-fat diets should be introduced gradually to allow the digestive tract to acclimate, which will decrease the risk of diarrhea or steatorrhea.

The amount of food fed daily initially should be modified in accordance with any increase in energy density resulting from a diet higher in fat. That is, if the energy density is 25% higher, 25% less food should be fed. During training the amount fed daily should be sufficient to keep the working dog in the desired body condition. If the work is very hard, the dog should be lean (BCS 2/5). The amount of food needed should not be overestimated. For example, greyhounds that race only once or twice a week and do little other work may require only about a 25% increase in food intake. Hunting dogs in hard training may require two or three times their usual food intake, about the same increase required by bitches nursing large litters at peak lactation. It has been reported that racing sled dog teams may require as much as 4.5-fold increases in nutrient intake to sustain them during races. These extremes emphasize the need for the trainer to determine the requirements of hardworking dogs by daily evaluation of body weight, condition, and performance.

In addition to a dietary history, some additional specific information should be obtained for canine athletes. Detailed information on environment and housing should be collected—for example, whether the dog is housed indoors or outdoors, the size and type of housing, and how much opportunity exists for spontaneous activity. Information should be collected regarding any medications or supplements used to improve performance and stamina. The specific type, amount, frequency, and performance level of exercise should be noted. Listed in Table 2-2 are three common categories of exercise, their descriptions, and examples.

Table 2-2
Common Categories of Exercise

Type	Description	Example
Sprint	High intensity, sustained for <2 minutes	Racing greyhounds
Intermediate	Lasting a few minutes to a few hours	Hunting dogs
Endurance	Lasting many hours to days	Sled dogs

CLIENT COMMUNICATION TIPS: Performance Dogs

- Review the importance of the BCS with the client and discuss what differences might be noted at various times of the year (depending on exercise, training, and actual work the dog is doing).
- Review both the total energy intake and output (based on dietary history, body weight changes, BCS, and activity level) to determine if the dog is being overfed or underfed.
- Provide the client with the practice's top list of manufacturers of growth and adult maintenance products.
- Discuss with the staff the criteria for determining which diets everyone in the practice recommends, as well as diets to avoid recommending. Which foods are on the practice's "A list," and why. Which are on the practice's "B list," and why. Help staff identify clients who are receptive to learning more about dietary recommendations.

TECH TIPS: Performance Dogs

Working animals may require as much as two to ten times the recommended intake of sedentary domestic dogs. To best meet these dogs' nutritional needs, it is important to do the following.
- Obtain a complete dietary history (see Appendix C) to determine the actual number of kilocalories the animal is taking in.
- Obtain an accurate assessment of the pet's total activity level to appropriately assess energy demands.
- Teach clients how to assess the animal's body condition (see Figure 1-1).
- If a change in diet is recommended, instruct the client on the proper way to make the transition to the new food (see Appendix D).
- If activity level is inconsistent, instruct the client to adjust food intake as necessary.

The amount of energy required depends on the total work done. This equals intensity × duration × frequency. Sprinters need between 1.5 and 3 times the resting energy requirement (RER) and should be fed a high-carbohydrate, low-fat diet. Intermediate athletes need 1.5 to 6 times the RER and should be fed a diet that is higher in fat content. Endurance athletes need up to 10 times the RER and need diets that are very high in fat. See Appendix A for nutrient comparison tables for performance foods.

GERIATRIC DOGS

No definition of the word *old* is applicable to all dogs. In one survey veterinary specialists believed *geriatric* should be applied to dogs based on age within breed groups (see Table 2-3). Diseases associated with aging, such as cancer and cardiovascular, gastrointestinal, and renal disorders, were thought to begin to increase in frequency at the ages indicated in Table 2-3.

Table 2-3

Results of Geriatric Survey—Weight and Age at which Dogs Are Considered "Old"

Age (yr)	Weight (lb)
11.5	<20
10	21-50
9	51-90
7.5	>90

From Kealy RD, Lawler DE, Bllam JM et al: Effects of diet restriction on life span and age-related changes in dogs, *J Am Vet Med Assoc* 9:1315, 2002.

Great variation also exists among individual animals; as the saying goes, "it's not so much the age as the mileage." The physical signs of aging—graying of the muzzle, decreased activity, or loss of sight or hearing—are more reliable indicators of advanced age in any particular dog than is its chronologic age. Presence of these signs suggests loss of the reserve capacity of body systems that allow young animals to adapt to changes in their environment and should raise the index of suspicion for the presence of age-related diseases.

Dietary advice for owners of aging dogs depends on the animal's usual diet and its current health status. Although all clients should be asked about the specific brand and amount of food they feed to their pet, what "people food" it consumes, and the type and amount of supplements given, this information is even more useful for evaluating the nutritional status of older animals. The brand and quantity of food provides an indication of the dietary history of the pet. If a high-quality commercial diet has been fed, little cause for concern about the patient's nutritional status exists. If, however, the dog is fed an uncommon diet, or significant amounts of table scraps, treats, or additional items, the possibility of nutrient deficiencies, excesses, and imbalances is greater. For these clients, advice to gradually introduce a high-quality commercial diet formulated for geriatric patients may be a way to improve the pet's diet without offending well-meaning owners. Younger adult animals have sufficient reserves to adjust to a broad range of nutrient intakes and may tolerate seemingly inappropriate diets for years; older dogs cannot be expected to sustain this level of tolerance.

The practitioner should also inquire about the pet's eating habits and body weight and any recent changes in them. Decreased appetite can be due to problems in any system, whereas increased food intake may be a time-filling activity or may suggest the onset of diabetes or hyperadrenocorticism. Recent weight loss may also result from a wide variety of causes, whereas increases are commonly the result of endocrine disease or of energy intake that exceeds energy expenditure.

The physical examination should include a search for signs of malnutrition. The most common form of malnutrition in older dogs is obesity, which is as easy to diagnose as it is difficult to treat. Other physical signs that may result from poor nutritional status include dry, rough haircoat, delayed wound healing, pressure sores, edema (hypoproteinemia), and cachexia.

Laboratory evaluation of nutritional status is difficult. Serum albumin does not appear to decline with age in dogs as it does in humans, so hypoalbuminemia in the absence of organ dysfunction may indicate protein deficiency. Other laboratory parameters are presented in Table 1-4.

Results of the history and physical and laboratory evaluation should allow the clinician to decide if the current diet is adequate and to identify the presence of any chronic disease that may require dietary modification. If the dog is healthy the clinician should decide if the diet is appropriate for a normal geriatric patient.

Nutrient Needs of Healthy Old Dogs

Many studies of the effects of nutrient intake on longevity have been conducted, usually with rodents. Restricting food, energy, protein, fat (and its constituents), and vitamin intake appears to prolong life in some cases, with the significance of the effect depending on the magnitude of restriction, the composition of the diet, the age at which restriction is instituted, and the rodent strain used. The applicability of these findings to dogs, which rarely develop primary hyperlipidemia and atherosclerosis (the subject of much of the work), is unknown. Nestlé Purina recently completed a 14-year study on effects of moderate food restriction on longevity as well as other health concerns of laboratory-housed dogs (Kealy et al, 2002). How these results will apply to client-owned dogs remains to be seen. Moreover, once dogs are old, the time for strategic manipulation of the diet to promote longevity has largely passed.

Owners should be reminded that great variability in energy needs exists among dogs and be advised to feed to a moderate body condition. Dogs become less active as they grow older, so they need less dietary energy to maintain normal weight and condition than when they were younger. Owners should be counseled to monitor the dog's body condition and adjust food intake to avoid obesity as energy needs decline.

The appropriate amount of protein to feed dogs has been intensely debated in recent years. Argument arose when it was proposed that a lifetime of consumption of excessive amounts of dietary protein were damaging to the kidney. Most of the evidence to support this hypothesis came from experiments conducted in rodents. The applicability of these findings to dogs in general has been challenged, and few results of studies of old dogs are available. Studies of the effects of diets differing in protein (and fat, sodium, phosphorus, and so on) on renal function of young dogs with induced kidney damage concluded that diets did affect renal function. Which, if any, single nutrient was responsible for the effect was not determined.

Other studies in rats have shown that when experiments control for the decrease in food intake that occurs when rats are fed low-protein diets, the effect of protein restriction is very small. Dogs appear to benefit from consuming at least 1 g of dietary protein per pound of body weight per day to maintain protein reserves and to maintain normal renal function. One gram is equivalent to 3.5 kcal as protein per day. If the dog consumes 15 to 20 kcal per pound per day to maintain moderate body condition (as many older, sedentary dogs do), the diet should contain *at least* 20% of energy as protein. Some geriatric diets contain less protein than this, and the status of protein reserves of dogs fed these diets is not known. We use 1 g per pound per day as a threshold level when decreased protein nutrition becomes a concern. We teach owners of dogs consuming less than this how to recognize signs of protein depletion—loss of muscle mass, poor coat quality, thin skin—by assessing for these signs in the owners' presence and encouraging them to be vigilant for deterioration in any parameter. Identification of the protein intake level at which preservation of renal function and maintenance of protein reserves are balanced awaits future research.

Fat generally improves diet palatability, supplies a concentrated source of energy, provides essential fatty acids, and enhances absorption of fat-soluble vitamins. Only small amounts of fat are needed to meet essential fatty acid requirements, so palatability must be balanced against the risk of obesity. Overweight animals should be fed diets containing less than 20% of energy as fat. Fat levels higher than 30% of total dietary energy are of value only for underweight dogs. In one study, geriatric dogs maintained at normal body weight and regularly exercised were found to be more alert and "spirited" than the sedentary controls. Exercise may also have beneficial metabolic effects.

No studies have shown healthy aged dogs to benefit from vitamin, mineral, or fiber supplementation. Commercial pet foods contain enough of these nutrients to make supplementation unnecessary. Nutrient supplements are expensive and of questionable value; veterinarians deserve and should demand results of properly conducted trials demonstrating the safety and efficacy of any supplement before recommending it.

Choosing Foods for Geriatric Dogs

Dog foods must be complete, balanced, digestible, palatable, and safe to be satisfactory diets. Label guarantees that a product is "complete and balanced for all life stages based on AAFCO feeding trials" mean that the food should meet the nutrient needs of older animals. Digestibility is also not an important issue for most older dogs. In all studies reported to date, nutrient digestibility by 16- to 18-year-old dogs is at least as good as that found in 1- to 2-year-old dogs. Finally, diets need not be too palatable unless inadequate food intake is a problem, because obesity is by far the more common situation in normal older dogs. See Appendix A for nutrient comparison tables for geriatric foods.

Feeding Management

Older dogs should not be fed free choice. Although this method may be adequate for some younger animals, the importance of maintaining normal body condition and of regular observation of the animal's food intake make once- or twice-daily feeding advisable for older pets. Because of the increased incidence of disease in older pets, clients should be advised that sudden unexplained decreases in food intake could be an early sign of disease that should be investigated. Obese dogs may be fed small quantities of food three or four times each day to reduce begging. Salted snacks for humans should not be given to older dogs, especially if any degree of heart disease is present. If the owner enjoys offering the pet snacks, part of the daily ration can be reserved for this purpose.

SUMMARY

Pregnancy and Lactation

- The dam should maintain normal body weight and feeding schedule until the final 3 weeks of pregnancy. At that time her weight will increase by 25%, and she should be gradually switched over to a puppy growth diet.

CLIENT COMMUNICATION TIPS: Older (Geriatric) Dogs

- Review the importance of BCS and regular exercise at each healthy-pet visit.
- Review the dietary history carefully with the owner.
- Determine total daily energy intake and calculate protein intake to assess whether pet is consuming its minimum needs. This is especially important for older dogs whose daily food intake may vary.
- Educate clients about the important benefits of meal-feeding older dogs, rather than feeding free choice. Individual meals allow the owner to observe appetite and water consumption and identify potential problems more quickly.
- If the client feeds commercial treats, provide two to three options for low-calorie products.
- Recommend that any dietary change be performed gradually, over a period of several days.
- Discuss with the staff the criteria for determining which geriatric diets everyone in the practice recommends, as well as diets to avoid recommending. Which foods are on the practice's "A list," and why. Which are on the practice's "B list," and why. Help staff identify clients who are receptive to learning more about dietary recommendations.

TECH TIPS: Geriatric Dogs

- Obtain an accurate dietary history (see Appendix C).
- Calculate protein intake to determine whether pet is receiving its minimum needs (see Appendix F). This is especially important for older dogs whose food intake may vary daily.
- Teach clients how to assess the body condition of their animals (see Figure 1-1).
- If a food change is recommended, give the client instructions regarding the proper way to make the transition to a new food (see Appendix D).
- Make sure enough time is scheduled for each appointment to cover each area adequately.

- The nutrient needs of the dam will increase to three times that of maintenance by the third week of lactation. Therefore, she should be fed the best diet possible and water on a free-choice basis.
- After the puppies are weaned, the dam should be returned to her normal diet, but at half the amount measured before breeding. Slowly increase her intake over 2 to 3 days to this previously measured amount.

Neonates

- It is extremely important that the pups nurse to receive colostrum within the first 24 hours of life. It is also important to keep them very warm during their first few weeks, or they may not eat.
- Pups should be encouraged to eat on their own by the third week of life. This can be done by allowing them to play in a gruel of their mother's food and water.
- Pups should grow 1 to 2 g per day per pound of anticipated adult body weight and should be fed appropriately to maintain this growth.
- Orphaned pups should be fed milk replacers four times a day and can be introduced to normal food at the same time and in the same manner as mothered pups.

Growing Puppies

- The first 6 months of life is the time of most rapid growth and largest nutrient needs.
- Overfeeding may be a problem, especially in large and giant breeds, and can lead to orthopedic problems.
- Only high-quality diets that have been tested and that the veterinarian trusts should be fed at this time.
- Amount fed is more important than type of food, because overfeeding is often at the root of orthopedic problems.
- Teaching owners how to recognize body condition and to feed to keep the animal's body condition lean (BCS 2/5) is vital in the prevention of orthopedic problems. However, clients should be aware that genetic peculiarities and trauma can also cause DODs.

Adult Dogs

- Adult dogs have relatively small nutritional requirements compared with dogs at other life stages.
- Adult dogs can be maintained on a wide range of diets; however, commercial diets are still best because they have been carefully formulated (and many have been tested).
- Dogs may be fed on a free-choice basis or on a schedule, depending on the situation and the dog's susceptibility to overeating.

Performance Dogs

- Work increases all nutrient needs.
- "Weekend athletes'" increased needs can usually be met by increased consumption rather than supplementation.
- Hard work and maximum stamina require high digestibility and low bulk, with each energy-providing (protein, fat, and carbohydrate) nutrient comprising a specific percentage of total dietary energy.
- If an animal is fed a normal diet when not working, introduce higher-protein and higher-fat diets slowly, beginning 1 to 2 weeks before training.
- The amount of food fed daily should not be overestimated and initially should be restricted in accordance with any increase in energy density from a higher fat content. However, the amount fed should be sufficient to maintain the desired body condition.

Geriatric Dogs

- Presence of the physical signs of aging, such as graying of the muzzle, decreased activity, or loss of sight or hearing, should raise the clinician's suspicion for the presence of age-related diseases.
- Dietary advice depends on the animal's usual diet and current health status. The history should be taken, and physical and laboratory evaluations should be performed to determine patient's current status.
- Dogs become less active as they grow older and may lose muscle mass, so they need less dietary energy to maintain their normal weight and condition.

- Dogs need at least 1 g of dietary protein per pound of lean body weight per day to maintain normal protein reserves.
- Only small amounts of fat are needed to meet essential fatty acid requirements, so the trade-off associated with a high-fat diet is higher palatability versus greater risk of obesity.
- Older dogs should not be fed on a free-choice basis.
- Clients should be advised that sudden unexplained decreases in food intake could be an early sign of disease that should be investigated.

REFERENCE

Kealy RD, Lawler DE, Ballam JM et al. Effects of diet restriction on life span and age-related changes in dogs, *J Am Vet Med Assoc* 9:1315, 2002.

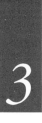

Normal Cats

GESTATION AND LACTATION

As with bitches, queens should be fit and in normal body condition before breeding. During gestation the queen's body weight increases linearly (in contrast to dogs, whose body weight gain is more rapid during late gestation). Queens fed free choice adjust their food intake to meet the increased food needs of gestation. Cats, like dogs, may stop eating for a day or two at around the thirtieth day of pregnancy. If the animal is normal in all other respects this is not a cause for alarm. Inappetence recurs approximately 24 hours before parturition.

Once the kittens are born, the owner ensures that they all ingest colostrum by putting each kitten up to a nipple to nurse if all kittens are not observed to nurse on their own. Queens and their kittens are left alone except by the one person designated to watch over them during lactation; a young, inexperienced queen may eat her offspring if she becomes nervous.

Normal kittens gain 5% to 10% of their birth weight per day, approximately doubling their body weight every 7 to 10 days during the first 3 weeks of life. Newborn kittens also must be kept warm; like puppies, they cannot regulate body temperature during the first week of life. The kittens' environment is maintained at approximately 90° F for the first 3 weeks of life. If the queen is not able to maintain this temperature, an external heat source that can be controlled within 1 to 2 degrees is provided. Weighing the kittens frequently is one of the best ways to evaluate their health and well-being; kittens are weighed every 2 to 4 days, and initially even more frequently. If kittens are small, cool, or not gaining weight, problems should be suspected immediately and the kittens evaluated carefully.

At approximately 3 weeks of age the kittens are old enough to start eating food on their own. The food they will be fed after weaning is moistened into a soft gruel, and a small amount is put into a shallow pan. The kittens are placed into the pan so they get the food on their paws and are introduced to it as they groom themselves.

Kittens can be weaned at 6 to 8 weeks of age. They are weaned in 24 hours. The queen is taken away from the kittens the morning before weaning. The queen is deprived of food, and the kittens are fed the gruel they normally receive. The queen and kittens are reunited overnight, and all are deprived of food so that the kittens will drain the queen's mammary glands. The next day the kittens are weaned abruptly and completely. Depending on the degree of mammary gland distention, the queen is returned to one half of her *prebreeding* intake. If she is still engorged with milk she is deprived of food for another day before she is "weaned" back to her normal food intake. Food intake increases as much as threefold during

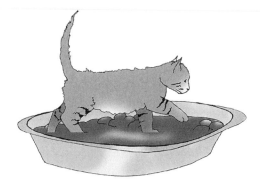

TECH TIPS: Gestating and Lactating Cats

Pregnancy is one of the most nutritionally stressful times in a cat's life. Client education is very important for a successful outcome. The following guidelines are recommended.

- Obtain a complete dietary history (see Appendix C), noting the type and amount of food eaten before pregnancy.
- Carefully evaluate body condition score (BCS), muscle condition score (MCS), skin, and haircoat, and teach the owner how to do the same (see Figures 1-1 and 1-2).
- If a change in food is recommended, instruct the client on the proper way to handle the transition to the new food (see Appendix D).
- Instruct the owner to always make sure that plenty of water is available and to add water to food if necessary to help keep up with milk production.

lactation, so the queen's nonpregnant nutritional needs are met with a significantly reduced amount of food. Owners should be advised to note the amount of food their cats are receiving at the time of breeding, so that after the kittens are weaned the owners know how much food their cat was receiving before pregnancy. If this precaution is taken, the owners will understand that apparently large decreases in food volume are not dangerous for queens.

The same recommendations made for kittens raised by queens apply to orphaned kittens. In place of queen's milk a commercial cat milk replacer that has been tested in kittens is fed. Volumes to be fed vary among individuals and with the environmental temperature (see Figure 2-2 for directions on building an incubator). Feeding is begun according to the manufacturer's directions, and the amount of food received is adjusted to achieve acceptable growth rates. Properly managed orphans behave similarly to queen-raised kittens, vocalizing and becoming restless only when in need of care or feeding. See Appendix B for nutrient comparison tables for kitten milk replacers.

GROWING CATS

Clients begin to receive dietary and nutritional advice when kittens are first presented for vaccinations. Most nutrition-related problems are avoidable if clients are taught early in their kittens' lives about cat nutrition and feeding. Veterinarians should explain to their clients that because cats are carnivorous they are eaters of *animals*, not just eaters of *muscle meat*. The distinction is important because muscle meat by itself is deficient in many nutrients. The fact that cats are carnivorous means that it is not safe to attempt to make "vegetarians" of them. Many of the nutrients they require—for example, taurine, arachidonic acid, and vitamin A—are present only in animal products. In addition, veterinarians should recommend only foods with which they have had some experience and in which they have confidence.

Cats vary widely in the amount of food they require to maintain a normal body weight, and they should be fed whatever is necessary to maintain a moderate body condition. Clients are shown how to recognize a moderate body condition: the ribs are easily palpable but not visible, the cat's waist is visible from above, and from the side the abdomen appears "tucked up." Because many clients do not have extensive experience with animals, their opportunities to evaluate the body condition of cats may have been limited. The elements of body condition scoring are explained to them, and they are advised to use body condition rather than the fullness of the food dish to determine the adequacy of food intake.

Clients occasionally ask if they may cook for their cats. Many pet food recipe books are available in bookstores. The probability that the diet is nutritionally inadequate, however, is much greater with home-prepared foods than it is with commercial diets that are of excellent quality. Reputable manufacturers quickly incorporate new nutritional information into pet food formulas, often before the information is published. For most owners, therefore, the use of commercial foods that have been carefully formulated and adequately tested is in the cat's best interest.

Clients should be told that cats are "nibblers." Domestic cats normally eat 12 to 20 meals a day, with the meals evenly spaced over the 24-hour period. This behavior pattern is quite different from that of the large cats, which, like dogs, consume large meals less frequently.

Owners commonly question the value of nutrient supplementation to a cat's diet. Cats that are receiving excellent-quality commercial diets do not require supplements. If the cat's diet is defective in any observable respect, then that food should not be fed. The diet may also be deficient in inapparent ways. No reason exists to support manufacturers who produce defective diets. Some clients do not understand that cat foods that support gestation, lactation, and early rapid growth contain as much as three times the nutrient density needed for adult maintenance. This differs somewhat from the situation in humans, who consume a variety of natural foods. Human nutritionists recommend supplements infrequently, but cat foods should be regarded as already "supplemented" with a significant surplus of most nutrients. To add more to such diets does not make sense nutritionally or economically. The excess of nutrients in high-quality commercial diets does, however, allow for provision of treats if the owner desires to give them. As long as treats constitute less than 20% of the daily energy intake of the cat they do not create a significant problem. Another option is for part of the regular dry diet to be set aside for use as treats.

Dietary recommendations can be made to owners when they present cats for neutering. At the time of suture removal the veterinarian explains that the cat's energy requirements have been lowered with removal of the gonads; neutered animals are less active and have a slightly lower metabolic rate. If an owner has been feeding a diet formulated for kittens, the diet may be changed at this time to one formulated for adults, and the owner is reminded how to evaluate the cat's nutritional status by its body condition. If the owner understands that the animal's body condition depends on its food intake and knows how to identify a

CLIENT COMMUNICATION TIPS: Growing Cats

- Review the importance of BCS at each well-kitten visit.
- Provide the client with the practice's list of preferred manufacturers of kitten growth products and adult maintenance products.
- Provide the client with two or three options for commercial treats, and discuss replacement of energy rather than addition of energy to the total number needed daily by the kitten.
- Discuss exercise and environmental enrichment for indoor cats (see Appendix G).
- Talk to clients about the decrease in metabolic requirements that results from neutering, when to switch from a growth-formulated to an adult-formulated food, and how that transition should occur.
- Discuss with the staff the criteria for determining which diets everyone in the practice recommends, as well as diets to avoid recommending. Which foods are on the practice's "A list," and why. Which are on the practice's "B list," and why. Help staff identify clients who are receptive to learning more about dietary recommendations.

TECH TIPS: Growing Cats

When asked how much a new kitten should be fed the practitioner should teach clients how to assess an animal's body condition (see Figure 1-1).

- Provide a body condition scoring sheet and an 8-ounce measuring cup. These can be obtained from most pet food manufacturing companies.
- A cat's energy requirements are reduced by 25% after neutering. Nutritional counseling is needed regarding the proper type and amount of food required by animals after spaying and neutering to avoid unnecessary weight gain.
- At least one follow-up appointment is scheduled during the cat's growth stage to ensure that weight and body condition match the established guidelines.

moderate body condition, the risk for obesity is reduced. See Appendix B for nutrient comparison tables for growth foods.

ADULT CATS

Healthy adult cats have relatively low nutrient requirements compared with cats in the reproductive stages of life. Adult cats may be maintained for years on a wide range of commercial diets with apparently few consequences, which may seem to support the fervent beliefs of some owners that an apparently peculiar diet is beneficial. The risk of a diet-related problem, however, is lower in animals fed properly formulated commercial diets because such diets have been thoroughly tested and fed to millions of animals successfully for generations. Because no adverse consequences are observed in a single animal does not mean that the diet provides superior nutrition.

Adult cats may be fed on a free-choice basis, with food available at all times, or they may be fed at designated mealtimes, with the owner determining the size of each meal. Self-feeding is more convenient and ensures that timid animals are not denied access to food in group-feeding situations. Self-feeding has the disadvantages of reducing owner contact with

CLIENT COMMUNICATION TIPS: Adult Cats

- Review the importance of BCS at each healthy-pet visit, and discuss the benefits of regular activity.
- Provide the client with the practice's list of top manufacturers of adult maintenance cat foods.
- Provide the client with two or three options for commercial treats, and discuss replacement of energy rather than addition of energy to the total amount needed daily by the cat.
- Discuss options for environmental enrichment for indoor-housed cats (see Appendix G).
- If the client would like to feed a homemade diet, recommend the service provided at www.petdiets.com. Ask that the e-mail address of the practice be included, so that a report and updates will be received.
- Discuss with the staff the criteria for determining which diets everyone in the practice recommends, as well as diets to avoid recommending. Which foods are on the practice's "A list," and why. Which are on the practice's "B list," and why. Help staff identify clients who are receptive to learning more about dietary recommendations.

TECH TIPS: Adult Cats

At this stage clients are familiar with their pets' eating habits. Type and amount of food are noted for future reference; if an animal's eating habits change because of a health problem the owner may be able to identify it early. It is also recommended that the proper way to assess a BCS be discussed (see Figure 1-1).

The following materials are available from most major pet food companies, and should be provided to the client.
- A body condition scoring sheet to which the client can refer at home
- An 8-ounce measuring cup

the pet and decreasing the number of opportunities for evaluation of the animal's body condition and general health. Pets that tend to overeat are fed once or twice daily in amounts sufficient to maintain a moderate body condition. See Appendix B for nutrient comparison tables for adult cat foods.

GERIATRIC CATS

Nutritional needs can change as an animal ages, but few studies have investigated the nutrient requirements of cats during the last third or quarter of their lives. Until more information is available, only tentative recommendations can be offered beyond sound general advice based on a dietary history, a physical examination, and indicated diagnostic testing. The dietary history is obtained from the person who feeds the cat.

Healthy Geriatric Cats

Healthy geriatric cats should be fed diets that have been made by reputable manufacturers, that have passed feeding trials approved by the American Association of Feed Control

Officials (AAFCO), and with which the veterinarian has had positive experience ("satisfactory" diets). The index of suspicion for a diet-related problem increases if an unknown, an untested, or especially a homemade diet is fed.

Adequate water intake is encouraged; providing bottled, tap, or fountain water may increase intake in cats that seem predisposed to dehydration. Some cats prefer water that is flavored with small ice cubes made from chicken, fish, or other broths. If a cat's vibrissae seem unusually sensitive, providing fresh water in filled, wide-mouthed bowls may facilitate drinking. Placing several bowls throughout the house may facilitate access.

There is no evidence that "geriatric" diets are necessary if a cat is healthy and consumes a satisfactory diet. If a dietary change is needed, a gradual transition over the course of a week or more may accommodate the sluggish physiologic adaptive responses associated with aging. Some cats accustomed to continuous access to food may resist dietary changes. For such cats feeding is limited to two meals per day. When the cat has adjusted to the modified feeding schedule, the amount of food can be reduced and the new diet offered in a separate bowl adjacent to that containing the old food (see Appendix D).

Activity generally decreases as cats age, so fewer calories may be required to maintain moderate body condition, and fewer may be consumed. One report found that nearly 20% of owners of cats older than 14 years regarded their cats as underweight, compared with less than 10% who believed their pets were overweight. Digestibility also affected food intake in older cats. Digestibility of a standard canned diet declined from approximately 84% in 14-month-old cats to 75% in 14-year-old cats. The older cats accommodated to the decreased digestibility by increasing intake to maintain energy balance.

The protein requirements of older cats compared with those of younger cats are not known, but relative to other species, cats of all ages appear to have higher protein needs. The vitamin and mineral requirements of healthy geriatric cats do not appear to differ from those of younger cats, so dietary supplementation is not necessary if a satisfactory diet is being fed. If the diet is unsatisfactory, the owner should change the diet rather than attempt to compensate for the deficiencies. Dietary antioxidants may retard the progression of normal aging processes, but no benefits of supplementation have been documented in controlled clinical trials. Moreover, antioxidant preservatives are present in most cat foods.

Most commercial diets have restricted amounts of magnesium and contain acidifying ingredients to produce an acidic urine pH and thereby reduce the risk of struvite urolithiasis. Although the risk of struvite urolithiasis decreases in older cats, the incidence of oxalate urolithiasis increases; cats older than 10 years are at greatest risk. Because cat foods formulated for the prevention of struvite crystals may contribute to the risk of calcium oxalate formation, diets that are not magnesium restricted and maintain a more neutral urine pH may be more appropriate for older cats.

To ensure that nutrient intake is adequate, the food intake of geriatric cats is monitored. Some cats may benefit from a more nutrient-dense diet that promotes adequate intake of essential nutrients. For example, cats seem to need at least 1.5 g of protein per pound of body weight per day. In a cat that consumes 21 kcal per pound per day a diet containing 25% of energy as protein would meet requirements, whereas if 18 kcal per pound per day were consumed a diet containing 30% of energy as protein would be necessary. Thus the food intake of geriatric patients is assessed on an individual basis to determine the appropriate dietary nutrient densities. Advising clients to monitor food intake also provides an "early warning system" for health problems, because decreased food intake is a common early sign of disease. See Appendix B for nutrient comparison tables for geriatric cat foods.

Feeding Considerations

Owners should monitor the daily food intake of geriatric cats. A decrease in appetite often is an early sign of worsening of a problem or development of complications. Owners may encourage sick geriatric cats to eat by feeding favorite foods, feeding from wide and shallow bowls, warming or moistening the food, offering fresh food frequently and in a quiet environment, and petting the cat during feeding. Learned aversions—avoidance of a food because its presence has been associated with an aversive experience—can be induced in sick hospitalized cats by offering them novel foods (including veterinary foods). The risk of inducing a learned aversion can be minimized by delaying introduction of new diets until medical therapy has succeeded in improving a sick cat's condition. Patient health may be compromised by insistence on using a veterinary food formulated to accommodate the patient's condition; it is better for a sick cat to eat something than to eat nothing at all. For patients being given medication, interactions among drugs and nutrients may influence dietary intake or nutritional requirements.

Nutritional recommendations, as all recommendations made by the veterinarian, require consideration of the individual patient. Extreme care must be taken when attempting to extrapolate results of studies conducted on other species; how similar old rats, dogs, and people are to old cats remains to be proved. Normal aged pets are not nutritional cripples. Keeping geriatric animals in moderate body condition, feeding them a satisfactory diet, and keeping them active go a long way toward helping them reach their genetic life expectancy.

CLIENT COMMUNICATION TIPS: Geriatric Cats

- Review the importance of BCS at each healthy-pet visit, and discuss the benefits of regular exercise.
- Review the dietary history carefully with the owner, and provide the practice's list of top manufacturers for adult maintenance and geriatric cat foods.
- Determine total daily energy intake and calculate protein intake to determine whether the pet is consuming the minimum amount required. This has particular significance in older cats, whose daily food intake may vary.
- Educate the client about the benefits of monitoring the cat's appetite and its water consumption.
- If the client feeds commercial treats, provide two or three options for low-calorie products.
- Recommend that any dietary change be performed gradually over a period of several days.
- Discuss options for environmental enrichment for indoor-housed cats.
- Discuss with the staff the criteria for determining which "geriatric" diets everyone in the practice recommends, as well as diets to avoid recommending. Which foods are on the practice's "A list," and why. Which are on the practice's "B list," and why. Help staff identify clients who are receptive to learning more about dietary recommendations.

TECH TIPS: Geriatric Cats

Client education is crucial for owners of geriatric pets. Make sure enough time is scheduled for each appointment to adequately address all concerns. When a cat has reached the geriatric stage, an accurate dietary history is essential to future care (see Appendix C). A change in the animal's eating habits may help in identification of an illness early in its course.
- After the total daily food intake is calculated, the protein intake is calculated to determine whether the pet is receiving the minimum amount required (see Appendix F). This determination is particularly important with older cats, whose food intake may vary daily.
- Owners of geriatric pets are taught to assess the body condition of their animals (see Figure 1-1).
- If a dietary change is recommended, the owner is instructed regarding the proper way to make the transition to the new food (see Appendix D).

NUTRIENT NEEDS SPECIFIC TO CATS

The nutrient requirements of cats differ qualitatively and quantitatively from those of dogs. The felids diverged from the canids more than 30 million years ago. The felids evolved into metabolic carnivores and developed unique strategies for metabolism of protein, amino acids, fat, and vitamins that can have clinical significance (Figure 3-1). The minimum protein requirement of cats for growth is twice, and for maintenance three times, that of dogs. The higher requirements result for the most part from the inability of cats to control the activity of liver enzymes responsible for ureagenesis in response to changes in dietary protein intake.

This inability in cats does not mean that normal cats are less able to survive starvation than are dogs (in the absence of hepatic lipidosis). Rather, cats use a different strategy to control the urea cycle. In many species, including dogs, rats, and humans, flux through the

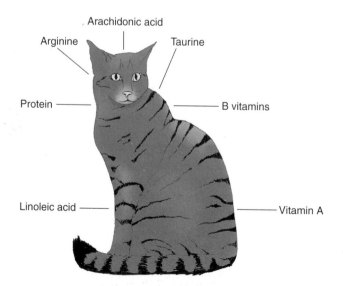

Figure 3-1 Nutrient needs specific to cats.

urea cycle is controlled by the amount of enzyme present. When protein intake is high, the enzyme activity increases, whereas during periods of food deprivation the activity decreases. This strategy decreases the rate of acid generation during protein catabolism and excretion of ammonium ion in the urine conserves sodium and potassium. If members of these species are fed a diet high in protein after a period of food deprivation, ammonia generation during amino acid catabolism may overwhelm the reduced capacity of the urea cycle, resulting in ammonia intoxication. Because cats normally consume a high-protein diet this strategy would not be successful. Cats survive extended periods of food deprivation as successfully as other species do, but by decreasing the concentration of urea cycle *intermediates*. This mechanism is successful because cats, in contrast to other species, do not convert glutamate to arginine in the intestine. Although cats are more susceptible to ammonia toxicity if fed an arginine-deficient diet, they are protected from ammonia intoxication when a high-protein diet is fed after a period of food deprivation because the enzyme concentration is adequate to metabolize any ammonia generated, and the urea cycle intermediates are contained in the diet. Cats require more arginine than most other animals do because they lack an intestinal enzyme, pyrroline-5-carboxylate synthase. This enzyme synthesizes ornithine, which is converted to arginine in the kidney. Arginine is present in sufficient quantities in most of the food proteins that cats eat (except casein) that an arginine deficiency in normal cats fed commercial cat food would not be expected. Signs of arginine deficiency have been observed in sick cats fed casein-based liquid diets, however, and plasma arginine concentrations in cats fed such diets have been reported to be low.

Taurine, a β-amino acid present only in animal tissues, is essential for cats. Although not incorporated into protein, taurine sustains normal cardiovascular, reproductive, and visual performance. Cats require a dietary source of taurine because they cannot synthesize enough taurine from dietary precursors to compensate for obligatory intestinal losses. Most mammals produce both glycine and taurine conjugates of cholesterol for secretion as bile acids, but cats can use only taurine. Bile reabsorption is not 100% efficient, so some taurine is continually lost via the intestine. Clinical signs of taurine deficiency have been reported in cats fed cereal-based dog foods, which are particularly likely to contain amounts of taurine that are inadequate for cats. Cats possess the two enzymes necessary for taurine synthesis, but the activities of these enzymes are low. The low enzyme activities limit endogenous synthesis of taurine, and cats cannot retain taurine as well as other species because taurocholic acid is the only bile acid produced by cats. The extent of recovery of taurine by enterohepatic circulation depends on the diet. Diets containing large amounts of protein (such as in canned foods), particularly if digestibility is reduced by processing, result in increased bile secretion and promote the presence of intestinal microflora that break taurine down. Therefore the amount of dietary taurine needed to meet cats' taurine requirement depends on the ingredients and the method of processing. For example, cats fed canned diets need approximately twice as much dietary taurine as cats fed dry diets do to sustain normal taurine status.

The industry response to the report in 1987 of taurine-deficiency–induced dilated cardiomyopathy in cats was rapid. Most manufacturers immediately began adding taurine to their foods to overcome the negative effects of processing on availability of taurine. Availability of sufficient amounts of taurine in cat foods resulted in a dramatic decline in the occurrence of dilated cardiomyopathy in cats (see the section on heart disease in Chapter 5).

Cats require dietary sources of both linoleic acid (18:2n6) and arachidonic acid (20:4n6), whereas dogs appear to require only linoleic acid. The requirement for both fatty acids arises from cats' inability to synthesize arachidonic acid from linoleic acid.

In the liver in most species of mammals arachidonic acid synthesis from linoleic acid occurs by addition of another double bond (Δ-6 desaturation), then a two-carbon fragment (elongation), and finally another double bond (Δ-5 desaturation). Cats and other carnivores cannot add the double bonds. Although the arachidonic acid requirement of cats has been widely reported, the probability that a cat will have the deficiency is very small. In the study demonstrating the essentiality of arachidonic acid, consumption of purified diets devoid of arachidonic acid for months to years was necessary to elicit signs of deficiency.

Cats also need more of the B vitamins thiamin and niacin than most species do. Although part of the niacin required by other animals may be met by tryptophan, niacin from this source is not available to cats because of the rapid removal of a pathway intermediate. Cats also lack the intestinal enzyme dioxygenase, which converts carotene, a plant precursor of vitamin A, into the vitamin A molecule. Therefore cats require preformed vitamin A, which is found only in animal tissues.

The feeding behavior of cats does not appear to follow the daily rhythmicity seen in dogs and many other species; when fed on a free-choice basis cats generally eat 12 to 20 meals per day, evenly spaced over the 24-hour period. The meals of feral cats consist of small birds, mammals, and insects; mice are a common prey and provide approximately 30 kcal per mouse. The average adult cat would therefore need to consume 8 to 15 mice to meet daily energy requirements.

Cats also appear to be more sensitive to the taste and physical form of the diet than are other species. Cats generally choose foods with a flavor or physical character that is novel to them. Some cats, however, refuse to eat novel foods, particularly under threatening circumstances or if they have been fed a single type of food previously. Palatability of cat foods is enhanced by moisture, animal fats, protein hydrolysates, meat extracts, the amino acids alanine, histidine, proline, and lysine, and acid. The preference for protein-breakdown products and acidity may explain the use of *digest* as an ingredient in dry and semimoist cat (and some dog) foods. Digest is a microbiologically stable material resulting from digestion of animal tissues. It is produced by enzymatic hydrolysis of animal tissues and byproducts, which yields a viscous solution of amino acids, peptides, and fatty acids. Digest also contains significant quantities of phosphoric acid, which is added to stop the enzymatic degradation process and to preserve the product. Digest is sprayed onto the outside of cat foods at 4% to 10% of the final finished product or is incorporated directly into the food. Digest can enhance the palatability of foods as much as two to three times that of the uncoated product. See Appendix B for nutrient comparison tables for cat foods.

SUMMARY

Gestating and Lactating Cats

- Queens fed on a free-choice basis adjust their food intake to meet the increased nutritional demands imposed by gestation.

- Queens may stop eating for a day or so at approximately the thirtieth day of pregnancy and again approximately 24 hours before parturition.
- The kittens must be made to ingest colostrum if they do not begin to nurse on their own.
- The queen and her kittens are left alone as much as possible.
- Normal kittens gain 5% to 10% of their birth weight per day during the first 3 weeks of life.
- Kittens are kept warm; the temperature of their environment is maintained at 90° F for the first 3 weeks of life.
- Kittens are weighed every 2 to 4 days to ensure that growth rate is adequate.
- At approximately 3 weeks of age kittens are exposed to a gruel made of water and the food they will receive after weaning.
- Kittens are weaned at 6 to 8 weeks of age.
- Depending on the degree of mammary gland distention the queen's food intake is returned to one half the prebreeding level and slowly increased back to normal.
- The recommendations for queen-raised kittens apply to orphaned kittens.
- Milk replacers tested on kittens are used to replace queen's milk for orphaned kittens.

Growing Cats

- Cats need to eat whole animals, not just muscle meat, if nutrient deficiencies are to be prevented.
- Cats are fed whatever amount is necessary to maintain moderate body condition during growth.
- Domestic cats normally eat 12 to 20 meals a day, evenly spaced over the 24-hour period.
- Commercial cat foods should be regarded as already "supplemented" with significant excesses of most nutrients.
- A cat's energy requirements are reduced after neutering or spaying.

Adult Cats

- Healthy adult cats have relatively small nutrient requirements compared with those of cats in the reproductive stages of life.
- Adult cats may be fed on a free-choice basis, or they may be fed on a meal schedule.
- Pets that tend to overeat are fed once or twice daily in amounts sufficient to maintain moderate body condition.

Geriatric Cats

- Few studies have investigated the nutrient requirements of cats during the last third of their lives.
- Only tentative recommendations can be offered beyond sound general advice based on a dietary history, a physical examination, and diagnostic testing as indicated.
- Healthy geriatric animals should consume diets that are made by reputable manufacturers and that have been tested by the AAFCO.
- Adequate water intake is encouraged.

- No evidence has shown that "geriatric" diets are necessary for cats that are healthy and consume a satisfactory diet.
- If dietary changes are needed, they are made gradually.
- As cats age their activity decreases and less energy is required to maintain moderate body condition.
- Protein requirements of older cats compared with those of younger cats are not known.
- Vitamin and mineral requirements of healthy geriatric cats do not appear to differ from those of younger cats.
- Food intake of geriatric cats should be monitored closely.

4

Diet and Feeding Factors

COMMERCIAL DIETS

Characteristics of a Satisfactory Diet

Pets require a satisfactory diet to maintain normal structure and function at all stages of life. A satisfactory diet is complete, balanced, digestible, palatable, and safe. A diet is complete if it provides adequate amounts of all required nutrients; a diet is balanced if the nutrients are present in the proper proportions. Balance is crucial, because excesses of some nutrients may cause deficiencies of others. The completeness and balance of a diet can be evaluated by comparing the chemical composition of the diet with the pet's nutrient requirements. Regardless of the chemical composition of the diet, however, the nutrients must be digestible enough to become available to the animal. Nutrient digestibility is measured by subtracting the amount of the nutrient found in the feces from that present in the food. Even if a diet is complete, balanced, and digestible, it must also be sufficiently palatable to be eaten in quantities great enough to support normal function. A food is useless if a pet refuses to eat it. In addition, diets must be safe—that is, free of toxins. Whereas completeness and balance can be estimated chemically, the determination of digestibility, palatability, and safety requires live animal feeding studies.

A diet that is appropriate for an animal in one stage of life may not be appropriate for an animal in another. As shown in Figure 4-1, nutrient requirements vary according to stage of life; lactating animals or those in early growth may need four times the nutrients that are required for maintenance of older, sedentary adults. Deficiencies in the nutrient content of diets often become evident only during the periods of greatest nutritional stress, so during these times the veterinarian must take care to recommend the highest quality diet available to the client.

Pet Foods

Pet foods are available in three physical forms: dry, semimoist, and canned. Each form is associated with a standard method of food preservation, and each has advantages and disadvantages. Quality, however, is not dependent on physical form; satisfactory and unsatisfactory diets can be made in any of these forms. See Appendixes A and B for nutrient comparison tables for commercial dog and cat foods.

Dry pet foods are predominantly extruded, expanded products. Extrusion is a process whereby dry ingredients are cooked with steam and pressure to kill microorganisms and to

39

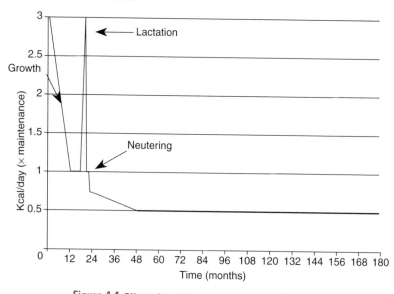

Figure 4-1 Effect of the life stage on energy requirements.

increase digestibility of the ingredients. For example, starch in the mixture is partially degraded, or "gelatinized," during the process, which enhances the digestibility of the starch. The heated food is then forced (extruded) through a small opening in a plate at the end of a high-pressure chamber. The sudden reduction in pressure causes the gelatinized carbohydrate to expand when the food exits the chamber. The shape of the opening in the plate is varied to produce food of different shapes.

Advantages of dry foods include potentially lower cost and greater convenience. Dry foods may be left out for longer periods than foods in other forms without spoiling, allowing an animal to self-feed, although unopened packages of dry foods tend to spoil more quickly than semimoist or canned foods in humid climates. Disadvantages of dry foods may include lower energy density, palatability, and digestibility of the dry ingredients commonly used in these formulas. The amount of energy available in some dry foods may make it difficult for some pets to eat enough food to meet caloric needs during periods of nutritional stress, such as rapid growth and lactation.

Semimoist foods are produced by processes similar to those used to produce dry foods. The primary difference is that chemical preservatives are added to prevent spoilage and to retain a soft, moist texture. Compounds used to preserve semimoist foods include acids and sugars. Phosphoric, hydrochloric, and malic acids are added to bind water and to increase the acidity of the food to inhibit bacterial growth. Sorbitol is added to decrease fungal growth. In the past, propylene glycol was added to bind water in semimoist cat foods, but recent concerns regarding the safety of propylene glycol (which induces increases in Heinz body and reticulocyte numbers and a decrease in erythrocyte survival in some cats) have halted its use in these foods. Like dry foods, semimoist foods may be self-fed. They are digestible and palatable and, like dry and canned foods, can be formulated to include fresh animal tissue. The main disadvantage of semimoist foods is that they may be expensive.

Canned foods also are palatable and digestible. Any ingredient can be included in canned foods because heat and pressure are applied to the sealed cans to ensure sterility. This method of processing generally results in the greatest loss of nutrients, and the product formulation must compensate for this loss. Two major forms of canned food are produced for pets: "ration" type diets, which are made up of animal tissue, soy, and cereal grains, and "gourmet" diets, which primarily are made from some form of meat with vitamins and minerals added to produce a satisfactory diet. Gourmet products must be carefully formulated because meat alone is a poorly balanced, incomplete food. Animals in the wild also eat the viscera and bone of their prey, which results in a more balanced diet. Advantages and disadvantages of canned foods are similar to those of semimoist foods, with the additional disadvantage that if a can is opened and left out for a prolonged period, the food may spoil.

Some pet food manufacturers use what is known as *least-cost formulation* to compound their diets. This means that the proportion and quality of ingredients may fluctuate with ingredient prices. The final formula at any given time depends on a computer program, which may or may not generate exactly the same formulation as the one actually tested during feeding trials. Although variations generally are minor, this method may explain why some variability may be noted among batches. Manufacturers of premium pet foods commonly use fixed formulas, which do not change based on ingredient prices. This is one reason for the higher price of these foods, which often are sold only in specialty pet stores. Neither of these methods clearly is preferable to the other. Although the variation in nutrient composition is greater with the least-cost formulation, changing ingredients may reduce the risk of a deficiency of a nutrient in one of the "fixed" ingredients. Moreover, healthy animals are sufficiently resilient to survive minor changes in nutrient intake.

Direct comparisons of nutrient content among foods of different types may be quite misleading because of the different amounts of water and energy in the three forms. For example, the amount of protein guaranteed on the label of dry cat foods is approximately 35% and on that of canned foods is approximately 10%. Canned foods, however, contain more water than dry foods do. For products of differing moisture content but similar energy density a more appropriate way to compare the nutrient content is on a "dry matter" basis (Box 4-1), that is, based on the dry matter content of the diets.

For example:
* *Dry food*

10% moisture: 100% − 10% = 90% dry matter
35% protein: 35% protein ÷ 90% dry matter = 0.38
0.38 × 100% = 38% protein on dry matter basis

Box 4-1
Calculating Dry Matter Basis

1. Percent dry matter = 100% − percent moisture (or water, given on the label).
2. Percent of nutrient is divided by percent of dry matter.
3. Answer from step 2 is multiplied by 100; result is percent of nutrient on dry matter basis.

• *Canned food*

78% moisture: 100% − 78% = 22% dry matter
10% protein: 10% protein ÷ 22% dry matter = 0.45
0.45 × 100% = 45% protein on dry matter basis

Calculated on a dry matter basis the canned food in this example contains 18% more protein than the dry food.

Another way to compare dietary constituents is on the basis of the energy contained in the diets. This method is most useful for foods differing in fat content, because the energy density of fat in pet foods is approximately 8.5 kcal/g, versus 3.5 kcal/g for carbohydrate and protein. Many commercial diets contain an energy (metabolizable energy [ME]) density of 350 kcal per 100 g for dry food and 100 kcal per 100 g for canned food as fed. The foods in the dry matter example can also be compared on an energy basis:

• *Dry food*

35 g of protein per 100 g of diet ÷ 350 kcal ME per 100 g of diet = 1 g of protein per 10 kcal

• *Canned food*

10 g of protein per 100 g of diet ÷ 100 kcal ME per 100 g of diet = 1 g of protein per 10 kcal

If we compare two diets of differing fat content, however, the result is quite different, because fat contains 2.25 times the energy per gram of protein or carbohydrate. The fat content of commercially available pet foods ranges from less than 6% to greater than 45% on a dry matter basis. The foods in the example above can be used to illustrate the effect of differences in energy density on dietary protein content:

• *If the dry food contains 350 kcal/100 g (~10% fat on a dry matter basis)*

35% protein = 35 g protein/100 g diet ÷ 350 kcal/100 g diet = 0.10 g protein/kcal
0.1 × 100 = 10 g protein per 100 kcal

• *And the canned food contains 120 kcal/100 grams (~30% fat on a dry matter basis)*

10% protein = 10 g protein/100 g diet ÷ 120 kcal/100 g diet = 0.083 g protein/kcal
0.083 × 100 = 8.3 g protein per 100 kcal

Calculated on an energy basis the canned food in this example contains 17% less protein than the dry food.

Because of differences in energy and moisture content among diets, nutrient comparisons among foods are most meaningful when made on an energy basis. Recent changes in Association of American Feed Control Officials (AAFCO) regulations permit the addition of ME estimates to pet food labels, but manufacturers have been slow to provide this information on labels. The information can be obtained by calling the manufacturer or visiting their home page on the World Wide Web.

If economy is a consideration, food costs are compared on an energy basis. Cost per kilocalorie ME is the most relevant comparison if the ME content of the food is known. If the ME content is not listed on the food label, the manufacturer can be contacted for the information. A simple way to determine the economic value of a food is to note the price of the food and the date it is purchased. When all the food has been consumed, divide the price of the food by the number of days fed to determine the feeding cost per day.

Pet Food Labeling

Pet food labels are legal documents. Pet food labeling in the United States is based on rules established by the AAFCO to ensure compliance with federal and state feed regulations. Regulations that apply to pet food labeling and testing of foods for nutritional adequacy are published in the AAFCO manual. This manual, updated annually, also provides definitions of terms. For example, the AAFCO defines *complete* as "a nutritionally adequate feed for animals other than man; by specific formula [it] is compounded to be fed as the sole ration and is capable of maintaining life and/or promoting production without any additional substance being consumed except water." *Balanced* is defined as "a term that may be applied to a diet, ration, or feed having all the required nutrients in proper amount and proportion based upon recommendations of recognized authorities in the field of animal nutrition, such as the National Research Council, for a given set of physiological requirements. The species for which it is intended and the functions such as maintenance or maintenance plus production (growth, fetus, fat, milk, eggs, wool, feathers, or work) shall be specified."

Pet food labels must include the food type and product name, net weight, guaranteed analysis, ingredient content, manufacturer's or distributor's name and address, and "a claim that the pet food meets or exceeds the requirements of one or more of the recognized categories of nutritional adequacy: gestation, lactation, growth, maintenance, and complete for all life stages, as those categories are set forth in AAFCO regulations PF2 (l) and (m) ... [U]nless another scientifically substantiated claim is made, the food is designated solely for intermittent or supplemental feeding, or is to be used on the advice of a veterinarian."

The phrase *food type* means that the label must identify the species for which the food is intended (e.g., *dog food* or *cat food*). This statement is intended to help guide consumer purchase, although dogs can eat cat food, and many high-protein, high-fat dog foods probably are relatively safe for cats. In addition, dogs with decreased appetites may be fed diets labeled for cats to improve nutrient intake. Many phrases used in product names are designed to appeal to consumers (e.g., *dinner, platter*). Table 4-1 shows the AAFCO labeling rules.

The net weight is the amount of food in the container, often indicated on the label in pounds and in grams. As mentioned previously the label may give a rough estimate of the energy density of canned foods, many of which contain approximately 1 kcal/g as fed. One

Table 4-1
Labeling Rules of the Association of American Feed Control Officials

Wording on Label	The Product Must Contain
Beef (or other meat) dog or cat food	At least 95% beef (minus water for processing)
Beef *dinner* (entree, etc.)	25%-94% beef
With beef	At least 3% beef
Beef *flavor*	A "detectable" amount of beef

reason to read the net weight when comparing foods is that manufacturers sometimes reduce the size of containers without changing the price. For example, what many consumers think of as a "16-oz can" really weighs 13.2 ounces, and a package thought of as "6 oz" may weigh only 5.5 ounces.

The guaranteed analysis lists minimum amounts of crude protein and fat and maximum amounts of crude fiber and moisture present in the product. Although it is a legal requirement, the guaranteed analysis is of little value. The analytic methods were developed in Germany in the mid-nineteenth century to evaluate ruminant animal feeds; the methods of analysis for fat and protein are nonspecific, and the crude fiber method used underestimates the indigestible fraction of the food for pets. Furthermore, the numbers are not meant to represent the amount of nutrient present, only the minimum or maximum. More accurate analyses are often available from manufacturers on written request or on their World Wide Web sites.

A list of ingredients must also be present on the label. Listed ingredients fall into four major categories: water, energy sources, protein sources, and vitamins and minerals added to balance the food. Table 4-2 shows the ingredients listed on commonly purchased pet foods in the United States and the function of these ingredients in the diet.

Ingredient names have specific legal definitions, which are also presented in the AAFCO manual. The definitions are somewhat imprecise to allow for normal variation in feeds and processing procedures. The AAFCO requires that ingredients be listed "in descending order by their predominance by weight." Descending order must be evaluated carefully, however, because ingredient lists can be misleading. For example, a meat protein source followed on the list by two or three grain sources may indicate that grain, not meat, is the primary ingredient. This is especially true if the adjective *fresh* is used to describe the meat, because it means that the meat contains its natural water content, which often is removed during processing. Moreover, there is no way to know the quality of the ingredients used, which could affect nutritional adequacy.

The manufacturer's or distributor's name and address are required on the label to identify the source of the product and permit the consumer or other interested persons to contact the producer of the food. Many commercial foods also provide toll-free telephone numbers and World Wide Web addresses that can be used to gain information concerning the food.

The phrase *complete and balanced* must appear on the label. This claim may be met in any of three ways. The first is by calculation. A manufacturer can calculate that the combination of ingredients used meets or exceeds the nutrient levels recommended by the National Research Council (NRC) in published nutrient composition tables. The second method is by analysis of the diet. If chemical analysis shows that the food contains levels of nutrients that exceed the minimums recommended by the NRC, the manufacturer can claim nutritional adequacy. Unfortunately, these methods are of very little practical value in the veterinary evaluation of pet foods. The analytic profile of many pet food ingredients is too variable for "book values" to be useful and provides no measure of nutrient availability. Moreover, nutrient *excesses* or unmeasured toxic substances could be present. The third, and best, method of establishing a nutritional claim is by "protocol testing." Protocol testing requires that the food be fed to pets during the period for which the claim is made—often gestation, lactation, or growth.

Table 4-2
Pet Food Ingredients and Their Functions

Ingredient	Function
Animal fat, vegetable oil	Sources of energy, essential fatty acids; increase palatability of products
Meat by-products; meat and dried whey products; egg, meat, and bone meal; beef digest; chicken; beef; cheese; liver; DL-methionine (an essential amino acid); whole wheat; whole ground corn; soybean meal; soy flour; soybean grits; textured soy protein	Sources of animal protein (essential amino acids), animal fat and energy; sources of vegetable protein (essential amino acids), fiber, and vegetable fat
Calcium carbonate, monocalcium phosphate, dicalcium phosphate, salt, zinc oxide, ferrous sulfate, copper sulfate, copper oxide, ethylenediamine dihydriodide	Supplemental sources of calcium, phosphorus, sodium, chloride, zinc, iron, copper, and iodine (other minerals are supplied by the major ingredients)
Vitamin A supplement, vitamin D supplement, vitamin E supplement, thiamin mononitrate, riboflavin supplement, pyridoxine hydrochloride, calcium pantothenate, vitamin B_{12} supplement	Sources of vitamins A, D, E, B_1, B_2, B_6, pantothenic acid, and B_{12} (other vitamins are supplied by the major ingredients)
Soybean hulls, rice hulls, wheat middlings, wheat shorts, bran	Sources of fiber (for proper intestinal action and feces formation); influence textural qualities of the product
Onion and garlic powders, white pepper, artificial flavor	Added to enhance flavor and aroma
Sucrose, propylene glycol, corn syrup, sodium carboxymethylcellulose, guar gum	Sources of carbohydrate for energy; contribute to product texture; preservatives (by binding water)
Potassium sorbate	Preservative used to inhibit mold formation (also used in bread)
Ethoxyquin, butylated hydroxyanisole	Preservatives used to prevent destruction of vitamin A and protect fat from oxidation
Artificial color, caramel color, titanium dioxide	FDA-approved additives for coloring
Water sufficient for processing	Amount of water necessary for proper cooking and preparation

FDA, Food and Drug Administration.

A problem with AAFCO label guarantees is that there is currently no requirement for retesting. Despite this limitation, feeding tests are the most valid way to ensure that a food can actually meet the nutritional needs of pets to which it is fed.

Despite the required amount of information, evaluation of the label may not be sufficient to predict the quality or price of the food. The label information from four diets, varying in feeding cost per day from $0.22 to $0.91, is presented in Table 4-3. It is impossible from the data presented to determine which diet is which.

A relatively recent development in labeling is the use of so-called "descriptive" terms. For example, the terms *light*, *lean*, and *low* or *reduced* with regard to calories or fat content have

Table 4-3

Label Information for Four Diets for Dogs

	Diet A		Diet B		Diet C		Diet D	
Analysis—.	Protein	23 (5.7)	Protein	21 (6.6)	Protein	26 (7.5)	Protein	21 (6.4)
percent of diet	Fat	14	Fat	9	Fat	15	Fat	8
as fed (grams	Fiber	1.6	Fiber	4	Fiber	5	Fiber	4.5
per 100 kcal)	Water	12	Water	12	Water	10	Water	12
First five	Corn		Corn		Chicken BPM		Corn	
ingredients	Poultry BPM		MBM		Corn		SBM	
	SBM		SBM		Rice		MBM	
	Animal fat		Wheat middlings		Sorghum		Tallow	
	Natural flavor		Animal fat		Animal fat		CGM	
Claim basis	Feeding studies		Feeding studies		Feeding studies		Feeding studies	
Life stage	Maintenance		All		All		All	
Cost per 1000 kcal	$0.91		$0.22		$0.67		$0.48	

Data from *Consumer Reports* 63:12, 1998.
BPM, By-product meal; *CGM,* corn gluten meal; *MBM,* meat and bone meal; *SBM,* soybean meal.

been approved by the AAFCO for use on pet food labels. The terms refer to energy density in kilocalories per kilogram of diet, calibrated by the percentage of moisture. The definitions as they apply to dog and cat foods are presented in Table 4-4.

The use of these terms permits manufacturers to draw attention to foods with reduced calorie and fat contents. Unfortunately, as is the case when they are used on labels of human foods, these terms do not address the fact that energy and fat intake are feeding issues rather than dietary issues. The increase in "low-fat" human foods during the last two decades has been accompanied by a relentless increase in the number of obese humans. Unless food intake is controlled, a change in the nutrient density of the diet cannot produce a moderate body condition, seductive as the suggestion is.

Similarly, claims such as "promotes urinary tract health" on commercial cat food labels have little veterinary value. This expression, coined in the 1980s, is intended to convey that a diet is formulated to reduce the risk of struvite urolithiasis. The subsequent increase in the prevalence of calcium oxalate urolithiasis and the recognition that struvite urolithiasis is not a common cause of lower urinary tract disease render the descriptive value of this term limited and questionable.

Table 4-4

Descriptive Terms Used on Pet Food Labels

			Water Content of Food	
Term	Type of Food	<20%	20%-65%	≥65%
Light, "lite,"	Dog	≤3100 kcal/kg	≤2500 kcal/kg	≤900 kcal/kg
low-calorie	Cat	≤3250 kcal/kg	≤2650 kcal/kg	≤950 kcal/kg
Lean, low-fat	Dog	≤9% fat	≤7% fat	≤4% fat
	Cat	≤10% fat	≤8% fat	≤5% fat

FEEDING FACTORS

The amount of food required to maintain normal body weight varies widely among pets, and animals should be fed whatever is necessary to maintain moderate body condition (see Figure 1-1). Pets may be fed on a free-choice basis, with food available at all times, or they may be fed on a meal basis, in which the owner determines the size of each meal. Self-feeding is more convenient for many owners and ensures that timid animals are not denied access to food in group-feeding situations. Self-feeding has the disadvantage of reducing owner contact with the pet. If pets tend to overeat, they are fed on a meal basis, with feeding frequency dictated by the owner's schedule and the behavior of the pet.

Although diets are appropriately compared on an energy basis, and manufacturers tout the percentages of various nutrients and ingredients present or absent in their diets, animals do not eat percentages of nutrients and ingredients; they eat amounts of food. Comparisons of food analyses with tables of nutrient requirements are based on the presumption that an animal is eating enough of the diet to meet its energy needs. In veterinary practice this often is not the case. Owners may limit food intake to sustain moderate body condition, and the food intake of older animals may decline for a variety of physiologic and medical reasons. For these reasons the food intake of patients may need to be measured to confirm that the actual amount of diet consumed is sufficient to provide the required amounts of nutrients.

This is particularly important when animals with reduced intake are fed diets with restricted nutrient content. The most common example, discussed previously, is protein. The food intake of sedentary adult animals commonly is restricted to maintain moderate body condition, and older animals commonly have relatively small intakes of food. When reduced intake is combined with consumption of a protein-restricted diet, protein depletion of the patient may result, with the attendant detrimental effects on physiologic function. The most appropriate diet for a particular animal therefore may depend on the physiologic status of the animal.

Changing the Diets of Finicky Eaters

Many pets choose foods with a flavor or physical character (e.g., shape, size, texture) that is novel to them. Some pets, however, refuse to eat novel foods. This aversion to new foods can make it extremely difficult to introduce new foods into the pet's diet. These pets often have been fed high-quality, very palatable diets on a free-choice basis and have come to expect unlimited food availability. If a dietary change is necessary, the animal must first be made dependent on the owner for its food intake. This can be accomplished by offering the pet as much food as it wants for an hour twice daily. The pet soon learns to consume its daily nutrient requirements in two feedings. Once the pet is maintaining itself on two feedings a day, the old diet is restricted to approximately 75% of the previous food intake, and the new diet is offered in a separate bowl adjacent to the old food. Animals are much more likely to switch over to new diets when the transition is made by this method rather than by an abrupt dietary change. This method is particularly useful for cats, in which hepatic lipidosis may occur if they refuse to eat for prolonged periods. More strategies to change diets may be found in Appendix D.

If the diet cannot be changed by means of this method, the client may be resistant to making the change for some reason that must be identified and addressed. It is sometimes helpful to ascertain whether the client agrees with the necessity for the change and to soliciting his or her advice regarding strategies that may work.

SUMMARY

Characteristics of a Satisfactory Diet

A satisfactory diet is all of the following.
• Complete—provides adequate amounts of all required nutrients
• Balanced—the nutrients are present in the proper proportions
• Digestible—nutrients can become available to the animal
• Palatable—appealing enough to be eaten in quantities great enough to support normal function
• Safe—free of toxins and antinutrients

Pet food is available in three physical forms: dry, semimoist, and canned. Each form is associated with a standard method of food preservation, and each has advantages and disadvantages. Satisfactory and unsatisfactory diets can be made in any of these forms. Both least-cost and fixed formulation may be used to compound diets. Neither of these methods is clearly preferable to the other.

Direct comparisons of nutrient content among foods of different types may be quite misleading because of the different amounts of water and energy in the three forms. Because of differences in energy and moisture content among diets, nutrient comparisons among foods are most meaningful when made on an energy basis.

Pet Food Labeling

Pet food labeling in the United States is based on rules established by the AAFCO to ensure compliance with federal and state feed regulations. Pet food labels must include the food type and product name, net weight, guaranteed analysis, ingredient content, manufacturer's or distributor's name and address, and a claim that the pet food meets or exceeds the requirements of one or more of the recognized categories of nutritional adequacy. One limitation of the AAFCO label guarantees is that there is currently no requirement for retesting. Despite this limitation, feeding tests are the most valid way to ensure that a food can actually meet the nutritional needs of pets to which it is fed.

Feeding Factors

The amount of food required to maintain normal body weight varies widely among pets, and animals should be fed whatever is necessary to maintain moderate body condition. Although diets are appropriately compared on an energy basis, animals do not eat percentages of nutrients and ingredients; they eat amounts of food. For this reason the food intake of a patient may need to be measured to confirm that the actual amount of diet consumed is sufficient to provide the required amounts of nutrients. This is particularly important when animals with reduced intake are fed diets with restricted nutrient content.

5

Clinical Dietetics

$Three\ types\ of$ nutrition-related problems can affect animals: those related to the presence of a nutrient-sensitive disease, those induced by diet, and those related to feeding. A nutrient-sensitive disease is one in which the affected patient has a defect that prevents it from consuming diets appropriate for healthy animals. Treatment of nutrient-sensitive diseases requires provision of a diet specifically modified to accommodate the disease-related nutritional limitations of the patient.

A diet-induced problem originates with the diet rather than with the animal. Formulation errors, processing problems, and postprocessing mistakes all may result in diet-induced diseases. Formulation errors include deficiencies and excesses of nutrients, imbalances in nutrient content, and the presence of toxins or antinutrient compounds. Problems that occur during processing include alterations in nutrient availability and destruction of nutrients. Postprocessing mistakes include improper storage, which can result in stale, moldy, or infested foods. Treatment of diet-induced disease consists of switching to a satisfactory diet, preferably one in which the caregiver has confidence based on personal experience.

A feeding-related problem is related to the way in which an animal is fed. Feeding-related problems include an excessive or inadequate amount of an appropriate diet and the feeding of a diet that is inappropriate for an animal's physiologic condition. Examples of feeding-related diseases include obesity, cachexia, developmental orthopedic disease, growth failure, and reproductive failure. Treatment for feeding-related diseases usually consists of client education to effect a change in feeding practices.

Preliminary results of an epidemiologic survey of 54 primary care veterinary practices in the United States are presented in Table 5-1.

According to these data, diet-induced and feeding-related diseases do not appear to be common in cats of any age (although some cases of dermatopathy may be diet induced). Nutrient-sensitive diseases appear to increase in frequency with age, as they do in most species. Some oral diseases may be nutrient sensitive, in that some animals may be predisposed to oral disease, or may be diet induced.

Conditions commonly diagnosed in dogs are shown in Table 5-2. With respect to nutrition-related diseases, these data are similar to those seen in cats.

Table 5-1

Top Diagnoses in Cats by Age Category

Age 0-7 Years (n = 9148)	Percent of Total	Age 7-10 Years (n = 1795)	Percent of Total	Age 10-25 Years (n = 2981)	Percent of Total
Healthy	34.2	Oral disease	20.1	Oral disease	19.5
Oral disease	9.9	Healthy	18.9	Healthy	11.9
Ear mites	4.4	Cat bite abscess	2.5	Chronic renal failure	2.4
Fleas	2.7	Dermatopathy	2.3	Weight loss	2
Cat bite abscess	2.6	Obesity	1.6	Cardiac murmur	1.8
Upper respiratory infection	2.2	Fleas	1.5	Hyperthyroidism	1.8
Tapeworms	2	Animal bites	1.5	Tumor	1.7
Conjunctivitis	1.7	Ear mites	1.4	Diabetes mellitus	1.4
Roundworms	1.4	Upper respiratory infection	1.3	Cat bite abscess	1.4
Dermatopathy	1.3	Vomiting	1.3	Vomiting	1.3
All others	37.6	All others	47.6	All others	54.8

Modified from Lund EM, Armstrong PJ, Kirk CA: Health status and population characteristics examined at private veterinary practices in the United States, *JAVMA* 214:1336 1999.

Table 5-2

Top Diagnoses in Dogs by Age Category

Age 0-7 Years (n = 24,165)	Percent of Total	Age 7-10 Years (n = 6699)	Percent of Total	Age 10-25 Years (n = 8692)	Percent of Total
Healthy	32.4	Healthy	15	Oral disease	13.6
Oral disease	5.8	Oral disease	13.7	Healthy	6.9
Otitis externa	5.8	Otitis externa	5.8	Nuclear sclerosis	3.1
Dermatopathy	3.6	Dermatopathy	3.2	Arthritis	3
Lameness	1.3	Tumor	2	Tumor	2.8
Roundworms	1.2	Lipoma	1.9	Otitis externa	2.7
Conjunctivitis	1.2	Conjunctivitis	1.2	Cardiac murmur	2.4
Fleas	1.1	Arthritis	1.2	Lipoma	2.3
Lacerations	1	Anal sac disease	1.2	Cataract	2.2
Anal sac disease	1	Lameness	1.1	Dermatopathy	1.5
All others	45.6	All others	53.7	All others	59.5

Modified from Lund EM, Armstrong PJ, Kirk CA: Health status and population characteristics examined at private veterinary practices in the United States, *JAVMA* 214:1336, 1999.

CANCER

Cancers are common causes of disease in dogs and cats. They usually affect older animals, and so have become more common as pets live longer. As longevity continues to increase in the pet population, this trend can be expected to continue. The role of nutrition in prevention and treatment of cancers varies with the type of tumor and the stage of progression of the disease. Because cancers are common among humans, a wealth of data are available from epidemiologic and laboratory studies of the effects of a wide variety of nutrients and foods on numerous cancers. Unfortunately, few clinical trials have documented that these results can readily translate into improved patient care.

Some epidemiologic studies found differences in the distribution of cancer types between industrialized and nonindustrialized populations. For example, breast, colon, lung, and prostate cancers were found more commonly in industrialized populations, whereas cancers of the cervix, esophagus, liver, oral cavity, and stomach were identified more often among members of nonindustrialized populations. These findings led to the idea that diet may play a role in prevention of cancer, although it was recognized that many features of these populations other than diet differed.

Estimates of the prevalence of common cancers in dogs are presented in Table 5-3.

A comparison of estimates of the prevalence of the most common types of cancers in humans, dogs, and cats in the United States is presented in Table 5-4.

With the exception of breast cancer, the prevalence of common tumor types in humans is generally higher than in dogs or cats. Diet and feeding may play a role in both prevention and treatment of cancers. Some of the factors thought to influence cancer risk in humans are shown in Table 5-5.

Based on the information presented in Table 5-4, the risk of mammary tumors in dogs might be expected to be increased by rapid growth rate before puberty. (In fact, studies of dogs generally have found that common risk factors for humans also apply to canines.) Epidemiologic studies of dogs suggest that a thin body condition at 9 to 12 months of age reduces the risk of mammary tumors in spayed dogs by more than 90%. Even in intact dogs the risk is reduced by 40%. Although early spaying has a greater effect on reducing mammary cancer risk than does lean body condition, the additional reduction in risk

Table 5-3
Prevalence of Common Cancers in Dogs

Type of Cancer	Percent of Total Cancers	
	Females	Males
Breast	30	0
Connective tissue	9	17
Testicle	0	16
Melanoma	8	14
Lymphoma	6	10
Oral	5	10
Bone	2	4
Gastrointestinal	2	3
Others (difference)	38	26
TOTAL	100	100

Modified from Kelsey JL, Moore AS, Glickman LT: Epidemiologic studies of risk factors for cancer in pet dogs, *Epidemiol Rev* 20(2):204, 1998.

Table 5-4

Approximate Prevalence of Common Cancers in Humans, Dogs, and Cats*

Type of Cancer	Prevalence in Humans	Prevalence in Dogs	Prevalence in Cats
Breast	23	30	5
Prostate	17	<1	0
Colon	11	<1	<1
Lung	4	1	1

Data for human subjects from http://cancercontrol.cancer.gov/ocs/prevalence/prevalence.html#allsites.
*With the exception of breast cancer, the common tumor types in humans are not common in dogs or cats.

Table 5-5

Nutritional Effects on Cancer Risk in Humans

	Risk Factor or Protective Factor	Type of Cancer for Which Risk Is Increased or Decreased
Factors that increase risk of cancer	Rapid growth rate before puberty	Breast (and probably other cancers)
	Excessive energy intake	Breast, colon, kidney, uterus, and gallbladder
	Animal fat independent of total energy intake and red meat	Breast (no); colon (slight); prostate
	Inclusion of red meat in the diet	Colon
	Low intake of fruits and vegetables	Lung, stomach, colon, others?
	Alcohol consumption	Breast
	Alcohol consumption plus smoking	Oral cavity, larynx, esophagus, liver
Factors that decrease risk of cancer	Physical activity	Colon
	Lean-to-moderate body condition	Breast, colon, kidney, uterus, gallbladder
	Consumption of fruits and vegetables	Lung, stomach, colon, others?

Modified from Kelsey JL, Moore AS, Glickman LT: Epidemiologic studies of risk factors for cancer in pet dogs, *Epidemiol Rev* 20(2):204, 1998.

supports recommendations that a lean body condition be maintained in young dogs during the period of growth. For adult dogs the recommendations to avoid excessive energy intake, keep the animal in a moderate body condition, and avoid excessive intake of animal fats may be pertinent.

Comparable information regarding cats is currently not available. Given the differences in metabolism among cats, dogs, and humans, predicting which guidelines may apply to feline patients is difficult. The recommendations to maintain a moderate body condition and avoid excess animal fat may pertain to cats as well as to humans and dogs because some carcinogens are fat soluble. Thus, they may be contained in the fat of animals exposed to them and also retained in the adipose stores of animals consuming this dietary fat.

Beyond the important reduction in mammary cancer risk associated with a lean body condition in growing puppies, the potential reduction in cancer risk obtained by following dietary recommendations has not been well documented in veterinary medicine. According to studies in humans, however, "eating right," staying physically active, and maintaining a healthy weight can reduce cancer risk by 30% to 40%. This reduction may be even more achievable in pets, whose diet and food intake can be carefully controlled.

Nutrition also may play an important role in the treatment of cancer. Beyond the possibility of increasing survival, nutritional intervention might improve quality of life for the patient and client satisfaction with therapeutic efforts. The utility of recommendations depends on the risk-benefit ratio of the intervention and the cost of the therapy.

Historically, the interest in the role of nutrition in cancer therapy has been motivated in part by concern about cancer cachexia. Cancer cachexia, the wasting of body substances that is observed in some cancer patients, occurs relatively commonly in people, especially those with pancreatic and gastric cancers. Loss of both fat and muscle mass occurs, and depletion of muscle mass often exceeds that of viscera. Weight loss usually occurs early in the course of disease and is often apparent at the time of presentation. Food intake usually is normal at this stage, suggesting that decreased food intake is not likely to be a primary cause.

The cause of cancer cachexia in humans is not known. Tumor-host competition is not the most likely cause of cancer cachexia; some patients with very large tumors show no signs of cachexia, whereas cachexia has been reported in patients with tumors that are only 0.01% of the host's weight. In dogs the resting energy needs of patients with nonhematopoietic malignancies were not different from normal and were not altered by removal of the tumors. Cancer researchers have conducted an extensive search for a "catabolic factor," but to date no single factor has been identified. Cytokines (tumor necrosis factor [TNF]-α, interleukin [IL]-1 and IL-6, and interferon [IFN]-γ) do not seem to be responsible, but recently identified lipid- and protein-mobilizing factors may play a more direct role, at least in mouse-model systems.

Although common in humans with cancer, cachexia is *not* common in veterinary cancer patients. Moreover, nutritional intervention in humans with cancer cachexia does not appear to be successful in replacing muscle mass, with weight gains occurring only in fat and water.

Most of the research investigating the role of diet in veterinary cancer patients has focused on lymphoma in dogs. Some of these studies have focused on analytic variables, and one study investigated the effect on outcome in dogs with lymphoma of a diet modified in a variety of ways. Many of the analytic variables examined, such as serum lactate and amino acid concentrations, were found to be altered in dogs with lymphoma. Unfortunately, the differences identified, although "statistically significant," were unlikely to have been clinically important. Moreover, the differences persisted in dogs in remission after therapy, further diminishing the likelihood of their relevance to the cancer itself.

A variety of nutrients at "nutriceutical" intakes have been investigated to determine their potential value as cancer chemotherapeutic agents. For example, supplementation of diets with n-3 fatty acids and arginine has been investigated in humans with cancer. Unfortunately, although reduced infection rates and duration of hospital stay were identified, the interventions did not improve survival times.

Several years ago, Hill's Pet Nutrition introduced an interesting diet designed specifically for dogs with lymphoma. One published clinical trial reported promising results, but data from randomized controlled trials comparing this diet to diets of similar composition are not yet available for evaluation. Because of the preferences of the oncologists at our institutions, we have not had sufficient experience with this diet to comment on its efficacy.

Given the current state of knowledge of nutrition and cancer in veterinary medicine, we agree with The American Cancer Society's *Cancer Facts and Figures 2003*, which states the following.

"The scientific study of nutrition and cancer is highly complex, and many important questions remain unanswered. It is not presently clear how single nutrients, combinations of nutrients, overnutrition and energy imbalance, or the amount and distribution of body fat at particular stages of life affect one's risk of specific cancers."

The same is equally true of the role of nutrition and cancer treatment. Pending clinically relevant developments, our recommendations for nutritional care of cancer patients are the same as those for hospitalized and critical care patients, and for those with chronic diseases.

In summary, we believe the most important role we can provide (in our respective practices) is to encourage and support our colleagues (clinicians, students, and technicians) as they discuss quality of life issues with clients. One of the most obvious concerns for owners of cancer patients is making sure their pet eats every day. This is not always physically possible for patients who have undergone surgery, chemotherapy, or radiation. The ability of the veterinary health care team to provide short-term or long-term nutritional support through feeding tubes has greatly enhanced the quality of life for many terminal patients, and thereby maintained the human-pet bond that is so crucial for our clients. Training in how to place and manage feeding tubes should be a part of any hospital staff that is caring for cancer patients. We are also advocates of pet support hotlines and pet loss support groups, and recommend them for both colleagues and clients who are working through the grieving process.

CRITICAL CARE

The ultimate goal of nutritional support of sick animals is for the patient to eat its own food in its own environment. Until this goal can be achieved, the next best thing is for the patient to eat its own food in the hospital. Obtaining an accurate and complete dietary history from the client is very important with regard to attaining this goal. If the patient is offered a food to which it has never been exposed, the animal may not recognize it as food. This is particularly true for cats, which are often exclusively fed one cat food. The owners of patients that spend 1 or more nights in the hospital should be asked to provide the food that is typically offered at home, and they should be encouraged to feed the pet during hospitalization (many pets eat more willingly for their owners than for strangers). The most relevant question for caregivers to consider before starting nutritional support for hospitalized patients is not, "Should this patient be fed?" but rather, "Should this patient be starved?"

Nutrition and Sick or Injured Animals

Animals that cannot or will not eat enough to meet their nutrient needs require nutritional intervention. Poor nutrient intake has a number of adverse consequences, including impaired

CLIENT COMMUNICATION TIPS: Cancer

- Teach clients how to monitor the pet's food intake each day and how to watch for signs of wasting. Reference Fig. 1-2 on lean muscle scoring.
- Review the dietary history carefully. If a client does not know how much food the pet consumes in a given day or week, instruct the client regarding completion of a 5-day food diary. A piece of notebook paper can be used, with columns created for the date, time, type of food or treat offered, quantity or serving size, and initials of the person who offers the food. Everything consumed by the pet is recorded in the food diary. Follow up with clients after the food diary has been completed to identify factors that can potentially be modified (e.g., products, serving sizes, behaviors).
- Review total daily caloric needs. If the pet is unable or unwilling to consume adequate calories to maintain its body condition, the practitioner may discuss with the client the need for a feeding tube that can be maintained at home (see the discussion on feeding tube placement in this chapter).
- Educate clients regarding the important benefits of meal-feeding pets rather than feeding on a free-choice basis. Individual meals allow the owner to observe appetite and water consumption and identify potential problems.
- Recommend that any dietary change be made gradually over a period of several days or longer. If food aversions are to be avoided, dietary changes should not be made in the hospital setting, but in the home and after the pet is feeling better.
- Communicate clearly with clients regarding the type, dosage, and cost of any nutritional supplements that may be recommended.
- Tell clients to call the veterinarian if they have problems or questions.
- Discuss with the staff the criteria for evaluating "cancer" diets and "nutraceutical" products marketed for cancer patients. Which products are on the practice's "A list," and why. Which are on the practice's "B list," and why. Help staff identify clients who are receptive to learning more about dietary recommendations.

TECH TIPS: Cancer

Owners whose pets have been diagnosed with cancer often need some extra time to discuss the best way to feed their pets. Many homemade diets geared toward pets with cancer are described on the Internet, and this variety may cause confusion on the owner's part when it comes to deciding which diet is "best."

Following are some suggestions for enhancing preparation for assisting these clients.

- Make a copy of each new cancer-related diet that is discussed, date it, and write relevant notes regarding the results if the diet was given to a pet. Place these notes in a file for future reference.
- Have a variety of complete and balanced homemade recipes available for use for finicky or sick patients.
- Keep up with the current literature regarding nutrition and cancer, and have copies of articles available for interested owners.
- Obtain from the owners a complete dietary history (see Appendix C).
- Calculate protein intake to determine whether the pet is receiving its minimum needs.
- Teach clients how to assess the animal's body condition (see Figure 1-1).
- Give the owner written instructions on the proper way to make the transition to a new pet food (see Appendix D).
- See Appendixes H and I for a selection of nutrient-dense diets for dogs and cats.

cell-mediated and humoral immunity; decreased resistance to infection; inability to withstand shock, surgery, and the effects of cytotoxic drugs; decreased wound strength; muscular weakness; organ failure; and death. The consequences of malnutrition become more severe as time passes, and anorexia (complete loss of appetite) associated with disease must be recognized and treated. Decreased food intake and anorexia can be caused by a wide variety of medical problems, and also by the fear and anxiety associated with hospitalization. Patients with chronic disease often lose their appetite and become malnourished as the disease progresses. Animals with facial injuries or obstruction of the gastrointestinal (GI) tract may not eat because they are physically incapable of taking in, chewing, or swallowing food.

Illness and injury can significantly affect the need for many nutrients. Dogs and cats that are eating food require 50 to 100 ml of water per kg of body weight for daily maintenance, depending on environmental temperatures, type of food, and level of activity. Part of this water requirement is provided by the diet; how much depends on the type of food being fed. Dogs and cats eating canned foods can obtain most or all of their total daily water intake from food. When anorexia is present, absence of the renal solute load of the diet (minerals and urea generated from protein breakdown) causes water needs to decline significantly. The amount of water required to maintain hydration of anorectic animals is only approximately 10 ml per kilogram of body weight per day, much less than that required by animals that are eating. In addition to water in the food and any consumed orally, water also is produced from the metabolism of nutrients. This "metabolic water" provides approximately 10% of the total daily water intake. In food-deprived animals, approximately 500 to 700 g of water is produced for every 1 kg of weight lost.

Water loss takes place via three different routes: in the urine, in the feces, and by evaporation from the respiratory tract, mucous membranes, and skin—the "insensible losses." Approximately 70% of the daily water intake is excreted in the urine. Excessive water loss via the urine can occur in patients with diabetes or polyuric renal failure and as a result of the use of osmotic diuretics. In addition to the normal losses, water loss in ill animals also can result from vomiting, diarrhea, burns, and hemorrhage. Approximately 7% of total water intake is excreted in the feces. In the absence of diarrhea, fecal water loss from animals that are not eating is minimal. Insensible losses account for approximately 25% of total water intake and production. In normal animals the rate of loss is determined primarily by the environmental temperature and amount of exercise. Water losses by insensible routes increase in the presence of fever, hyperventilation, increased metabolic rate, and burn wounds in ill animals.

The caloric intake required by sick or injured animals depends on the rate of energy use for basal metabolism (resting), nutrient assimilation, body temperature maintenance, and activity. Recent data suggest that the energy needs of resting critically ill, postoperative, and severely traumatized dogs were not higher than basal needs for healthy animals, as had previously been suggested. Based on these results and the risks associated with overfeeding, we provide hospitalized patients with their basal energy needs. Graphs of the basal energy needs of dogs and cats over a wide range of body weights are presented in Figures 5-1 and 5-2. These graphs were constructed using an exponential expression: $97 \times$ kg of body weight$^{0.665}$ per day. An exponential equation is required to estimate basal caloric needs for animals that weigh less than 2 kg and more than 50 kg. For animals weighing between 2 and 50 kg, the following linear equation can be used.

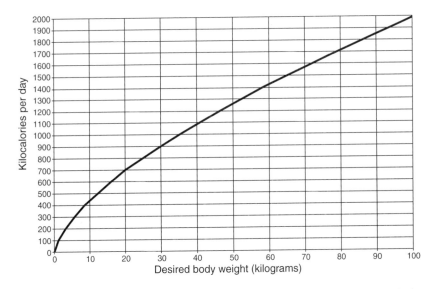

Figure 5-1 Energy needs graph for dogs. The graph was drawn using the equation 97 × body weight$_{kg}$$^{0.665}$, which estimates basal energy needs of adult dogs.

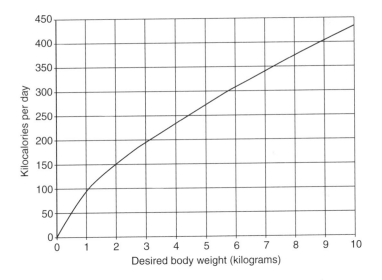

Figure 5-2 Energy needs graph for cats.

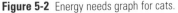

(30 × kg body weight) + 70 = kcal/day

Although activity makes up the largest portion of the maintenance energy requirement of healthy dogs and cats, sick, hospitalized patients are not active, so energy is not required to support this function.

These estimated energy needs are conservative and may be lower than the number of calories required by some patients during the course of disease. The immediate goals are to support protein synthesis and to attempt to reverse disease-induced catabolism. Repletion of lean muscle mass and fat stores is deferred until convalescence (after the patient goes home), when the disease process is under control. The recommendations regarding energy intake are also intended to avoid adverse consequences of overfeeding; we believe that it is better to err by providing slightly less food than needed than by having to stop nutritional support completely because of a complication of overfeeding.

The estimated caloric needs of a patient can be converted to food needs by assuming that canned foods contain approximately 1 kcal/g and that dry foods contain approximately 350 kcal/8 oz. More accurate values can be obtained for foods commonly fed by consulting with representatives from the pet foods' manufacturers. Based on the caloric estimate and observation of voluntary food intake, the index of suspicion for the need for nutritional support can be established.

Protein makes up 15% to 20% of the body mass, and approximately half the body protein provides structural support—bones, tendons, and cartilage. The rest constitutes muscle, plasma, and visceral protein. Proteins in metabolically active tissues are maintained in a "dynamic steady state" of constant synthesis and breakdown. These "labile" proteins, such as enzymes and hormones, turn over much more quickly than structural proteins do, which ensures prompt response to changing situations and enables a limited amino acid pool to be used with optimal efficiency. Rapid turnover is metabolically expensive; during growth or healing, protein turnover and related processes can account for as much as 40% of the total basal energy expenditure. During early stages of anorexia, labile proteins present in the liver, kidney, and GI tract maintain plasma glucose and amino acid concentrations. After the first 2 or 3 days of anorexia, muscle proteins begin to be broken down as well.

Injury also stimulates synthesis of a variety of acute-phase proteins, including C-reactive protein, haptoglobin, ceruloplasmin, and fibrinogen. This may be mediated, at least in part, by cytokines such as IL-1. After a lag phase of a few hours the plasma concentrations of these proteins increase as a result of increased synthesis, the extent of which is proportional to the severity of the insult. While acute-phase protein synthesis and plasma concentrations are increasing, the plasma concentration of other proteins, including transferrin and albumin, are declining. Hypoalbuminemia in severe injury and sepsis states is often related to large, sustained increases in extracellular, extravascular water content and *not* to enhanced catabolism or depressed synthesis. Enhanced acute-phase protein synthesis, however, cannot account for all the amino acids released during muscle protein catabolism. Some amino acids are deaminated and burned for energy to support leukocytes, regenerating wounds, and other glycolytic tissues, which places significant additional demands on gluconeogenesis. The increased use of amino acids for gluconeogenesis is reflected as increased nitrogen excretion in the urine.

Severely stressed patients may be unable to provide sufficient amino acids for high-priority protein synthesis, which results in decreased wound healing, erythropoiesis, and immune function. Animals with chronic diseases may be protein depleted at the time of presentation because of decreased food intake along with ongoing or increased nitrogen losses that result from the disease process. Calculation of precise protein needs in disease is difficult because of uncertainties in the previous nutritional status of the patient, the effects of the particular disease on protein metabolism, and the severity of the insult. In a number of conditions (e.g., fever, fracture, burns, surgical trauma), protein is lost extensively during the acute phase of the disease, with losses decreasing during convalescence. Protein needs often are measured as a percentage of total calories administered; the provision of 18% to 25% of kilocalories as protein usually meets requirements for growth in young dogs and cats, and has been used for estimating protein needs of ill patients. Unfortunately, these estimates were made in animals consuming four to six times the energy needed by hospitalized patients and therefore cannot be directly extrapolated for use in this population. In patients with no disease-related limitations on protein intake, consumption of diets that contain 7 to 10 g of protein per 100 kcal of metabolizable energy seems to be adequate. Patients with advanced liver and kidney disease require careful use of limited amounts of high-quality protein. Dietary protein needs in animals with these diseases are not well studied but are probably in the range of 2 g (in dogs) to 3 g (in cats) of a high-quality protein per kilogram of body weight per day. Animals consuming these amounts or less should be monitored carefully for signs of protein depletion. Although some practitioners prefer to add the amount of protein required to the established energy needs, by preference we estimate these requirements separately; the differences are not likely to be clinically significant in most patients.

Specific vitamin and mineral needs of hospitalized patients depend on the type and severity of the disease process. For short-term nutritional support, at least sodium, chloride, potassium, phosphate, calcium, and magnesium should be provided. Provision of supplemental zinc should also be considered, especially in anorectic patients with GI disease, where losses may be increased. Zinc is also important because of its role in protein synthesis, immune function, in vitro phagocytic activity, and taste and smell. Very little research has been conducted on the effect of various diseases on vitamin requirements in any species. At present, provision of vitamin levels at or near the National Research Council requirements for growth seems reasonable in the absence of a specific contraindication.

Nutritional Assessment

The purpose of nutritional assessment is to determine whether malnutrition is present as an independent problem. If malnutrition is not present initially, the patient should be reevaluated periodically during hospitalization to ensure that malnutrition does not develop secondarily to an ongoing disease process, administered drugs or treatments, a persistent inability to eat, or food deprivation. Nutritional support should be instituted as part of the primary therapy for malnourished patients and when voluntary food intake is impossible for prolonged periods. However, nutritional support should not be initiated until the goals of fluid therapy—rehydration, electrolyte replacement, and normalization of acid-base status—have been achieved. The steps in making a nutritional assessment include the taking of a complete dietary history, performance of a physical examination, and evaluation of any supporting laboratory data (see Chapter 1 for definitions of low-, moderate-, and high-risk factors).

A recent history of greater than 10% weight loss, decreased food intake, increased nutrient needs because of trauma or surgery, increased nutrient losses resulting from vomiting, diarrhea, or burns, and acute exacerbation of a chronic disease problem are important risk factors for malnutrition. A dietary history (see Appendix C) should be taken to determine the quality and appropriateness of the diet fed and the total daily intake of food. Clients should specifically be asked if drugs such as corticosteroids, cancer chemotherapeutic agents, antibiotics, or diuretics, all of which may adversely affect nutritional homeostasis, have been prescribed recently.

Any historical evidence that suggests malnutrition can be confirmed by a thorough physical examination. Underweight animals have loss of subcutaneous fat and muscle wasting. Patients in moderate or overweight body condition also may be tissue depleted; however, they may not appear so because of an "overcoat" of fat. This situation occurs because metabolic changes associated with critical illness cause lean body mass to be broken down more quickly than adipose tissue. Affected patients usually can be recognized by a poor haircoat, easily pluckable hair, thin, dry skin, and abnormal prominence of the bones of the head, and by using the techniques described in the discussion of the muscle condition score (MCS) in an earlier chapter (Figure 1-2). Structural impediments to eating that decrease food intake also may be found during a thorough physical examination.

Laboratory findings of hypoalbuminemia, lymphopenia, and anemia support the diagnosis of malnutrition, but are nonspecific. Decreased resistance to the passage of a needle for blood collection because of loss of skin collagen is a reasonably sensitive indicator of peripheral protein depletion. Biochemical profiles provide information regarding visceral organ function, which may influence the composition of the diet or route of administration. For example, evidence of significant abnormalities of liver or kidney function may require protein restriction, and severe pancreatitis could necessitate parenteral administration of nutrients.

Routes of Nutrient Delivery

Once the decision to deliver nutritional support is made, nutrients may be provided in two ways: enterally or parenterally.

Oral feeding is successful a large percentage of the time and is the safest, least expensive, most beneficial physiologically, and most convenient method of feeding; it should be used whenever possible. Many methods to stimulate food intake have been suggested. One common recommendation is B-vitamin injections, but there is no compelling evidence that such treatment stimulates food intake in sick dogs or cats.

Nursing techniques to improve food intake (often referred to as *coax-feeding*) should be tried before proceeding to more aggressive methods of nutritional support. Hand-feeding, petting or stroking, vocally reassuring the animal, offering food when the animal is outside of the cage (during a walk around the building or in a quiet area of the hospital), warming the food to body temperature to enhance aroma, or changing the type of food may be sufficient. If the patient's nasal passages are occluded, cleaning them with warmed saline improves olfaction.

Drugs used to stimulate appetite include diazepam, oxazepam, and cyproheptadine (Table 5-6). No controlled studies are available in veterinary patients for any of these compounds.

Psychogenic (anxiety- or fear-induced) anorexia is common in hospitalized animals because of the stress of disease or trauma, the pain associated with surgery and treatments,

Table 5-6
Drugs Recommended to Stimulate Appetite*

Drug	Cat	Dog
Diazepam	0.2 mg/kg IV	Do not use
Oxazepam	2.5 mg PO	Do not use
Cyproheptadine	2 mg bid-tid PO	2-8 mg/dog bid-tid PO
Prednisolone	0.1-0.25 mg/kg IV, PO, sid both species	
Nandrolone decanoate	5 mg/kg maximum dosage, or 200 mg/week IM both species	
Stanozolol	1-2 mg PO bid or 25-50 mg IM both species	

*No controlled studies are available in veterinary patients for any of these compounds.
bid, Twice per day; *IM*, intramuscular; *IV*, intravenous; *PO*, by mouth; *sid*, once per day; *tid*, three times daily.

and the unfamiliar sights, sounds, animals, and humans. Although the drugs listed in Table 5-6 are sometimes effective for treating psychogenic anorexia, they do not appear to resolve disease-induced (pathologic) anorexia. Moreover, the sedative effects of these drugs are undesirable in depressed patients, and the drugs are contraindicated in patients with liver disease.

Other drugs, including glucocorticoids and the anabolic steroids nandrolone decanoate and stanozolol, also have been recommended to stimulate appetite. Pharmacologic appetite stimulation often motivates an animal to eat small meals immediately, which may lead the veterinarian or technician to conclude that the patient's food intake is adequate. Because of the inconsistent response, these drugs should be restricted to cases in which food intake is being measured.

It is not in the best interest of most patients with inappetence or anorexia to offer novel foods to stimulate the appetite. When new diets are introduced to sick animals, the possibility of creating a learned food aversion must be minimized. For this reason, placement of a "smorgasbord" of foods in a cage to entice a sick animal to eat is not recommended. We prefer to offer 15 to 30 g of a food familiar to the animal at a time. If resistance is observed, all food is removed and a subsequent attempt is made in 1 or 2 hours. If food is kept in the cage, only one variety is chosen and a very small amount is offered. If no intake is observed within 1 or 2 hours, or if the food hardens, it is removed immediately and a different food offered, preferably a favorite food the patient is most likely to eat.

When the objective is to institute a particular dietary therapy for long-term patient management, the diet should not be introduced during hospitalization if at all possible. Offering the diet after the patient is home and feels better improves the probability of long-term acceptance and success. Learned aversions in veterinary patients have not been studied in any systematic way, but they may be one reason why some veterinary foods are difficult to institute as diets for sick animals.

If attempts to restore food consumption fail, force-feeding via a syringe may be tried for 1 or 2 days. Force-feeding provides some nutrition, but the inconvenience and the stress imposed on the patient during feeding limit the usefulness of the technique. Another invasive method involves the passage of a feeding tube through the mouth into the stomach for each feeding. Passing an orogastric tube is relatively simple, and the most important criterion for success is the gentleness with which the maneuver proceeds. Limited restraint and the opening of the animal's mouth just far enough to introduce the tube minimize the patient's opposition to this procedure.

The equipment required for orogastric intubation of large dogs consists of a double-action rubber bulb connected to rubber tubing of an appropriate size and length. This type of bulb ensures a continuous forward flow of material. A three-way stopcock that connects the food container and feeding tube via a 12- or 20-cc syringe may be used to feed small dogs and cats. For passage of an orogastric tube, the distance from the mouth to the last rib is measured and the tube is marked with a piece of tape at 25% of the distance from the oral end. The animal's head is restrained by grasping it with a free hand, a mouth gag designed for the passing of stomach tubes is inserted, and the mouth is closed around it. The tube also may be passed through a disposable syringe case with the closed end cut off and smoothed or through a roll of tape. If necessary, the mouth may be tied shut with the gag in place. The first 4 to 6 inches of the tube are lubricated with a water-soluble lubricant and then the tube is passed through the gag and into the oropharynx. When the animal swallows, the tube is pushed progressively downward into the esophagus and stomach to the depth of the premeasured mark. The animal's head should be held in the normal static angle of articulation; if the head is extended or flexed, the likelihood of endotracheal intubation increases. During passage of the tube, care must be taken to avoid damage to the pharyngeal and esophageal mucosa, and intubation of the trachea must be avoided.

Nasogastric and Nasoesophageal Tubes

If the patient is too debilitated to tolerate repeated tube feedings, or if nutritional support is required for more than 2 days, a nasogastric (used synonymously here with nasoesophageal) tube may be placed. Nasogastric tube placement is a simple procedure that does not require anesthesia or sedation and allows provision of fluid and nutrients for extended periods of time (days to weeks). Techniques for passing a nasogastric tube have been described for both cats and dogs. A feeding tube of appropriate size (Table 5-7) and, if necessary, a stylet are selected. Unlubricated feeding tubes must be flushed with 1 or 2 drops of mineral oil before the stylet is introduced to allow its removal after insertion of the feeding tube. Polyvinyl chloride tubes are the least expensive and work well for intragastric feeding. These tubes may harden if left in the stomach for prolonged periods, and therefore they should be changed approximately every 2 weeks. Polyurethane or silicone tubes, although more expensive, are resistant to gastric acid and may be used for prolonged nutritional support.

A topical anesthetic (four or five drops of 0.5% proparacaine hydrochloride for cats and 0.2 to 0.5 ml of 2% lidocaine hydrochloride for dogs) should be instilled into a nostril. Before the tube is passed, the distance from the tip of the nose to the last rib is measured and a butterfly tape-tab is placed on the feeding tube to mark the length to be inserted. When the tube is passed, the animal's head is held at the normal static angle of articulation to avoid tracheal intubation. For intubation of medium and large dogs the tube is passed through the nose by directing it medially, then ventrally as the nasal planum is pressed upward. Pushing the tip of the nose upward (the "pig-nose" technique) as the tube is passed guides the tube into the ventral meatus (Figure 5-3).

Passage through the nasopharynx and esophagus into the stomach is then much the same as in the horse, with very little risk of intubation of the trachea if the head is held at a

Table 5-7
Nasogastric Tubes

Tube Size	Tube Length	Patient Type
3.5 French	15 inches	Puppies, kittens
5 French	15 inches	Cats, small dogs (<15 lb)
5 French	36 inches	Dogs (15 to 30 lb)
8 French	36 inches	Cats (>15 lb), dogs (15 to 30 lb)
8 French	42 inches	Dogs (>30 lb)

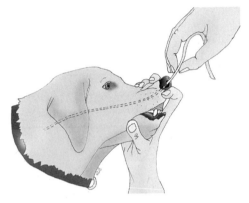

Figure 5-3 Placement of nasogastric tube.

Figure 5-4 Placed nasogastric tube.

normal angle and not pushed too far up or too far down. Once the tube is installed, the stylet, if present, is removed and the position of the tube in the stomach is confirmed. Placement is assessed by infusion of a small amount of sterile water through the tube, which causes the animal to cough if the tube has been placed into the lungs. If no reaction results, a small bolus of air is injected through the tube while the practitioner auscultates for borborygmus in the cranial abdomen. Most nasogastric tubes are radiopaque, and a plain radiograph should be taken to confirm the position of the tube if uncertainty persists. Some small tubes may be difficult to see on radiographs; their visibility can be enhanced by flushing the tube with a small amount of water-soluble contrast medium. Once the tube is passed and its position in the stomach confirmed, the butterfly tape-tab is sutured or glued (surgical skin glue is recommended) to the upper lip, as close to the nostril as possible (Figure 5-4). An Elizabethan collar should be placed to prevent the animal from removing the tube. Cats and small dogs are intubated by passing the tube directly through the ventral meatus without manipulating the nose; in other respects the technique is similar to that described above. The most common complication associated with this type of feeding tube is inadvertent tube removal. Although we prefer to place nasal feeding tubes into the stomach, others prefer to leave the distal tip in the esophagus. No studies of the relative clinical efficacy of the different placement sites have been published, and the choice of site of tube placement appears to be a matter of personal preference.

Esophagostomy and Pharyngostomy Tubes

If the nature of the problem prevents use of the nasogastric route, or if a prolonged course of enteral feeding is anticipated, a feeding enterostomy may be created. Pharyngostomy or esophagostomy tubes permit feeding of patients that have a functional GI tract and no history of vomiting or regurgitation, but that are unwilling or unable to consume nutrients orally. For placement of an esophagostomy tube the patient is anesthetized with either a short-acting injectable or inhalant anesthetic (endotracheal intubation is not essential) and placed in right lateral recumbency. The feeding tube can be placed on either the right or left side; however, because the esophagus lies slightly left of the midline, left-sided placement is more desirable. The hair of the midcervical neck is clipped from the vertical ramus of the mandible to the thoracic inlet. The skin is aseptically prepared for surgery. The mouth is held open with an oral speculum, and the head and neck are extended. A 16-Fr or 18-Fr polyvinyl chloride feeding tube is premeasured by holding the distal end at the seventh or eighth intercostal space and marking the proximal end where the tube will exit the esophagus and skin. Using curved Kelly or Carmalt forceps, the clinician places the instrument into the esophagus to the level of the midcervical region, and the tip is palpated as it creates a visible bulge in the skin along the lateral aspect of the neck. A 0.5-cm incision is made through the skin and subcutaneous tissues, directly over the end of the forceps. The incision is enlarged in the subcutaneous tissues, cervical musculature, and esophageal wall with the tip of a no. 15 scalpel blade. The distal end of the feeding tube is grasped with the forceps and drawn through the incision into the oral cavity to the predetermined measurement. The tube is lubricated and gently placed into the esophagus by extending the tongue and flexing the tube 180 degrees; the tube is then advanced through the esophagus until the oral portion disappears. A minimum of 4 inches of feeding tube should remain exterior to the skin. Tubes can be secured to the cervical skin with a Chinese finger-trap suture; the point of exit of the tube can be left exposed or lightly bandaged.

The distal end of larger feeding tubes (≥12-Fr red rubber or mushroom-tipped catheters) should *not* be placed in the stomach. Gastroesophageal reflux may occur if the feeding tube disrupts the integrity of the lower esophageal high-pressure zone. Esophageal dysfunction may also occur, and chronic esophageal irritation by refluxed gastric acid may cause esophageal stricture. Placing the distal end of the tube in the midthoracic region of the esophagus permits secondary peristaltic waves to move the food bolus into the stomach. Complications associated with the use of esophagostomy feeding tubes are minimal, but local infection or swelling at the tube site and scarring of the esophagus may occur. Reported complications associated with pharyngostomy feeding tubes include hemorrhage, local infection and swelling, recurrent laryngeal nerve injury, epiglottic entrapment, laryngeal obstruction, respiratory stridor, coughing, vomiting, aspiration of food, esophageal erosion or esophagitis, gastroesophageal reflux, and premature displacement or occlusion of the tube. When feeding is no longer necessary, the tube can be removed without sedation. The wound is left open to heal by second intention.

Gastrostomy Tubes

When nutrient intake proximal to the stomach cannot occur in patients with normal GI function, a gastrostomy feeding tube may be placed. Gastrostomy feeding tubes are specifically indicated in patients that are comatose or that require bypass of more proximal structures because of neurologic or neuromuscular diseases, dysphagia, neoplasia, obstruction, inflammation, or stricture. Surgical gastrostomies are the safest, but the most expensive and difficult to place. Alternatively, a feeding tube (20-Fr to 24-Fr mushroom-tipped catheter) can be placed by means of an endoscope or a blind technique with a placement device. Gastrostomy tubes can be maintained in patients for months with good nursing care, but should remain in place for at least 14 days to allow adequate adhesions to occur between the stomach and the peritoneum. Gastrostomy tubes are easily removed by gentle traction or, if necessary, with the patient under anesthesia and by means of an endoscope. The wound is left open to heal by second intention.

If an endoscope is available, it may be used to place the gastrostomy tube percutaneously. Most of the materials and procedures are similar to those described below when a blind, nonendoscopic, percutaneous placement device is used. Mushroom-tipped catheters, 16 Fr to 24 Fr, are used for percutaneous gastrostomy tubes and are prepared before placement. The flared connecting end of the catheter is removed with scissors. This discarded end can be cut into a 3-cm length of tubing to serve as an internal or external flange. Once placed on the feeding tube, these flanges prevent the feeding tube from pulling out of the gastric lumen.

The patient is anesthetized with a general inhalant anesthetic and placed in right lateral recumbency. The left paracostal region is clipped, and the skin aseptically prepared for surgery. An oral speculum is placed in the patient's mouth, and a fiberoptic endoscope with a biopsy port is passed through the mouth and esophagus into the stomach. The stomach is insufflated with air until distension of the left abdominal wall is externally visible; this displaces any abdominal viscera that may be located between the stomach and the left body wall. The endoscope is then positioned so the illuminated end is located within the stomach directly caudal to the last rib. A no. 11 scalpel blade is used to make a small stab incision through the skin at this site. An 18-gauge intravenous cannula with a needle stylet is placed through the skin incision and through the abdominal and gastric walls into the gastric lumen. The endoscope is repositioned within the stomach to allow visualization and confirmation of the presence of the cannula within the gastric lumen. The stylet is removed from the cannula, and the end of a length of 0 or 2-0 suture material is passed through the cannula into the gastric lumen. The length of suture material required for this procedure can be estimated by measuring from the rostral end of the patient's nose to the greater trochanter of the femur. The biopsy snare is passed through the biopsy channel of the endoscope to grasp the suture material. The biopsy instrument with the suture attached should not be retracted through the biopsy channel of the endoscope. Instead, while the biopsy snare is held in a closed position to retain the suture material, the entire endoscope is withdrawn from the stomach through the mouth. The suture material extends through the left abdominal wall, stomach, and esophagus and exits the oral cavity. The cannula can then be removed from the abdominal wall, with care taken not to remove the suture. The suture end that exits from the mouth is passed retrograde through this cannula. An 18-gauge hypodermic needle is passed through the end of the feeding tube. The suture is then passed through the hypodermic needle and tied securely to the feeding tube. The gastrostomy tube and cannula are fitted together and well lubricated before the retraction of the suture through the abdominal wall begins. The cannula and feeding tube pass through the mouth, oropharynx, esophagus, and stomach and exit through the gastric and abdominal walls. The cannula is then removed from the tube, which is gently retracted to pull the mushroom tip

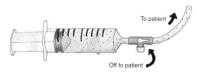

Figure 5-5 Feeding syringe.

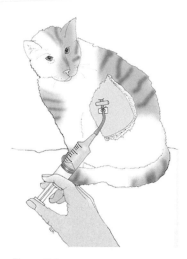

Figure 5-6 Gastrostomy tube feeding.

securely against the gastric mucosa. Replacement of the endoscope into the stomach allows visualization of the positioning of the gastrostomy tube. An external flange should be placed around the feeding tube next to the skin to prevent separation of the stomach from the abdominal wall until a permanent adhesion forms. The remaining end of the gastrostomy tube is capped and fixed to the skin with an antitension suture and abdominal bandage. Feeding is accomplished with use of a feeding syringe (Figures 5-5 and 5-6).

Gastrostomy feeding tubes can be maintained in patients for months with good nursing care, but should remain in place for at least 14 days to allow adequate adhesions to occur between the stomach and the peritoneum (see Appendix K for client instructions for home gastrostomy tube care). These adhesions prevent the leakage of food and fluid into the peritoneal cavity. The skin surrounding the feeding tube should be kept clean and dry, and bandages should be changed as needed. At the conclusion of gastrostomy tube feeding the sutures between the skin and the feeding tube are removed. If a Foley catheter was surgically placed, the balloon is deflated. Both mushroom-tipped and Foley catheters are easily removed by gentle traction. The paracostal wound is cleaned and left open to heal by second intention. Complications associated with the placement and maintenance of gastrostomy feeding tubes include leakage of food or fluid around the feeding tube, which may result in peritonitis, necrotizing fasciitis, or subcutaneous abscess; vomiting; regurgitation; gastroesophageal reflux; aspiration pneumonia; and premature tube displacement.

Jejunostomy Tubes

A needle catheter jejunostomy or gastrojejunostomy may be performed when gastric atony, gastroduodenal obstruction, neoplasia, regurgitation, or vomiting prevent feeding via more proximal sites. Jejunostomy tubes (5-Fr to 8-Fr human pediatric feeding tubes) are typically placed at the time of surgery. Patients requiring extensive surgical procedures of the stomach, duodenum, pancreas, or hepatobiliary system also can be provided with immediate postoperative nutritional support by means of this technique. Jejunostomy feeding tubes also can be threaded through surgically placed gastrostomy tubes at the time of surgery if the patient will not be able to eat orally for a prolonged period. The patient can be fed immediately postoperatively via the jejunostomy tube, which can be removed from the gastrostomy tube to permit gastrostomy feeding once motility returns to the stomach. Contraindications to jejunostomy feeding include ileus, persistent diarrhea, and intestinal obstruction distal to the feeding tube. Complications associated with jejunostomy feeding tubes include diarrhea, excessive hemorrhage, infection, premature displacement of the feeding tube, and the leakage of bowel contents or feeding solutions around the catheter into the peritoneal cavity or subcutaneously. Jejunostomy feeding tubes should remain in place for at least 7 days to allow adhesion formation. When enteral feeding is no longer necessary, the external skin suture and catheter can be removed without pain or discomfort to the patient.

Diet Selection

Diets for enteral feeding should supply the nutrients required by the patient without causing digestive disturbances. Nutrients should be easily digested, readily assimilated, and efficiently metabolized with a minimum of waste. Diets should be sufficiently well tolerated by the GI mucosa that they can be administered to animals with gastritis, enteritis, or colitis without producing additional irritation. They should be easy to administer, yet palatable enough to be eaten, and patients should not lose weight when diets are fed at the prescribed quantities. For a selection of enteral foods for dogs and cats see the dietary tables in Appendixes H and I.

Many diets fulfill these criteria reasonably well, so the choice of the appropriate diet for a given patient depends for the most part on any disease-related nutrient modifications that are required; secondary factors include both size and location of the feeding tube. Liquid diets specifically formulated for veterinary use (Canine and Feline CliniCare) are available and may be fed through a tube of any size. To maximize success and minimize the incidence of clogged tubes, we recommend that only liquid diets be used in nasogastric tubes smaller than 12 Fr. For tubes larger than 12 Fr, veterinary foods that have been processed in a blender or commercial canned pet foods (with water added as needed) may be efficiently and economically used. See the dietary tables in Appendixes H and I.

Commercial nutritional products (liquid diets) for humans are available at large public pharmacies, at hospital pharmacies, and through vendors of health-care products. Although some of these products may be less expensive and may be nutritionally adequate for short-term feeding of dogs, they may contain not enough arginine or taurine and too much soluble carbohydrate for sick cats. Since veterinary liquid diets have become available, we no longer attempt to modify products formulated for human patients for use in veterinary patients.

Feeding

Food or water may be provided soon after the patient recovers from anesthesia. Total fluid and nutrient needs are estimated and delivered in four to six feedings over a 24-hour period. We recommend small volumes distributed over several meals during the first 24 to 48 hours of feeding to avoid overdistention of the stomach, vomiting, and regurgitation. Slow constant rates of administration, particularly in severely ill patients, also help minimize incidents of diarrhea and cramping and maximize uptake of the nutrients. Reservoirs and delivery tubes for feeding solutions are available from a number of manufacturers. Hanging small volumes of liquid diet (approximately a 12-hour supply) in a fluid therapy burette or a gavage set for gravity-assisted constant infusion minimizes the possibility of "overdosing" patients with the feeding solution during continuous feeding. To avoid occlusion of tubes with food or mucus, tubes should be flushed with water before and after each feeding.

The most common problems associated with enteral feeding are tube clogging, inadvertent tube removal, and diarrhea. Clogging may be prevented by flushing the tube after each bolus feeding and capping the tube with a column of water inside. The use of feeding tubes for administration of nonliquid materials should be discouraged. Flushing clogged tubes with a variety of solutions, including cranberry juice and cola beverages, has been recommended. The use of acidic solutions is effective only if the clogging material is more soluble in acid; if it is not, acidic solutions will only exacerbate the obstruction. Tubes usually can be unclogged by the injection of a slurry of warm water and pancreatic enzymes into the tube and the flushing of the tube after a 30-minute waiting period. Another method that may be successful is the threading of a Venocath through the tube to dislodge the clog.

Nasogastric tubes are inadvertently removed by approximately 30% of veterinary patients, a much lower rate than that occurring in human patients. Tubes that are removed by accident usually can be readily replaced. Patients often remove tubes when they are feeling better, so when a tube is removed we offer food to the animal, if no food has been recently offered, to determine if the animal will eat on its own. We do not sedate patients to reduce the risk of tube removal.

The diarrhea (usually small amounts of soft, pasty feces) that sometimes occurs in enterally fed patients is generally more of a nuisance than a threat to the patient and usually results from overly rapid administration of the bolus meal and rapid gastric emptying. We manage these problems by reducing the feeding rate and by feeding diets that contain fiber or higher concentrations of fat (>50% of total kcal) to delay gastric emptying.

General guidelines regarding nutritional support are provided for students and staff who are managing critically ill patients in our respective hospitals. These guidelines include the following.

- Determine and record patient's body condition score (BCS) and MCS (see Figures 1-1 and 1-2).
- Determine resting energy needs and document them in the medical record.
- Identify and record the patient's usual diet and favorite foods.
- Avoid introducing novel diets, which may induce a learned food aversion.
- Measure the patient's body weight and food intake every day and document it in the medical record.
- If food intake is less than calculated caloric needs, determine the most appropriate route of support (enteral vs parenteral), and make a plan for instituting it. If necessary, provide owners with a handout that contains instructions for use and maintenance of a feeding tube. Explain all the steps carefully to the client when the patient is discharged.

Parenteral Nutrition

Most patients that require nutritional intervention can be fed enterally, but parenteral nutrition (PN), or intravenous feeding, allows the provision of short-term metabolic and immune system support to animals with severe GI disease or pancreatitis. Because PN therapy is relatively expensive and more dangerous than feeding through the GI tract, enteral feeding should be used whenever the GI tract can tolerate it. PN is also not indicated when the patient's prognosis is hopeless.

The high osmolality of most PN solutions requires the use of a central venous catheter in the external jugular vein or a peripheral catheter placed in the medial saphenous vein and advanced into the caudal vena cava. Intravenous catheter placement should be treated as a surgical procedure, with appropriate aseptic technique used. If well cared for, catheters may be used for prolonged periods and should not be removed unless a specific indication for their removal exists. Proper insertion and maintenance of the PN catheter is one of the keys to successful PN therapy. Once a catheter is placed and designated for PN therapy, it should not be used for other purposes, such as drawing blood samples, administering medications, or measuring central venous pressure. Adverse drug-nutrient reactions and clogged catheters are serious potential complications of these practices.

We formulate PN solutions based on the patient's estimated nutrient needs (Figures 5-1 and 5-2). Calories may be provided as either glucose or lipid. Glucose is a readily metabolized source of energy that mixes easily with other constituents of PN. It is also required for the nervous system, red and white blood cells, fibroblasts, bone marrow, the renal medulla, and some phagocytic cells. The utilization of glucose requires insulin from endogenous or exogenous sources. The most commonly used PN solution for patients at The Ohio State University (OSU) contains 17.5% glucose. Examples of two different PN formulas provided at OSU and Michigan State University (MSU) are shown in Table 5-8.

The other major energy source for PN is lipid; solutions consisting of 10% and 20% safflower and soybean oils (emulsified with egg phospholipid in water) are currently available. Some controversy exists regarding whether glucose or lipid should be used as the primary energy source for PN. Advantages of glucose are that the solutions are filterable; they

Table 5-8
Parenteral Nutrition Formulas

Ingredients	The Ohio State University Glucose-Based Formula	Michigan State University Lipid-Based Formula
Travasol 8.5% amino acids + electrolytes	500 ml	460 ml
50% Dextrose	350 ml	290 ml
20% Intralipids	N/A	240 ml
Calcium gluconate 10%	1 ml	1 ml
MulTE-Pak-4 (trace elements)	0.5 ml	N/A
B-complex vitamins	1 ml	1 ml
Magnesium sulfate (not for patients with renal disease)	2 ml	N/A
Kilocalories	Approximately 1 kcal/ml	Approximately 1 kcal/ml

are bacteriostatic because of the high osmolality; they are relatively easy to prepare; and they are relatively inexpensive. On the other hand, the hyperosmolality of the solutions necessitates central venous access, and thrombophlebitis may result if solutions are infused at high rates into small veins. Hyperglycemia, usually less than 600 mg/dl, is also more common with glucose-based solutions than with lipid-based solutions, but no pathophysiologic significance has been established for this in parenterally fed veterinary patients.

Lipid-based PN, by contrast, is lower in osmolality, so it can be administered via peripheral veins. Lipid-based PN solutions provide an alternate source of calories for patients that are glucose intolerant; the solutions are also a source of essential fatty acids (EFAs). The disadvantages of lipid-based PN include an inability to filter the solution, a higher cost, a greater propensity for bacterial growth in the solution, the possibility of development of pathologic hyperlipidemias (necessitating the monitoring of serum triglycerides), and the fact that lipids, particularly linoleic acid, have been reported to be immunosuppressive and proinflammatory in dogs (although these problems have not been reported in clinical practice). Given the increased cost and complexity associated with addition of lipids to PN formulations, glucose-based systems are adequate unless a specific contradiction to their use exists.

Energy needs of PN patients are estimated as shown in Figures 5-1 and 5-2. Parenteral administration of nutrients in excess of resting energy needs is attempted only after the initial goal has proved tolerable for the animal. We usually provide 2.5 g of protein per kilogram of body weight. We restrict protein intake to approximately 2 g/kg/day in animals with severely compromised liver or kidney function.

The macromineral portion of the parenteral solution is provided by an amino acid–electrolyte solution. Minerals such as zinc, copper, manganese, and chromium, as well as water-soluble vitamins, are routinely added to PN solutions for patients at OSU. However, the fat-soluble vitamins and minerals necessary for prolonged PN therapy (such as selenium, molybdenum, iodine, and iron) are not thought to be necessary for the short-term PN that is more typically required in veterinary patients.

The apparatus required for PN administration includes the solution, the solution container, an administration set, a 0.22-μ filter (for glucose-based solutions), a dedicated central venous catheter, and, preferably, an infusion pump (Figure 5-7). We provide PN at a rate intended to meet basal (resting) energy needs (approximately 45 kcal/kg/day by the end of the first 24-hour period). Patients are then advanced to slightly higher caloric goals, if necessary, over the next 24 to 48 hours as their tolerance allows. During the initiation phase, blood glucose is measured every 4 to 6 hours until stable. Once goals are reached, we monitor the patient as described subsequently. At the end of nutritional therapy, patients are weaned from the solution over 4 to 24 hours as tolerance permits by progressive halving of the infusion rate to avoid hypoglycemia, particularly if insulin has been infused. If the patient should be able to eat, we periodically offer food and record the food intake. As soon as signs of appetite are observed, the PN administration rate is decreased to approximately half the previous rate to encourage the animal to begin eating on its own.

For patients receiving the glucose-based PN solution, the most important monitoring parameter is blood glucose, which is monitored closely during initiation of therapy. We treat patients with hyperglycemia with intramuscular administration of 0.25 U of regular insulin per kilogram of body weight approximately every 4 to 6 hours as necessary when blood

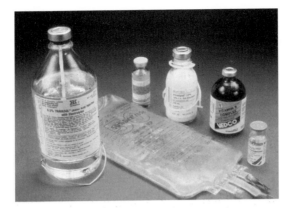

Figure 5-7 Parenteral solution ingredients.

glucose concentrations exceed 250 mg/dl. In our experience, insulin therapy is not commonly required for dogs, although we sometimes administer it to cats during the first 36 hours to control hyperglycemia. When insulin is used, caution must be exercised with regard to the central venous catheter, which is presumed to be in place continually. If insulin is given and then vascular access is lost, a 5% glucose infusion via a peripheral vein should be instituted immediately to prevent severe rebound hypoglycemia.

The most common PN-related complications we experience are mechanical, technical, and related to glucose abnormalities. Other metabolic complications, although reported in the literature in human medicine, are not serious problems in our patients. We recommend use of a strict protocol for prevention, diagnosis, and treatment of sepsis, and have seen PN-related infections occur only rarely. It has been shown in human medicine that sepsis is a problem better avoided than treated. When sepsis prevention protocols are in place, infection rates are approximately 3% to 5%. Infection rates when protocols are not in place and when breaks in protocol technique occur are approximately 10 times higher.

Returning to Normal Food Intake

Each animal is unique with regard to when the weaning from enteral nutrition or PN should be started and normal feeding resumed. In general, however, patients should be eating a quantity of food that contains at least one half of the calculated basal (resting) energy needs before the feeding tube is removed or the PN pump rate is reduced. Factors influencing the decision include the patient's short-term recovery and long-term prognosis, as well as the owner's financial situation. Coax-feeding may be used for most ill patients, in conjunction with enteral or parenteral support methods. Amounts of food consumed orally should be monitored and recorded on a daily basis. Ideally, the weaning process should not be abrupt, but should take place gradually over 2 or 3 days before a feeding tube is removed or a parenteral solution is stopped. With proper training, technical organization, and high-quality nursing care, the challenges of providing enteral or parenteral nutritional support can be minimized, and the health benefits to most critically ill patients can be maximized.

DENTAL DISEASE

Oral disease is the most common problem of adult dogs and cats presented to veterinarians. In 1999, 14% of dogs and 20% of cats aged 7 to 25 years reportedly were seen by primary care veterinarians for oral disease. Although dental caries (cavities) are not commonly seen in pets, periodontal disease is considered the most common oral disorder of dogs and cats. This disease is thought to result when plaque and calculus accumulate at the gingival margin, which induces an inflammatory reaction called gingivitis. Odontoclastic resorptive disease is another common oral disease of cats and occurs infrequently in dogs.

Oral health affects systemic health, so a healthy oral cavity may promote longevity and quality of life. The goals of promoting oral health in dogs and cats include the following.
- Assessment of the level of plaque control necessary to prevent gingivitis
- Determination of the owner's ability to accomplish home oral health care
- Selection of the methods of oral health care that are most likely to ensure compliance

Although the awareness of the importance of oral care for pets is increasing, some pet owners are unable to comply with stringent home health-care routines that require active, ongoing participation. Because of this, veterinary and commercial pet foods and treats designed to benefit oral health have become available (Table 5-9). Some people choose natural diets to help control problems related to oral health, whereas others choose to feed only dry foods. Which diet-related method best promotes oral health in a particular patient may be confusing; the following information is intended to help in making the best choice.

Natural Diets

Historically, natural diets of carnivores consisted of prey animals. Today the phrase *natural diet* more commonly refers to a mixture of ingredients such as raw meats with or without bones, vegetables, and fruits. Some people believe that the acts of ripping meat from and

Table 5-9
Dental Treats

Name of Treat	Manufacturer
Treats for Dogs	
Chew-eez	Friskies
Tartar Check	Heinz
CET Chews	VRx Products
Tartar Chew Treats	Waltham
Tartar Control Biscuits	Nutro
Pedigree Dentabone	Waltham
Treats for Cats	
Pounce Tartar Control	Heinz
Whisker Lickin's Tartar Control Treats	Purina
CET Forte Chews	VRx Products

chewing bones cleans the teeth. Unfortunately, no currently published reports compare the oral health of domestic dogs or cats that consume a natural diet with that of animals that consume commercially available foods. Early literature reported that the natural diets of wild canids and felids had a plaque-retardant effect, and that these dogs and cats were not affected by periodontal disease. Recent reports suggest the contrary. One study followed 67 English foxhounds, 1 to 9 years of age, that were routinely fed raw carcasses consisting of the bony skeleton, muscle, and associated tissues. Oral examination revealed that all the dogs had varying signs of periodontal disease, and many had tooth fractures.

Soft versus Hard Foods

Many people feed only dry food to their animals in the belief that the act of chewing and breaking down the food helps scrape plaque from their pets' teeth. Some owners believe that feeding only canned or soft food promotes oral disease. Many studies have investigated these claims. The studies are difficult to compare because different methods were used to assess substrate accumulation and gingival health, and different populations of animals were studied, but the results are reasonably consistent. No independent, clinically significant benefit to oral health of consuming dry food, or avoiding wet food, has ever been demonstrated.

It appears more likely that the diet interacts with the anatomy of the animal, because breed and familial tendencies play a role in oral health. Animals with a predisposition toward problems with oral health may develop them even with the best preventative care. These include smaller, brachycephalic breeds such as Shetland sheepdogs and toy poodles; the smaller the dog, the worse the plaque, because less space is present between the teeth. The reduced space may promote retention of substrate for bacterial growth. In large breeds, facial bones are longer, so there is more space between teeth. One exception to this is the greyhound breed; despite being large-breed dogs, greyhounds are known for developing a genetic juvenile periodontitis. In cats, Persians and Himalayans may be at increased risk for periodontitis because of their brachycephalic tendencies and because less space is present between the teeth.

Textured Food

Dry foods with altered textural characteristics (textured food) may promote oral health. A textured food combines fiber of a particular orientation with a size, shape, and pattern that promote chewing and maximum contact with teeth. Hill's Prescription Diet t/d is a veterinary diet that consists of an oversized kibble that has been specially extruded to form a fiber pattern of transverse striations that will not break apart until the tooth penetrates it. This provides removal of plaque up to the gum line of teeth distal to the canine teeth.

Treats and Biscuits

Many treats that are claimed to have a variety of dental benefits are now available to consumers. Plain baked biscuits are often given to help remove plaque from teeth but provide little additional benefit compared with feeding dry food alone. Some treats for cats are claimed to reduce tartar buildup, but no data demonstrate their effectiveness. There are also treats available for dogs and cats that have an "enzymatic" coating. These have been shown to be effective in helping to reduce plaque and tartar buildup when given as directed. Refer to Table 5-9 for a partial list of treat manufacturers.

Nonnutritional Dental Aids

Flat rawhide chews, not those that are formed into the shape of bones and other large objects, help clean the teeth. In one study regular consumption of up to three rawhide strips per day was effective in helping to remove dental calculus in dogs. Large "knots" of simulated beef hide, bones, and other objects may become lodged in airways, however, and are not recommended. Some toys that are made of synthetic materials also help clean the teeth. Regular chewing of Gumabone toys (Nylabone Products, Division of TFH Publications, Neptune City, NJ) has been shown to reduce dental calculus in dogs, and chewing Nylafloss (Nylabone Products) has been shown to reduce supragingival calculus buildup. The Plaque Attacker (Nylabone Products) has been recommended to reduce dental calculus, and the Dental Ring (Omega Paw Inc., St. Marys, Ontario, Canada) has been recommended to remove plaque and tartar to help prevent tooth decay.

Feeding

It is not necessary to provide a dental treat or toy every day, although the rate of plaque accumulation is approximately 36 hours for the pellicle to attach to the teeth. Feeding an animal twice daily and providing some type of dental aid every other day should be sufficient.

Conclusion

A thorough oral examination by a veterinary dental technician and a veterinarian is necessary at each checkup to ensure that the owner receives the best advice regarding the pet's oral health. If periodontal disease is diagnosed and treated at the early stages (grades 1 and 2 [Table 5-10; Figure 5-8]) the damage may be reversible. Aftercare and continued dental hygiene determine the overall success of dental therapy; if continued dental hygiene is not possible, then it may be necessary to feed a "dental" food with textural characteristics daily to help control plaque, calculus, and gingivitis.

For a selection of dental diets for dogs and cats, refer to Appendixes H and I.

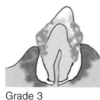
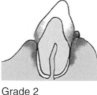
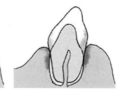

Grade 4   Grade 3   Grade 2   Grade 1

Figure 5-8 Grades of dental disease.

Table 5-10
Grades of Dental Disease

Grade	Definition
Grade 1 (initial)	Minimal plaque and tartar accumulation; slight gingival redness; breath may be mildly unpleasant; reversible
Grade 2 (early)	Greater amounts of plaque and tartar accumulation that extend under the gum line; gingival redness accompanied by inflammation; some bleeding may occur; reversible
Grade 3 (established)	Moderate to heavy accumulation of plaque and tartar that extends under the gum line; pocket formation and bone loss around the teeth; gums are red and inflamed and bleed easily; painful; not reversible
Grade 4 (advanced periodontitis)	Most of the supporting bone around the teeth is destroyed; large pockets are formed around the teeth; large accumulations of tartar may be present; possible pus formation in the mouth; very painful; not reversible

CLIENT COMMUNICATION TIPS: Dental Disease

- Conduct a thorough examination of the entire oral cavity at each healthy-pet visit, and educate clients regarding the importance of this examination.
- If commercial treats are recommended, educate clients regarding the caloric content of treats and snacks. No more than 10% of the pet's total caloric needs should be met with commercial treats.
- Provide clients with a list of top manufacturers of appropriate dental treats and foods; discuss the pros and cons of each product.
- Discuss with the staff the criteria for determining which dental diets and treats the veterinarians in the practice recommend, as well as which foods they avoid recommending. Which foods are on the practice's "A list," and why. Which are on the practice's "B list," and why. Help the staff identify clients who are receptive to learning more about dietary recommendations.

ENDOCRINE DISEASE

A variety of endocrine disorders occur in dogs and cats. The role of nutrition in the care of patients with diabetes mellitus and hyperlipidemia has been extensively studied and is described in the subsequent section. Patients with other endocrine disorders, such as hyperadrenocorticism and hypothyroidism, may benefit from obesity therapy. The principles of nutritional support may apply to some cats with hyperthyroidism. Once patients have received treatment for their primary diseases, however, their nutritional needs do not appear to differ from those of healthy patients in comparable circumstances.

Diabetes Mellitus

Diabetes mellitus in dogs and cats is a complex disorder that cannot be explained by a single cause. Various researchers have suggested that the cause is related to genetic, infectious, or other diseases, is immune mediated, or is drug induced. Two types of diabetes are commonly recognized in dogs and cats. Type 1, or insulin-dependent diabetes mellitus (IDDM), is characterized by an absolute insulin deficiency resulting from destruction of the beta cells of the pancreas. Type 2, or non–insulin-dependent diabetes mellitus (NIDDM), results from a variable combination of beta-cell dysfunction and resistance to the effects of insulin by peripheral tissues. Type 1 appears to be the more common form of diabetes in both dogs and cats, and type 2 is more common in cats than in dogs. Both types of diabetes result in hyperglycemia, and sometimes in abnormal lipid and protein metabolism. The primary treatment for diabetes is insulin therapy, with dietary and feeding management playing an important supporting role. The objectives of nutritional support of dogs and cats with diabetes mellitus are to provide adequate nutrients for moderate body condition to be maintained if possible, to coordinate feeding with insulin administration to promote control of blood glucose concentrations, and to acknowledge and attempt to manage concurrent diseases or complications of diabetes.

Body weight and condition play an important role in determining the most appropriate diet for patients with diabetes mellitus. An animal with diabetes may have any BCS. After the animal's BCS and MCS are determined, the daily food intake is adjusted with a goal of attaining or maintaining a moderate body condition. Obesity can exacerbate the diabetic state in some cases, and some weight loss in obese diabetic cats may resolve the diabetic state in type 2 diabetes. In obese humans with Type 2 diabetes, weight loss of only 5% to 10% results in significant improvement in blood glucose control, and a weight loss of 15% may eliminate the need for insulin. Because of this, rather than prescribing a specific amount of weight to be lost, we recommend that weight-loss efforts continue until control of blood glucose has been achieved.

Some patients with diabetes may be underweight; managing diabetes in these patients also includes improvement of body condition toward moderate. Once the diabetic state has been controlled, the nutrient needs of patients with uncomplicated diabetes may not be different from those of normal dogs or cats.

A complete dietary history should be taken, and the animal's current nutrient intake evaluated. If the diet does not seem appropriate for patients with diabetes, a change to a more appropriate food may be indicated. Unfortunately, the most appropriate diet for dogs and cats with diabetes has not yet been identified. Specific considerations identified to date in pets relate to fiber, carbohydrate, and fat; the roles of a variety of other nutrients have been considered in humans with diabetes, but comparable data in veterinary patients are not available. As discussed in the section on GI diseases, fiber functions depend on the relative solubility of the fiber in the diet. Diets with fiber that exert gelling properties (relatively soluble) are recommended in humans because of the perceived ability of these diets to slow the rate of presentation of nutrients to the body, which moderates increases in postprandial blood glucose concentrations. In dogs and cats, however, the presence of some fiber seems to be more important than its form. Moreover, the most appropriate amount of fiber has not yet been identified, as can be seen in Table 5-11. We currently cannot accurately predict fiber function in patients with diabetes. Rational use of fiber depends on results of clinical trials of commercial products and consistency in formulation (dietary fiber is like wine in that the soil, weather, harvest, and postharvest practices all affect the quality and consistency of the final product). For a selection of modified-fiber diets for dogs and cats, refer to Appendixes H and I.

Table 5-11
Amounts of Fiber in Various Foods

Food	Amount per Tablespoon (g)	Total Fiber (g)	Insoluble (Bulking) (g)	Soluble (Fermenting) (g)
Wheat bran	5.3	2.7	2.3	0.3
100% Bran cereal	6.4	1.8	1.6	0.2
All-Bran cereal	5	1.4	1.2	0.2
Oat bran	6.7	1	0.5	0.5
Metamucil	5.8	3.4	0.7	2.7
Canned pumpkin	0.6	5*	NA	NA

*5 grams in each half-cup serving; 4 servings per 16-ounce can of Libby's canned pumpkin (Nestlé).

Table 5-12
Differences Between a "High-Fiber" and a "High-Protein" Feline Diet

	Carbohydrate		Protein		Fat		Fiber	
Diet (Hill's)	DM (%)	g/100 kcal	DM (%)	g/100 kcal	DM (%)	g/100 kcal	DM (%)	g/100 kcal
w/d	25	6.5	41	11	17	4.4	10.7	2.9
Feline growth	7.5	1.6	49	11	34	7.3	0.6	0.1
DIFFERENCE	70% ↓	75% ↓	20% ↑	0%	100% ↑	66% ↑	94% ↓	97% ↓

DM, Dry matter.

A greater consensus seems to exist regarding the type of carbohydrate to be provided. More-soluble carbohydrates, such as those contained in semimoist foods, do not promote blood glucose control, so these diets should not be fed to patients with diabetes. The amount of carbohydrate in the diets of cats with diabetes recently has come under scrutiny, with some endocrinologists suggesting that reduced-carbohydrate diets may be preferable. Some initial confusion resulted concerning the relative importance of protein and carbohydrate when diets were compared on a dry matter basis. As shown in Table 5-12, when foods are compared on an energy basis, it can be readily seen that cats consuming a growth diet ingest an amount of protein equal to that consumed by cats fed the veterinary food. The cats fed the growth diet also ingest 75% less carbohydrate and 66% more fat. This difference in nutrient intake may slow gastric emptying in the cats fed the growth diet, resulting in an effect comparable to that of soluble fiber in humans. More clinical trials are currently underway to determine whether alteration of nutrient intake in cats with Type 2 diabetes leads to a better outcome.

The most appropriate amount of fat in the diet depends on the situation. In obese animals, and particularly in those prone to pancreatitis or hyperlipidemia, restriction of fat to <2 g per 100 kcal may be prudent and may contribute to weight loss; in other patients the situation is far less clear.

Because insulin is usually administered in conjunction with meals, the feeding method plays an important role in helping to control blood glucose concentrations. The goal is to have nutrients slowly absorbed when insulin levels are adequate, thereby minimizing rapid increases in blood glucose concentrations. The most common approach is to feed the patient just before the insulin injection. If one insulin injection is used, half the daily food is provided before the injection (to be sure the patient has eaten before the injection), and the rest is given 8 to 10 hours later. If injections are given twice daily, half the daily food should be provided before each injection. If the patient has poor blood glucose control, the food may be divided into three or more smaller meals to help reduce the effects of diet on blood glucose concentrations.

In addition to coordination of feeding with insulin injections, consideration should be given to the pet's activities. Because activity affects glucose utilization, playing with the pet closer to the time of insulin injection may be preferable, although this has not been well studied. Once a therapeutic plan has been established and an insulin dose chosen, adherence to the regimen should be as strict as possible from day to day. Significant changes in diet, activity, and environment all may necessitate adjustment of the glucose dose.

Obese cats are at much greater risk for development of Type 2 diabetes than are cats of normal body condition, and they may be more sensitive to environmental stressors such as indoor housing. For this reason, we try to treat obese cats on an outpatient basis as much as possible to avoid the stress of housing in the hospital for such things as serial blood glucose determinations. Clients are instructed to observe the cat's food and water intake, physical condition, and behavior. We also recommend consideration of the cat's environment as a potentially aggravating factor, and offer suggestions for environmental enrichment as appropriate (see Appendix G).

Careful follow-up, whether at home or in the hospital, is very important for ongoing assessment of the need for modifications to dietary or feeding recommendations resulting from changes in an animal's body weight, body condition, or overall health. Many factors other than diet may impair the effectiveness of insulin therapy in dogs and cats. Although no insulin dose clearly identifies insulin resistance, control of blood glucose can be achieved with approximately 1 U of insulin per kg of body weight per dose for most dogs with diabetes and less than 6 U per dose for cats.

Diseases that occur in diabetic patients and can adversely affect insulin therapy are presented in the following list. Adequate therapy for any concurrent diseases may be necessary if control of blood glucose is to be achieved.

- Obesity
- Hyperadrenocorticism or glucocorticoid therapy
- Increased progesterone during diestrus in intact animals
- Acromegaly
- Bacterial infections—urinary or pulmonary infection; pyoderma
- Chronic pancreatitis
- Exocrine pancreatic insufficiency (EPI; uncommon)
- Hyperthyroidism (cats) or hypothyroidism (dogs)
- Hyperlipidemia

In the absence of any concurrent diseases, the following list may be helpful in troubleshooting insulin resistance in patients with diabetes.

- Ensure that insulin is not outdated or overheated and that the proper syringe is used for the insulin prescribed.
- Verify proper injection technique.

- Ensure that the Somogyi phenomenon is not occurring.
- Switch to a more potent insulin. Insulin formulations, in order of least to most potent, are Ultralente, Lente, neutral protamine, Hagedorn, regular, and regular crystalline.
- Change route of administration. Insulin may be poorly absorbed after subcutaneous administration. This is most commonly seen in cats receiving Ultralente insulin.
- Ensure that excessive insulin-binding antibodies are not present. The structure of dog insulin is similar to that of the human and pig, and cat insulin is similar to cow insulin, so changing the source of insulin may be beneficial.

Hyperlipidemia

Abnormalities of lipid metabolism occur occasionally in dogs and rarely in cats (Table 5-13). Normal lipid metabolism includes digestion of dietary fat by pancreatic and epithelial lipases into fatty acids. Fatty acids are emulsified by bile salts into micelles, which dissociate at the epithelial surface to permit absorption into mucosal cells, where triglyceride resynthesis and chylomicron production occur. These products are released into the lymphatic ducts and enter the circulation via the thoracic duct. Once in circulation, lipoprotein lipase associated with endothelial cell surfaces in adipose, heart, lung, and muscle releases free fatty acids from triglycerides, chylomicrons, and very–low-density lipoprotein (VLDL) for tissue uptake and utilization. Lipoprotein lipase also can be activated by heparin.

Triglycerides and chylomicrons also undergo receptor-mediated uptake by the liver, where transformation to other lipoproteins occurs; these are released back into the circulation, where they undergo further metabolism. A summary of the characteristics of lipoprotein fractions in dogs and cats is presented in Table 5-14.

A cursory evaluation of the pet's lipoprotein status can be made by refrigerating a serum sample overnight. If chylomicrons are present, they float, forming a "cream layer" on top of the sample. If the serum below is clear, hyperchylomicronemia is present, which most commonly results from food deprivation for less than 12 hours before specimen collection or, uncommonly, may be primary hyperchylomicronemia. If the serum below is not clear, other lipoproteins are present in excess. Because hyperlipidemia can interfere with accurate

Table 5-13
Causes of Increased Serum Lipid Concentrations in Dogs and Cats

Physiologic Causes	Primary Causes	Secondary Causes	Drug-Related Causes
Hyperlipidemia normally exists for up to 12 hours after eating	Idiopathic hyperlipoproteinemia Idiopathic hypercholesterolemia Idiopathic hyperchylomicronemia (cats—rare) Lipoprotein lipase deficiency (cats—rare)	Hypothyroidism Hyperadrenocorticism Diabetes mellitus Pancreatitis Cholestasis Hepatic insufficiency Protein-losing enteropathy Nephrotic syndrome	Glucocorticoids Megesterol acetate (cats)

Table 5-14
Characteristics of Lipoproteins in Dogs and Cats

	Chylomicrons	Very–Low-Density Lipoprotein	Low-Density Lipoprotein	High-Density Lipoprotein
Size	Largest			Smallest
Triglyceride (%)	90	60	10	4
Cholesterol ester (%)	2	13	38	16
Free cholesterol (%)	7	7	8	6
Protein (%)	2	5	22	50
Phospholipid (%)	6	15	22	25
Electrophoretic migration	Origin	Prebeta, beta	Beta	Alpha
Density (g/ml) Dogs		<1.006	1.006-1.063	1.063-1.21
Cats		<1.019	1.019-1.063	

determination of a variety of serum analytes, a clinical pathologist should be consulted for interpretation of laboratory results from these patients.

The most common type of primary hyperlipidemia in dogs and cats is idiopathic hyperlipidemia, which affects miniature schnauzers, beagles, and occasionally other breeds of dogs; it is a familial disorder in miniature schnauzers and beagles. Lipid abnormalities in these patients include increased serum concentrations of chylomicrons, triglycerides, cholesterol, VLDL, and high-density lipoprotein (HDL). As the name implies, the cause of idiopathic hyperlipidemia is unknown. The condition is associated with varying combinations of abdominal pain, vomiting, diarrhea, and seizures; it may lead to or be exacerbated by pancreatitis and may resolve spontaneously and then recur. Common features include insulin resistance, fasting hyperinsulinemia, glucose intolerance, and hypertension. Hypercholesterolemia in Briard dogs and hyperchylomicronemia in cats are rare disorders of lipoprotein metabolism.

Secondary causes of hyperlipidemia include hyperadrenocorticism, diabetes mellitus, hypothyroidism, nephrotic syndrome, cholestasis, and pancreatitis; some of the more common lipid abnormalities are presented in Table 5-15. Serum for evaluation must be collected at least 15 hours after a meal to avoid misdiagnosis of postprandial hyperlipidemia.

Table 5-15
Lipid Abnormalities in Diseases that Cause Secondary Hyperlipidemia

	Cholesterol	VLDL	TG	HDL-1
Cushing's syndrome	↑	↑	↑	↑
Diabetes mellitus	↑	↑	↑	↑
Hypothyroidism	↑	↑	↑	↑
Nephrotic syndrome	↑ (early)	↑ (later)	↑	↑
Cholestasis	↑	?	?	↑
Pancreatitis	↑	↑	↑	±↑

HDL, High-density lipoprotein; *TG*, triglyceride; *VLDL*, very–low-density lipoprotein.

Primary nutritional management of hyperlipidemia includes treatment of underlying causes of secondary hyperlipidemia, provision of a low-fat diet (less than 2 g/100 kcal), and maintenance of adequate protein intake. A variety of other pharmaceutical and nutriceutical treatments, including fibric acid derivatives (clofibrate and gemfibrozil), nicotinic acid, and omega-3 fatty acids have been suggested, but none has yet been tested for effectiveness in veterinary patients with hyperlipidemia.

CLIENT COMMUNICATION TIPS: Endocrine Disease

- Discuss with clients the importance of using an accurate dietary history, BCS, and body weight to determine the most appropriate dietary plan for their pets.
- Review the dietary history carefully. If a client does not know how much food the pet consumes in a given day or week, instruct the client regarding completion of a 5-day food diary. A piece of notebook paper can be used, with columns created for the date, time, type of food or treat offered, quantity or serving size, and initials of the person who offers the food. Anything consumed by the pet is recorded in the food diary. Follow up with clients after the food diary has been completed to identify factors that can potentially be modified (e.g., products, serving sizes, behaviors).
- Determine the total daily caloric intake of the pet. When necessary, calculate the daily intake of specific nutrients of concern, such as dietary protein or dietary fat, to assess whether the amount being consumed meets minimum requirements. This is especially important for older dogs and cats, whose daily food intake may vary.
- Educate clients regarding the important benefits of meal-feeding pets rather than feeding on a free-choice basis. Individual meals allow the owner to observe appetite and water consumption and identify potential problems.
- Teach clients how to monitor food intake each day and how to watch for signs of inadequate consumption.
- Recommend that any dietary change be made gradually over a period of several days or longer. If food aversions are to be avoided, dietary changes should not be made in the hospital setting, but in the home and after the pet is feeling better.
- Instruct clients regarding whom to call if problems or questions arise.
- For owners of overconditioned or obese patients, discussion of the benefits of weight reduction and regular exercise is valuable. See the discussion on obesity for additional information regarding development of a weight-management program and for suggestions for increasing the activity of pets that live indoors.
- Discuss all the factors involved in maintaining good insulin control in patients with diabetes. Provide clients with educational brochures or handouts that include detailed instructions on insulin administration; when and how much to feed at each meal; suggestions for regular exercise or play; and when to contact the hospital with questions or concerns.
- Discuss with the staff the criteria for evaluating diets for patients with endocrine-related disease. Nutrients of interest in these patients may vary, and a single product is unlikely to be "right" for every patient receiving treatment for an endocrine disorder. Help the staff identify clients who are receptive to learning more about dietary recommendations.

TECH TIPS: Endocrine Disease

- Obtain a complete dietary history (see Appendix C) to see if the pet's condition may be caused or exacerbated by food choices.
- Supply the client with samples of modified-fiber pet foods. Make sure that the samples are of foods that are available for purchase by the client at a later time in the event that the pet likes the food.
- Give the client a list of common "people foods" that are high in fiber or fiber supplements that can be added to food in the event that a pet will not eat the pet food.
- Give the client written instructions on the proper way to make the transition to a new pet food (see Appendix D).
- Schedule a follow-up phone call, to be made after sufficient time has elapsed for the dietary transition to have occurred, to ensure that no problems have developed and to determine whether treatment has been effective.

GASTROINTESTINAL DISEASE

The GI tract is a massively complex, poorly understood system. Although diseases affect all portions of the GI tract, the causes of most of them are not understood, and most therapies are symptomatic and palliative. Nutrient-sensitive GI diseases include acute disease with diarrhea or vomiting, borborygmus and flatulence, chronic diarrhea, inflammatory bowel disease (IBD), pancreatic disease, and liver disease. Despite the limitations in understanding the mechanisms of GI disease, dietary and feeding modifications may be helpful in the management of many GI disorders.

Acute Gastroenteritis and Vomiting or Small Bowel Diarrhea

The most common sign associated with intestinal disease in dogs and cats, and one of the most frequent presenting complaints in small animal veterinary practice, is diarrhea. Diarrhea is defined as an abnormal increase in frequency, water content, or volume of feces. From the perspective of a nutritionist, diarrhea is an interesting problem in that diet may be the cause in some cases, may be used as the primary therapy in others, and be useful as adjunctive therapy in still others. Although diarrhea usually is abnormal, one nutritionist recently reported that "[in] normal dogs, feces quality varied from very hard to watery depending on the diet fed, time of day and how long a diet had been fed."

Vomiting and regurgitation are the other common signs of GI disease. As with diarrhea, these signs have many causes and a number of variably effective treatments. These two signs are common because they are evolutionarily conserved mechanisms for removing noxious agents from the GI tract, analogous to the withdrawal reflex that occurs in response to noxious somatic stimuli.

Acute-onset diarrhea or vomiting in a previously healthy dog often is the result of an abrupt dietary change or indiscriminate eating behavior and responds to brief modification of dietary and feeding management alone. Symptomatic therapy of patients with acute diarrhea includes depriving the patient of food for at least 24 hours. Food deprivation allows the tract to clear itself of luminal contents that may have caused the problem. Food deprivation also prevents mucosal cell abrasion, deprives opportunistic pathogenic organisms of luminal nutrients, prevents absorption of dietary antigens by a compromised mucosa, and may permit reestablishment of brush border enzyme function. After 24 hours the animal may be fed small, frequent meals (four to six per day) of a highly digestible diet (for a selection of reduced-fat diets for dogs and cats, see Appendixes H and I), such as lean meat or cottage cheese and rice. The amount fed is increased over 3 days to the patient's previous caloric intake, after which the animal is returned to its previous diet over approximately 4 days. In addition to the fact that digestibility is improved with the diet suggested, some gastroenterologists believe that allergy to constituents of the diet is more likely to occur with the diet that is consumed during periods of acute gastroenteritis. If so, feeding something other than the usual diet during such periods may reduce the risk of development of an allergy to the pet's usual diet. Clients should be instructed to avoid abrupt dietary changes and eliminate opportunities for their pets to eat garbage and nonfood items to minimize the recurrence of the problem.

Gastric Dilatation-Volvulus

Gastric dilatation-volvulus (GDV), or bloat, is a relatively uncommon disease of large-breed dogs. No single cause of bloat has been identified, and the disorder is thought to be the final common pathway of a variety of problems. Although diet may play some role in susceptible animals, no diet-related cause has been identified, so GDV is classified as a nutrient-sensitive disease. In the absence of definitive data, we follow the (adapted) recommendations of a 1990 Morris Animal Foundation panel for clients owning large-breed, deep-chested dogs, particularly of susceptible breeds (Doberman pinscher, German shepherd, Irish setter, Great Dane, and Saint Bernard). These recommendations are as follows.

- A good working relationship is established with the client; emergency measures to be taken in the event of bloat are discussed, including administration of antigas agents, passing of a stomach tube, or piercing of the abdomen with a hypodermic needle.
- The dog is fed two or three times daily, at times when the owner can observe the dog's behavior after it has eaten.
- Water is made available to the dog at all times, although access is limited immediately after feeding. If excessive drinking (more than 1 volume of water per volume of dry food) is a problem, mixing water and dry food in equal proportions also may reduce drinking after eating.
- Vigorous exercise, excitement, and stress are avoided for at least 1 hour before and 2 hours after meals. Leash-walking, however, may help stimulate normal GI function.
- Food changes are made gradually, over approximately 5 days, following the recommendations for dietary change outlined in Appendix D.
- Susceptible dogs are fed individually and, if possible, in a quiet location.
- Special care must be taken to apply these measures after dogs have returned home from the veterinary hospital, boarding facility, or any other potentially stressful environment.
- Clients are made aware of the warning signs of bloat. These include the appearance of abdominal distention after meals; glances from the dog toward its abdomen; whining; pacing; repeatedly getting up and down; stretching to extend the abdomen;

assumption of an anxious appearance (worried facial features, looking at owner); or unproductive attempts to vomit. Dogs showing any of these signs should be taken to a veterinarian as soon as possible.

- Clients are advised that dogs that have survived bloat are at increased risk for future episodes; therefore, owners should discuss the need for preventive surgery or medical management with their veterinarians.

Borborygmus and Flatulence

Belching and fetid flatus occur relatively commonly in dogs. In our experience, too-rapid consumption of food or consumption of a low-quality, poorly digestible diet usually is the cause. Initially, we recommend adding 1 volume of water per volume of dry food and increasing feeding frequency to reduce the rate of food consumption. If this does not solve the problem, a dietary change may be indicated. Commercial products that contain enzymes to reduce flatus are available, and the antifoaming agent simethicone reportedly is safe to use in dogs and cats. Unfortunately, to our knowledge, clinical trials of the efficacy of these products in dogs or cats have yet to be reported.

Hairballs in Cats

The vomiting of hairballs is so commonly observed by owners of indoor cats that it is a regular subject of newspaper and magazine cartoons. Clearly common, it is also a normal behavior and therefore might be expected to be reasonably randomly distributed among cats. Hairballs seem to be more common in indoor-housed cats (although this conclusion may result from observational bias), and we have noticed that cats with idiopathic cystitis (IC) are some 10 times as likely to vomit a hairball at least once a month. It is interesting to note that in cats with severe lower urinary tract disease donated to our colony at OSU, the frequency of occurrence declined dramatically once the cats were removed from their home environments and placed in the colony. Queries of veterinarians managing pet food companies and research catteries revealed that hairball production is uncommon in their facilities, does not seem to be related to haircoat length, and is observed regularly in the same very small number of affected individuals.

Many pet food companies market fiber-supplemented diets for cats with hairballs. Unfortunately, no clinical evidence of the effectiveness of these diets has yet appeared in the veterinary literature. Because of the associations between indoor housing and disease risk in cats, we ask specific or investigative questions regarding the environments of cats presented for treatment of recurrent vomiting of hairballs. For these patients, we also recommend offering a canned form of the preferred food and environmental enrichment as appropriate (see the discussion of IC in cats later in this chapter for more information).

Chronic Small Bowel Diarrhea

Chronic diarrhea is a sign of many different underlying diseases, and treatment is often difficult and frustrating. Clients commonly believe that the problem is caused by diet and that their pets may respond to dietary therapy. Because diarrhea is a nonspecific sign of so many diseases, effective management depends on identification and resolution of the inciting cause, if possible. We usually recommend low-fat (≤2 g of fat per 100 kcal), highly digestible diets as adjunctive therapy for patients with chronic small bowel diarrhea. As mentioned in the section on nutrition and the skin, dietary management is the primary therapy for adverse reactions to foods.

Adverse reactions to foods are divided into immune-mediated reactions, true food allergies, and non–immune-mediated reactions. Food allergies in small animal patients are not common; they are treated by removal of the source of the antigen, which is done by feeding a controlled diet. Resolution of signs after feeding of a hypoallergenic diet, followed by recurrence of signs after challenge with suspected antigens, confirms the diagnosis of food allergy. Non–immune-mediated adverse reactions to food are probably the most common and include dietary indiscretions (discussed previously) and food intolerance. Food intolerance includes pharmacologic, metabolic, and idiosyncratic adverse reactions to the diet. The treatment is to change the diet to one the animal tolerates. Highly digestible, reduced-fat commercial diets or homemade diets similar to the one presented in Appendix J are recommended for adjunctive therapy of other diseases that cause chronic small bowel diarrhea. The potential benefit of provision of novel protein (antigen) sources in the treatment of nonallergic diarrheal disease has not been tested. The rationale for recommendation of egg, cottage cheese, or tofu (soy) as the dietary protein source is based more on the digestibility of these foods than on their antigenicity. Low-fat cottage cheese may be used to reduce fat intake. We do not recommend yogurt or milk as alternatives to cottage cheese because of their higher lactose content. We also avoid gluten-containing carbohydrates—wheat, rye, barley, and oats—in case the patient is gluten sensitive.

Chronic Large Bowel Diarrhea

Recommendations for treatment of chronic large bowel disease are similar to those for chronic small bowel diarrhea, except that addition of fiber to the diet may be beneficial in some patients. Dietary fiber is the fraction of plant material that cannot be digested by mammalian GI enzymes. Although fiber often is classified as "soluble" or "insoluble," it is not a single chemical entity that can be so easily categorized. *Soluble* refers to fibers that form a gel when mixed with liquid, whereas insoluble fibers do not. Soluble fibers may form gels in the GI tract that influence intestinal transit and nutrient absorption. They also may be fermented to a variable extent by GI microbes. In contrast, insoluble fiber passes through the GI tract largely intact. It probably is more practical to refer to a soluble-insoluble ratio, because most foods exhibit properties of both types of fiber. Further complicating the situation is that the fiber content varies according to where the plant was grown, its maturity at harvest, the type and extent of postharvest processing, the volume and surface area of the fiber particles, and even the method of analysis.

In clinical nutrition, fiber-containing diets are of interest for their gelling, fermenting, and bulking properties. Unfortunately, it also is not possible to accurately predict the function of a diet from knowledge of the fiber added to it for all the reasons previously stated, plus the variability introduced by the effects of combination with other ingredients and additional processing. Even meal size can affect fiber function.

Table 5-16
Fiber in Common Foods and Pet Foods

	Amount of Food	Total Fiber (g)	Soluble Fiber (%)
Common Food Items			
Pectin	1 Tablespoon	?	100
Guar gum	1 Tablespoon	?	100
Metamucil	5.8 g	3.4	79
Oat bran	6.7 g	1	50
Bran flake cereal	1 cup	4	33
Cooked pasta	140 g	2	25
Kidney beans	1 cup	9	22
Whole-wheat bread	25 g	2.5	20
All-Bran cereal	5 g	1.4	14
Wheat bran	5.3 g	2.7	11
100% Bran cereal	6.4 g	1.8	11
Popcorn	1 cup	1	0
Corn	1 cup	3	0
White rice, cooked	205 g	1	0
Pet Food Ingredients			
Corn gluten meal	100 g	5.5	51
Beet pulp	100 g	68	50
Oat bran	100 g	13	31
Barley	100 g	31	29
Brewer's grains	100 g	59	11
Wheat midds	100 g	46	11
Wheat bran	100 g	42	8

Table 5-17
Effects of Dietary Fiber on Physiologic Function

Function	Soluble Fiber	Insoluble Fiber
Gastric emptying	↓	±↑
Pancreatic secretion	±→	→
Nutrient absorption	±→	±→
Small intestinal transit	↓	↑
Large intestinal transit	↓	↑
Intestinal mucosal mass	↑	→
Microbial growth	↑	→
Toxin binding	→	↑

↓, Decreased; ↑, increased; →, no effect; ±, more or less.

The fiber content of some common foods and pet food ingredients is presented in Table 5-16. Some functions commonly considered to be affected by dietary fiber are presented in Table 5-17.

Although the effects shown in Table 5-17 have been documented in a number of experimental studies, the clinical response of patients is quite variable. Clients should be educated regarding this variability and should not expect a "quick fix" from use of a fiber-containing diet or addition of fiber to the existing diet.

Dietary fiber should be introduced gradually, over the course of a week or so, to permit the GI microflora to adapt to the increased amount and probably different composition of the fiber. Changes that are made too rapidly can result in flatulence, bloating, and abdominal discomfort.

Constipation

Animals sometimes have difficulty defecating. Patients that pass stools infrequently or that strain to defecate may be constipated. Constipation is a clinical sign characterized by absent, infrequent, or difficult defecation associated with retention of feces within the colon and rectum. Constipation can result from a variety of diseases that must be investigated during the initial examination. For example, straining, or tenesmus, can result from colitis and urogenital disease, so these must be differentiated from constipation.

Once the presenting episode has been resolved, follow-up treatment of uncomplicated constipation may include dietary modifications and increases in activity. The two most commonly recommended dietary modifications are increased water and fiber intake. Before any dietary recommendations are made, however, an accurate dietary history must be obtained to determine the patient's existing intakes of water and fiber. Modification of the existing diet by addition of water or fiber or transition to a canned, fiber-supplemented food may be indicated if intakes of water and fiber from the existing diet do not match recommended intakes.

The recommended intake of water is 40 to 60 ml per kilogram per day. Maintenance of normal hydration is an important part of the management of constipated patients. A convenient and economic way to increase the water intake of dogs is to add 1 volume of water per volume of dry food fed. The water is as hot as the house faucet can supply and is added 10 to 20 minutes before feeding to soften the food. Several methods also may be used to encourage the pet to drink more water. These include providing several bowls of water in the pet's environment, feeding canned rather than dry food, providing fresh water more often in a given day, and using a device such as a pet water fountain.

The animal's fiber intake can be quickly estimated from the food label, which lists the crude fiber content of the diet as fed. For canned diets the percentage of crude fiber is multiplied by the number of grams fed (the net weight of the food in canned diets is provided in grams on the front of the label). Consider a 20-kilogram dog that needs to consume approximately 10 g of fiber per day. If the dog eats two cans (a total of 750 g, according to the labels) of a food that contains 0.5% crude fiber, it consumes fiber as follows.

$$750 \times 0.5\% = 3.75 \text{ g of fiber per day}$$

To get to 10 g per day, 6 g (approximately 1 tablespoon) of fiber (e.g., Metamucil) is added to the diet each day. If the diet is dry, the same dog might eat 2 cups (approximately 200 g) per day. If the diet contains 4% fiber, the dog consumes $200 \times 4\% = 8$ g fiber, so the quantity of fiber to be added is approximately 2 g (approximately 1 teaspoon) per day. Of course, the amount finally added is determined by the clinical response; more or less fiber may be needed to achieve the desired fecal consistency.

Which type of fiber is most appropriate for the treatment of GI disturbances has not been determined. The choices include the more insoluble bulking fibers (wheat, corn, and oat brans) and the more soluble bulking-fermenting fibers, such as psyllium. Canned pumpkin, which adds both water and fermentable fiber, has been recommended as a fiber source for constipated cats. If the fiber added produces flatulence, the amount may be reduced or another type chosen.

Addition of fiber to foods may make them unpalatable to the pet. If this occurs, choosing a commercially available fiber-supplemented diet may be a better alternative. A variety of veterinary foods for dogs and cats have increased fiber content (see Appendixes H and I). No clinical trials of any of these diets for treatment of constipation or comparisons among the available diets have yet been reported.

In humans, another factor that can aid in control of constipation is activity. Walking a dog immediately after feeding often causes the animal to defecate. For cats, a clean litter pan is an important environmental factor that helps encourage defecation.

Inflammatory Bowel Disease

The term *inflammatory bowel disease* refers to a group of chronic GI disorders, the causes of which currently are largely unknown. For all the disorders the diagnosis is based on the discovery of inflammation of the wall of some part of the GI tract. IBD is the most common cause of chronic vomiting and diarrhea in cats and dogs, depending on the region of the GI tract most affected. After a diagnosis of IBD is confirmed, the nutritional goals are to minimize clinical signs, provide adequate nutrient intake to meet requirements, and compensate for ongoing losses through the GI tract.

Before any dietary changes are made, a complete dietary and feeding history should be taken and evaluated by a veterinarian to determine whether diet or feeding practices may be contributing to the disease. Intervention may be useful if a diet high in fat or low in digestibility is fed, if large volumes are fed infrequently, or if the patient has access to other food sources.

If a dietary change is warranted, three kinds of modified diets may be useful in managing the clinical signs associated with IBD: highly digestible, low-fat diets; modified fiber diets; and novel protein diets. The most common initial step in the treatment of dogs with IBD is to provide a highly digestible, low-fat food to help reduce intestinal irritation or inflammation and normalize intestinal motility. Currently several varieties are available through veterinarians, or a homemade diet may be used. For cats, increasing the fat content may be beneficial in the slowing of gastric emptying, especially if diarrhea is the primary problem. Increasing the soluble-fiber content of the diet also may be useful to normalize intestinal motility, water balance, and microflora. The amount of fermentable fiber in the pet's food may be increased by providing a specially formulated veterinary food or by adding fiber as described in Appendixes H and I. Because one possible cause of IBD is allergy to a protein in the diet, a food that contains a novel protein source to which the patient has not been exposed previously may be offered to see if the clinical signs abate. Improvement of signs should be seen within 3 weeks of strict dietary management. (See the discussion in nutrition-related skin diseases for more details.)

Introduction of new diets for patients with IBD should occur slowly, over approximately 2 weeks, to avoid exacerbation of signs. We encourage owners to restrict their pets' access to other foods and to feed smaller meals more frequently to maximize digestion and absorption of the diet. As signs improve, the frequency may gradually be reduced.

At this time, no physical test findings, laboratory test results, or historical facts are predictive of which method will be successful in any particular patient; individual dietary trials and careful veterinary follow-up are necessary for successful nutritional management.

Megacolon in Cats

Cats occasionally suffer chronic recurrent constipation. When feces remain in the colon for a prolonged period, progressively more water is reabsorbed and feces become drier and harder. The animal eventually may not be able to defecate at all. The colon may become severely and irreversibly dilated and flaccid—a condition called *megacolon*. Although the cause of the condition is not known, veterinary gastroenterologists associate abnormal colon function with dietary factors such as inadequate fiber intake or ingestion of excessive hair, environmental and psychologic factors, painful defecation, obstruction of the colon or anorectum, neuromuscular diseases, dehydration, hypokalemia, and drug-related constipation.

In the early stages, episodes of constipation with mild to moderate impaction of feces and an absence of systemic signs (depression, vomiting, dehydration) can usually be treated on an outpatient basis by dietary adjustments and oral laxatives. Several commercial fiber-supplemented diets are available for cats. Beneficial effects of insoluble fiber in these patients include increased frequency of defecation and fecal water content, softer fecal consistency, decreased intestinal transit time, and reduction of the intracolonic pressure required for normal defecation. Because adequate water intake and hydration are required for these beneficial actions, as well as to prevent impaction of fiber in the colon, we recommend that the canned form of the diet be fed. In addition, because environmental factors may affect GI function in these cats, we also offer the owners the recommendations for environmental enrichment described in detail at the World Wide Web site of the Indoor Cat Initiative (www.nssvet.org/ici).

The most clinically useful laxatives for cats include fiber-supplemented diets, osmotic laxatives such as lactose or lactulose, and cisapride (Propulsid), a promotility laxative.

Unabsorbed disaccharides such as lactose and lactulose are fermented by colonic bacteria, thereby producing an osmotic diarrhea. Lactose (available as nonfat dry milk) and lactulose are excellent all-purpose laxatives for short- or long-term use in cats. Nonfat dry milk contains 50% lactose and may be used at an initial dose of 2 g of lactose per kg of body weight per day (approximately 1 tablespoon per day in cats) mixed in the food. Lactulose usually is started at 0.5 ml per kg, given orally every 8 hours. The dose of either of these is adjusted to produce an acceptable frequency of defecation of soft feces. If the dosage is too high, abdominal discomfort, flatulence, and diarrhea may occur. These side effects can be resolved by lowering the dosage.

Dietary adjustments alone usually fail to normalize colon function in cats with megacolon. Cisapride (Propulsid) given orally at 1 (tid) to 1.5 (bid) mg/kg is effective in many cats for treatment of megacolon that is unresponsive to all other forms of medical therapy. Cisapride is a promotility drug that stimulates propulsive motility of colonic smooth muscle by releasing acetylcholine in the myenteric plexus. The colon in cats with megacolon may even resume normal diameter (radiographically) with treatment with cisapride. Megacolon commonly becomes refractory to cisapride after several months of therapy, necessitating an increase in dosage to 2 mg/kg, or 7.5 mg per cat, every 8 hours. Promotility drugs are generally contraindicated in the presence of an obstructive lesion.

Severe constipation may initially require evacuation of impacted feces from the colon with enemas, manual extraction of retained feces, or both, with the patient under general anesthesia. In severe cases, complicating dehydration and electrolyte imbalances should also be corrected. For cases unresponsive to medical management, subtotal colectomy is the most effective method of treatment. This procedure involves the removal of 95% or more of the colon. In cats with obstipation from pelvic fracture malunion, pelvic reconstructive surgery can allow return of normal colonic function if obstipation has been a problem for less than 6 months; otherwise, subtotal colectomy is recommended. After subtotal colectomy, diarrhea and frequent defecation are common; however, bowel function gradually improves during the 2 to 4 weeks after surgery in most cats.

Lymphangiectasia and Exocrine Pancreatic Insufficiency

Lymphangiectasia is an uncommon disorder caused by obstruction of the intestinal lymphatic ducts in dogs and cats that prevents fat assimilation from the intestine. EPI occurs when the pancreas loses more than 90% of the ability to secrete the enzymes necessary for the digestion of luminal nutrients. EPI is the most common cause of maldigestion in dogs but is rare in cats. EPI usually is congenital, but also may occur secondarily to pancreatitis. Dogs with EPI typically have a chronic history of weight loss despite a vigorous, even ravenous, appetite. The client also may have observed the pet eating dirt or rocks (pica) or feces (coprophagia).

After the presence of intestinal lymphangiectasia or EPI has been confirmed, dietary therapy consists of providing a highly digestible commercial or homemade diet that is low in fat (≤2 g/100 kcal) and fiber (<2% dry matter basis). Because of the presence of fat malabsorption, the fat-soluble vitamins (A, D, E, and K) and vitamin B_{12} may need to be provided parenterally. More-frequent feeding of smaller meals enhances nutrient absorption. Each feeding regimen is tailored for the individual animal, to help it obtain its optimum body weight.

For patients with EPI, an additional goal is to compensate for the loss of pancreatic enzyme activity. This is achieved by supplementing the animal's food with a pancreatic enzyme powder at a dose of 1 teaspoon (approximately 5 g) per 20 lb of body weight per meal, with this dosage titrated to achieve the best possible feces quality. Reduced-fiber diets are recommended, because dietary fiber may impair enzyme activity. The addition of the enzyme powder can create challenges in some cases, especially if the animal refuses to eat the food with the powder on it. The following suggestions may be useful in the achievement of long-term success.

- Canned diets are the easiest for mixing with medications.
- When powder is mixed into the food, a small amount of the food should be tried first. If the dog will not eat the food-powder mixture, it will still have food left to eat.
- If dry food is fed, the powder is mixed with a small amount of water before being added to the food.
- If the dog refuses to eat the food with the enzyme powder in it, the powder can be put into gelatin capsules for direct administration.
- Medium-chain triglyceride oil may be added as a source of easily absorbable calories to improve weight gain if necessary.

Most dogs respond well to this method of treatment and have a favorable prognosis for a good-quality life.

Pancreatitis

Pancreatitis occurs when the pancreas becomes inflamed. Symptoms and signs of pancreatitis include depression, anorexia, nausea, vomiting, diarrhea, and behaviors that indicate abdominal pain. Many factors influence the development of pancreatitis, including breed, age, gender, neuter status, and body condition. In dogs the dietary history often reveals recent ingestion of a large fatty meal or an incident of getting into the garbage. This does not mean, however, that fat consumption per se causes pancreatitis. Given that many dogs eat very fatty meals without incident, it seems more likely that a fatty meal may unmask a predisposition to pancreatitis in susceptible individuals.

After the presence of pancreatitis has been confirmed, it is important before a feeding regimen is chosen to determine the severity of the condition and how long it has been since the animal's last meal. A validated clinical scoring system for pancreatitis in dogs recently was introduced; a modified form of this system is presented in Table 5-18.

For mild pancreatitis we provide fluid support and give nothing by mouth for at least 24 to 48 hours after the last episode of vomiting. We then give small amounts of water over 4 to 6 hours; if this is tolerated well, small amounts of a low-fat food are given, divided over

Table 5-18
Clinical Scoring System for Pancreatitis in Dogs

Score	Presenting Signs and Symptoms	Nutritional Support	Prognosis
0	Initial, mild signs	Nothing given by mouth; follow-up	Excellent
1	Significant dehydration, prerenal azotemia, discomfort	Nothing given by mouth; follow-up	Good to fair
2	Signs in 1 plus elevated white blood cell count and degenerative left shift, nausea, possible vomiting and diarrhea, pain	Nothing given by mouth; follow-up	Fair to guarded
3	Signs in 2 plus depression, vomiting, and diarrhea	Total parenteral nutrition	Poor
4	Signs in 3, with increased severity	Total parenteral nutrition	Grave

several meals (four to six) per day. If the water and food are tolerated without vomiting, the quantities of each are gradually increased, usually over 5 or 6 days, until the total daily requirements are being met.

For patients with severe pancreatitis, when the anticipated duration of withholding of food is expected to be greater than 72 hours, nutritional support via the enteral or parenteral route is considered. Severe pancreatitis seems to occur most commonly in older, neutered dogs with a history of pancreatitis, and it seems to occur much more commonly in dogs than in cats. In the most severe cases, PN allows the gut to rest completely and should be used for at least 5 days before the introduction of oral (enteral) nutrition is attempted. In cats, enteral support usually is adequate. Techniques for enteral and parenteral support are discussed in the section on nutritional support for hospitalized patients. One of the most common causes of relapse in dogs with pancreatitis is feeding too much too quickly. We prefer to return patients to their normal food intake slowly, with small amounts offered more frequently, rather than to risk the reoccurrence of vomiting and the consequent restarting of the feeding regimen. Once patients are discharged from the hospital, we consider them to be at high risk for recurrence of pancreatitis and recommend feeding a highly digestible, low-fat commercial or homemade diet at regular intervals.

Chronic Liver Disease

A variety of chronic liver diseases occur in dogs and cats. Energy needs for maintenance of patients with liver disease are assumed to be the same as those of normal, sedentary animals. Protein needs should be met with dietary proteins of high biologic value fed at levels close to the minimum recommended amount when animals show signs of ammonia intoxication—postprandial sleepiness, head pressing, or depression. We consider this minimum to be for dogs 2 g and for cats 3 g of protein per kilogram of body weight per day. When long-term intake is anticipated to be at this level or lower, clients are alerted to monitor their pets closely for signs of protein depletion (weight loss, decreased muscle mass, deteriorating skin or haircoat quality). This level of daily protein intake can be met by use of commercially available therapeutic diets, by dilution of commercial diets with fat and carbohydrates, or by formulation of a home-prepared diet. The diet should be fed as small meals over the course of the day to maximize utilization and minimize the amount of protein that escapes digestion in the small bowel. Undigested protein is fermented in the large bowel, with production and absorption of toxic metabolites such as ammonia and mercaptans, which are not detoxified by the diseased liver. The quantities of these substances may be reduced by substitution of dairy or vegetable proteins for meat proteins. In addition, provision of a carbohydrate source in the form of a soluble fiber of indigestible carbohydrate such as lactulose or lactose (~2 g or 30 ml of milk per kilogram of body weight per day) increases microbial mass in the colon and results in excretion of a significant portion of these metabolites in the feces. A diet specifically formulated for dogs with liver disease, Hill's l/d, recently became available; studies of its clinical efficacy are eagerly awaited.

Anorexia is a problem commonly associated with liver disease, and frequent feedings of small amounts of fresh food by the owner may help stimulate food intake. Changes in vitamin and mineral needs of animals because of liver disease are generally unknown, although restriction of sodium intake may be necessary to control ascites.

Idiopathic Hepatic Lipidosis in Cats

Excessive food restriction or anorexia may cause a syndrome called *idiopathic hepatic lipidosis* (IHL) in cats. IHL is a potentially fatal complication of prolonged food deprivation. Although anorexia is a common historical finding in nearly all cat diseases, most (but not all) cats that develop fatty liver syndrome were previously obese. Infiltration of the liver with fat may be a preexisting condition in these cats or may develop from a decreased rate of fatty-acid oxidation, increased rate of hepatic lipogenesis, reduced rate of triglyceride secretion from hepatocytes, or reduced clearance of circulating triglycerides associated with an unrelated disease process. Currently, insufficient information is available to allow distinction of the most probable site of dysfunction, which may not be the same in all cats with the syndrome. Cats with IHL often have variable combinations of anorexia, generalized weakness, muscle wasting, weight loss of variable duration, and icterus. Laboratory evaluation commonly reveals increased concentrations of ammonia, liver-specific enzymes, and bilirubin. Cholesterol and triglyceride concentrations are sometimes elevated. Plasma protein concentrations are usually normal. Pathologic findings include periacinal hepatocellular necrosis of variable severity, marked accumulation of fat in hepatocytes, and bile pigment retention.

Nutritional therapy for IHL consists of aggressive long-term support via an esophagostomy or gastrostomy tube. Feeding a diet that contains at least 30% of the

CLIENT COMMUNICATION TIPS: Gastrointestinal Disease

- Carefully review the dietary history of the pet with the client.
- Discuss any recent changes in the animal's body weight or BCS.
- If a client does not know how much food the pet consumes in a given day or week, instruct the client regarding completion of a 5-day food diary. A piece of notebook paper can be used, with columns created for the date, time, type of food or treat offered, quantity or serving size, and initials of the person who offers the food. Anything consumed by the pet is recorded in the food diary. Follow up with clients after the food diary has been completed to identify factors that can potentially be modified (e.g., products, serving sizes, behaviors).
- Determine the total daily caloric intake of the pet and calculate both protein and fat intakes to assess whether the animal is receiving the minimum (or maximum) requirement. This is especially important for sick or older dogs and cats, whose daily food intake may vary.
- Educate clients regarding the important benefits of meal-feeding pets rather than feeding on a free-choice basis. Individual meals allow the owner to observe appetite and water consumption and identify potential problems.
- Communicate clearly (both orally and in writing) about the type, dosage, and cost of any nutritional supplements that are recommended.
- Teach clients how to monitor food intake each day and how to watch for signs of wasting.
- Recommend that any dietary change be made gradually over a period of several days or longer. If food aversions are to be avoided, dietary changes should not be made in the hospital setting, but in the home and after the pet is feeling better.
- Tell clients to call the veterinarian if they have problems or questions.
- Discuss with the staff the criteria for determining which "GI" diets the veterinarians in the practice recommend, as well as those they avoid recommending. Which foods are on the practice's "A list," and why. Which are on the practice's "B list," and why. Help staff identify clients who are receptive to learning more about dietary recommendations.

kilocalories as protein is appropriate in the absence of hepatic encephalopathy. Cats respond to starvation by depleting urea cycle intermediates rather than urea cycle enzymes, as most omnivores do, so feeding higher-protein diets can be accomplished safely. Response to therapy is variable, likely because of differences in the stage of disease progression at the time of presentation. Nutritional support (enteral tube feeding) may be required for weeks or months. It recently has been suggested that the necessity for prolonged tube feeding may be the result of learned aversions conditioned by repeated early attempts to coax the animal to eat. If such attempts are made while the cat is ill and depressed, it may associate the feelings of ill health with the food. The tube-feeding period may be shortened by not offering the cat oral food for the first 2 weeks of therapy or until the cat's behavior suggests that it "feels better" and is interested in food again. Prevention of the disease through use of well-designed weight-loss programs, and attention to the food intake of hospitalized feline patients, should receive high priority.

HEART DISEASE

Chronic heart problems are relatively common in adult and older pets. The most common problems in dogs are diseases of the heart valves and dilated cardiomyopathy (DCM), whereas diseases of the heart muscle are more common in cats. Changing the diet to restrict sodium intake in the presence of a murmur but before signs of failure occur has been a mainstay of treatment for chronic heart failure. This recommendation has been made because patients with heart disease cannot excrete sodium normally, and excessive sodium and fluid retention adds to the workload of the heart.

More recently, however, the availability of angiotensin-converting enzyme (ACE)–inhibitors and improvements in understanding of the activation of the renin-angiotensin-aldosterone system have led to modification of the recommendation for early sodium restriction. ACE inhibitors block the production of angiotensin II and its stimulation of secretion of aldosterone. Both angiotensin II and aldosterone promote retention of sodium and water by the kidney, so inhibition of angiotensin II results in improved sodium and water excretion. Excessive sodium restriction can activate the renin-angiotensin-aldosterone system, which provision of ACE-inhibitors is designed to avoid, so sodium intake should be limited in proportion to the severity of the disease in an attempt to avoid depletion.

Congestive Heart Failure

Most dogs with congestive heart failure (CHF) that results from valvular disease are older, sedentary, small dogs, such as poodles, miniature schnauzers, dachshunds, Chihuahuas, terriers, and cocker spaniels. Obesity occurs commonly in many of these patients, which can exacerbate heart problems by further increasing the workload on an already failing pump. Some animals with chronic heart failure are also cachexic, so the BCS and MCS of the patient are noted and modifications to attain a more appropriate condition become part of the therapeutic goal. The severity of the disease—whether only a murmur signifies the presence of heart disease or the animal has developed the cough, shortness of breath, and exercise intolerance that are signs of heart failure—also should be assessed.

Table 5-19

Functional Classification* of Heart Failure and Corresponding Sodium Intake

Class	Description†	Sodium Intake (mg/lb body weight/day)
I	Normal; physical activity, including normal exercise, does not cause symptoms.	Unrestricted
II	Slightly limited physical capacity; ordinary physical activity leads to signs.	15
III	Markedly limited physical capacity; limited physical activity leads to signs.	10
IV	Unable to carry on any activity without signs; signs present at rest.	5

*Modified from New York Heart Association criteria.
†Signs include weight loss, exercise intolerance, coughing, respiratory distress, and ascites (occasionally).

Functional criteria for the severity of heart disease and corresponding recommendations for sodium intake are presented in Table 5-19.

The nutrients of concern in patients with heart failure include sodium, levels of which may be too high, and potassium and magnesium, levels of which may be too low. Before a diet is chosen, the food intake of the patient must be determined by means of a carefully obtained dietary history. The foods fed and their amounts should be determined so that an estimate of energy and sodium intake can be made. If questions regarding how much the patient eats cannot be answered, food intake should be measured for a few days in order to estimate the amount consumed. The energy and sodium content can be obtained from the manufacturer. These values are important because animals need amounts of nutrients per day rather than percentages in the diet. Older, sedentary animals often are maintained on intakes that are half of what would be determined from prediction equations. If such a patient is fed a severely restricted diet, the nutrient needs may not be met. For example, the minimum sodium requirement for dogs is approximately 10 mg per kilogram per day. If a dog eats 30 kcal per kilogram per day, the diet must contain 10 mg of sodium per 30 kcal, or 33 mg of sodium per 100 kcal. If the dog eats 60 kcal per kilogram per day, the diet must contain only half as much sodium per 100 kcal.

The client is asked what treats are fed to the dog. Many snacks contain relatively large amounts of sodium and should be avoided in patients with chronic heart disease. It also is essential that all medications be identified, along with the vehicles of their administration. These vehicles often are cheese, peanut butter, and delicatessen-type meat treats, which may contain large quantities of salt.

Once the sodium intake is estimated, it may be compared with the recommendations provided in Table 5-19. These are only general estimates; signs in individual patients may be controlled with intake of more or less sodium. As with other diseases, diets for patients with CHF should be compared on an energy basis. Knowing the caloric intake and desired sodium intake permits determination of how much sodium on a 100-kcal basis is desired and choice of a food that delivers this amount (dose). For example, a 20-lb dog with class III disease should consume approximately 200 mg of sodium per day. If the daily energy intake to maintain a moderate body condition is 20 kcal/lb, or 400 kcal, a diet that contains 200 mg of sodium per 400 kcal intake consists of 0.5 mg/kcal, or 50 mg/100 kcal. Once this value has been determined, a diet that contains sodium in this concentration (and any other desirable attributes, depending on the case) can be chosen. The sodium content of diets must be compared on an energy basis because so much variation exists in sodium content among dry and canned diets and among diets of differing energy densities. For example, the dry form of one veterinary food for animals with severe CHF contains 14 mg of sodium per 100 kcal, and the canned form contains 23 mg of sodium per 100 kcal, nearly twice as much. Variations in the fat content of diets also affect nutrient intake.

Potassium and magnesium may be lost because of diuretic use and decreased intake. Potassium may be retained in patients treated with ACE inhibitors. Because of the effects of these drugs, serum potassium and magnesium concentrations should be measured periodically, and the intake of potassium and magnesium adjusted as necessary.

The sodium intake of patients with chronic heart disease should be adjusted slowly. If the animal's existing diet is high in sodium, a lower-sodium diet can be blended slowly into the existing diet to gradually reduce intake. Abrupt changes in diet can cause a conditioned aversion to the diet, particularly if the new food is introduced when the animal is hospitalized and not feeling well. To avoid this problem, we recommend that dietary changes be made when the patient has gone home and the appetite has improved, so that the new diet is more likely to be associated with feelings of better health.

If the animal is obese, some weight loss may be helpful. In humans, gradual loss of approximately 10% of body weight leads to beneficial reductions in blood pressure. This suggests that the regaining of moderate body condition may be less important than previously believed, and that a modest weight reduction may be satisfactory. Although the benefits of sodium restriction in veterinary patients with hypertension have yet to be documented, intake of more-modest amounts than those present in some commercial foods may be appropriate.

The owner should monitor the animal's food intake daily during the course of therapy. Loss of appetite is an early sign of worsening of the disease, excessive drug (digitalis) intake, or fatigue with the diet. If the animal eats favorite foods readily, the diet is suspect; if it is generally inappetent, a drug problem or exacerbation of the disease is more likely.

In summary, recent evidence suggests that severe sodium restriction should not be instituted early in the course of heart disease, although avoidance of excessive sodium intake seems prudent. If sodium restriction becomes necessary to help control edema and hypertension, it should be instituted slowly and only to the extent necessary to control signs.

Dilated Cardiomyopathy in Dogs

DCM is a syndrome of impaired cardiac function, dilated ventricles, and, frequently, arrhythmia. Dogs with DCM may have exercise intolerance, weight loss, respiratory problems, weakness, or ascites, depending on the severity of the disease at presentation. Breeds predisposed to DCM include the Doberman pinscher, Great Dane, Scottish deerhound, Irish wolfhound, dalmatian, boxer, and American and English cocker spaniels. In 1991 a myocardial L-carnitine deficiency was identified in a family of boxers with DCM, and some affected dogs seemed to respond to L-carnitine supplementation. This led to the suggestion that DCM in these dogs might be a diet-induced disease. Unfortunately, all the affected dogs eventually died as a result of heart disease despite continued supplementation. Carnitine is synthesized in the liver from lysine and methionine, and myocardial depletion may occur for many reasons. L-Carnitine deficiency currently does not appear to be the cause of DCM in the majority of boxers or in other breeds. However, it is still considered a potential cause of DCM in boxers, and after consultation with a cardiologist, supplementation might be considered in these cases.

Fatty-acid supplementation also has been recommended for dogs with DCM. One study found that supplementation of Hill's dry h/d diet with 27 mg eicosapentaenoic acid (EPA) and 18 mg of docosahexaenoic acid (DHA) per kilogram of body weight per day improved the average cachexia score from 1.7 to 1.1 (2 indicates moderate, 1 indicates mild) in dogs with DCM but had no effect on survival time. This dose is comparable to 1 fish oil capsule per 10 to 15 pounds of body weight per day. The amounts of EPA and DHA in individual fish oil supplements vary widely, however, so in order to determine an appropriate dose, it is important to know the exact amount of EPA and DHA in the supplement.

DCM has been reported in a group of male dalmatians, most of which had been fed a low-protein diet for prolonged periods of time. Although the significance of this relationship was not documented, the protein intake of dalmatians that develop DCM should be maintained at 2 g per kilogram of body weight per day through supplementation or dietary change unless a specific clinical contraindication exists. If the patient also has urolithiasis, see the section on Urinary Diseases for recommendations for increasing water intake.

In some American cocker spaniels DCM has been associated with low plasma taurine concentrations (normal range is 44 to 224 nmol/ml). Taurine is a β-amino sulfonic acid synthesized from methionine and cysteine in the liver and other tissues of mammals. Supplemental oral taurine (500 mg twice daily with meals) may be provided pending results of measurements of circulating taurine concentrations and may be continued if a plasma taurine deficiency is identified. Supplementation may be needed for 3 or 4 months before significant improvement is seen; additional treatment is provided as needed for heart failure, arrhythmias, and other signs. Taurine supplementation may result in reversal of the disease and a significantly better prognosis. If plasma taurine concentrations are normal, the prognosis is poorer, but progression is fairly slow, and the dog may be kept comfortable through administration of heart failure medications for some time.

Dilated Cardiomyopathy in Cats

Taurine synthesis in cats occurs too slowly for taurine balance to be maintained in the absence of dietary taurine. Obligatory loss of taurine also occurs in cats because only taurine can combine with cholesterol during bile salt synthesis, whereas in most other species glycine can be substituted for taurine. Taurine is therefore required in feline diets, with the amount inversely proportional to the methionine and cysteine content of the diet. Taurine is present only in animal tissues, with 200 to 400 mg/kg present in fresh meat and up to 2500 mg/kg present in shellfish. The 1986 revision of *Nutrient Requirements of Cats* suggested a requirement of 400 mg of taurine for growth and maintenance, and 500 mg for reproduction, per kilogram (5000 kcal) of diet. For a 5-kilogram adult cat at maintenance that consumes 300 kcal per day, this translates to approximately 25 mg of taurine per day.

Experiences have demonstrated that the presence of National Research Council (NRC)–recommended amounts of taurine in commercial diets may not be adequate in all circumstances. For example, idiopathic DCM in cats was associated with low plasma taurine concentrations and was successfully treated with oral administration of taurine. Plasma taurine concentrations in cats diagnosed with DCM were only 10% of normal (7.5 ± 4.2 vs 109 ± 18 nmol/ml), and some cats had the eye lesions characteristic of taurine deficiency. These cats had been fed a variety of commercial diets, which by analysis contained adequate amounts of taurine. When the cats were provided supplemental taurine (500 mg twice daily) and drugs to control the signs of heart failure, all showed clinical improvement during the first 2 weeks of taurine supplementation. Echocardiographic signs of damage to the heart muscle began to diminish after 3 or 4 weeks of supplementation.

The low plasma taurine concentrations that occurred despite consumption of commercial diets that contained amounts of taurine in excess of the requirements were later found to result from excessive bile salt loss in feces caused by type of dietary processing (dry or canned), protein source, changes in location or numbers of intestinal microflora, and increased secretion of bile salts because of changes in cholecystokinin release. Manufacturers added more taurine to their diets, and DCM has become a rare occurrence in cats.

If collection of blood samples is required for plasma taurine determination, care must be taken to ensure that plasma is separated *before* the blood is chilled to avoid release of taurine from platelets. Alternatively, whole blood taurine may be measured by freezing the sample to ensure release of taurine from all the formed elements of the blood. Cats with taurine-deficiency–related DCM have plasma taurine concentrations below 20 nmol/ml and should receive taurine supplements (available as 500-mg capsules in health food stores) at 250 to 500 mg orally every 12 hours for 12 to 16 weeks or until echocardiographic parameters have returned to normal.

Plasma taurine concentrations fluctuate with food intake and stabilize after approximately 24 hours of food deprivation. Whereas the plasma concentration of taurine measures recent taurine status, the whole blood taurine concentration reflects the long-term history of taurine intake over the preceding weeks to months. The whole blood taurine concentration also approximates muscle taurine concentrations more closely than the plasma concentration does and therefore may be a better indicator of whole body taurine status. Until additional data on normal whole blood taurine concentrations become available, a concentration of 250 nmol/ml has been suggested to be satisfactory.

The response of the pet food industry to the problem of taurine inadequacy demonstrates that such problems usually are resolved by reputable manufacturers as soon as they are identified. Also demonstrated are the difficulties of extrapolating results obtained in studies of one diet to situations in which other diets are fed. In the case of taurine, for example, the "requirement" was established in unprocessed diets that used a protein source different from that used in most commercial diets.

Dietary therapy for heart disease has evolved from use of sodium-restricted diets to consideration of the intake of sodium and a variety of other nutrients. Early diagnosis and medical intervention have improved the quality of care for affected patients and, along with feeding recommendations based on the patient's condition and food intake, hold promise for improvements in patient quality of life and client satisfaction.

CLIENT COMMUNICATION TIPS: Heart Disease

- Determine the total daily caloric intake of the pet and calculate salt intake to assess how much is being consumed above the minimum requirement. This is especially important for older dogs and cats, whose daily food intake may vary.
- Review the dietary history carefully with the client, and discuss specific nutrient modifications that may necessitate a dietary change in the near future.
- Communicate clearly with clients about the type, dosage, and cost of nutrient supplements (such as L-carnitine, taurine, or fish oil capsules) that are recommended.
- If a client does not know how much food the pet consumes in a given day or week, instruct the client regarding completion of a 5-day food diary. A piece of notebook paper can be used, with columns created for the date, time, type of food or treat offered, quantity or serving size, and initials of the person who offers the food. Anything consumed by the pet is recorded in the food diary. Follow up with clients after the food diary has been completed to identify factors that can potentially be modified (e.g., products, serving sizes, behaviors).
- Educate clients regarding the important benefits of meal-feeding older pets rather than feeding on a free-choice basis. Individual meals allow the owner to observe appetite and water consumption and identify potential problems.
- Teach clients how to monitor food intake each day and how to watch for signs of wasting.
- Recommend that any dietary change be made gradually over a period of several days or longer. If food aversions are to be avoided, dietary changes should not be made in the hospital setting, but in the home and after the pet is feeling better.
- Instruct clients on when to call, if they have problems or questions.
- For owners of overconditioned or obese patients, it may be valuable to discuss the benefits of modest weight reduction and regular exercise.
- Discuss with the staff the criteria for determining which "heart-healthy" diets the veterinarians in the practice recommend, as well as those they avoid recommending. Help the staff identify clients who are receptive to learning more about dietary recommendations. Nutrients of interest in cardiac patients vary widely, so a single product is unlikely to be "right" for every patient being treated for cardiac disease.

TECH TIPS: Heart Disease

- Obtain a complete dietary history (see Appendix C).
- Offer appropriate literature for client education and samples of low-sodium pet foods. Make sure the samples sent are of foods available for the owner to purchase at a later time in the event that the pet likes the food.
- Give clients a list of common "people foods" that are low in sodium to aid clients in the event that pets will not eat the pet food.
- Discuss with clients the high sodium content of treats and foods used as vehicles for medications, and offer advice regarding low-sodium foods that can be used as alternatives if necessary.
- Give clients written instructions regarding the proper way to make the transition to a new pet food, if a change is necessary (see Appendix D).

For a selection of reduced-sodium diets for dogs and cats, refer to Appendixes H and I.

KIDNEY DISEASE

Chronic renal failure (CRF) is a relatively uncommon problem in dogs, but is one of the more common problems in old cats (see the discussion of CRF in the section on Geriatric Cats). As with many nutrition-related diseases, the cause of CRF usually is not known. Although the original cause of the renal injury may still be present (as in pyelonephritis or renal amyloidosis), an underlying cause for the initial renal insult usually cannot be found, despite the progressive loss of function. The goals of dietary therapy for patients with CRF include improvement of clinical signs, maximization of quality of life, and the slowing (if possible) of the progression of disease. In some instances, diet may be altered to decrease polydipsia and polyuria.

Patients with a decrease of up to 50% in glomerular filtration rate (GFR) are classified as having decreased renal reserve; those with a decrease in GFR of 50% to 75% have renal insufficiency; and those with a decrease in GFR greater than 75% have excretory renal failure. Measurements of serum urea nitrogen (SUN), serum creatinine (SCr), and serum phosphorus concentrations are commonly available laboratory tests that provide crude estimators of GFR in practice, but none is a sensitive indicator of the presence of kidney disease. More than 75% of the nephrons must be lost before the SUN or SCr increases beyond the normal range (azotemia), and more than 85% to 90% are lost before serum phosphorus concentrations increase. Once SUN and SCr become elevated, they tend to more accurately reflect further loss of kidney function as the disease advances. Therefore, the finding of normal SUN and SCr concentrations never excludes the presence of kidney disease. Figure 5-9 shows the severity of kidney disease.

Most diseases that affect the kidney result in progressive loss of urine concentrating capacity, and this often occurs earlier than an increase in SUN or SCr. At least 65% of nephrons must be lost before the decline in urine concentrating ability results in a urine specific gravity (USG) of 1.025. Cats and dogs with normal kidneys usually produce

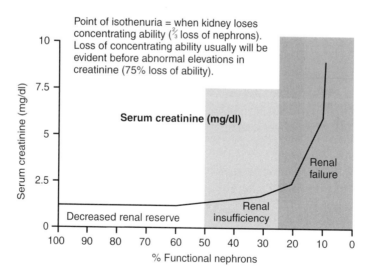

Figure 5-9 Severity of kidney disease.

concentrated urine. The USG of pets fed canned or other high-moisture foods often exceeds 1.035 (cats) or 1.02 (dogs) and is even higher in animals fed dry foods. Cats can retain urine-concentrating ability despite greater nephron loss than dogs can, and in cats, concentration of urine may occur normally even after the onset of azotemia. In cats with mild azotemia resulting from chronic primary renal failure, concentration of urine to a specific gravity greater than 1.04 often still occurs. Dogs and cats with azotemia and dilute urine (<1.03), however, are very likely to have primary renal failure.

At both OSU and MSU, we most commonly see patients with relatively severe disease. The average dog is 7 years old, weighs 12 kilograms, and has a SUN of 100 and a SCr of 6; the average cat is 16 years old, weighs 3 kilograms, and has a SUN of 75 and a SCr of 5. Most animals show signs of depression, inappetence, unkempt appearance, polyuria, polydipsia, and wasting. The average life expectancy is less than 6 months.

After diagnosis we ensure that patients with CRF are rehydrated, repair any electrolyte deficits and acid-base abnormalities, and institute nutritional support, often by feeding tube. The anorexia so commonly present probably results from varying combinations of GI ulcers, nausea, vomiting, stomatitis, oral ulcers, and necrosis of the tongue. Alterations in sense of smell and taste also may contribute to anorexia, as they do in humans with renal failure. Additionally, the phosphorus, protein, and salt restriction present in foods designed for the treatment of CRF may make them less palatable in general. Learned aversion to foods associated with hospitalization or forced feedings can contribute to anorexia.

Cimetidine, ranitidine, and famotidine, which inhibit histamine-2 (H_2) receptor–mediated gastric acid secretion, can be useful in the treatment of gastric ulcers and gastritis. The increased gastrin concentration in the serum that results during CRF from decreased renal degradation may be responsible for stimulation of excessive gastric acid secretion and ulcer formation. Some dogs and cats with uremia develop a dramatic increase in intake of and interest in food after one of these drugs is provided. Some animals with uremia may need to receive this medication for the rest of their lives. Our nephrologists usually prescribe cimetidine at an initial dose of 10 mg/kg followed by 5 mg/kg bid orally, or famotidine (Pepcid) at 1 mg/kg once daily. Omeprazole (a proton pump blocker in the stomach) may be an alternative to the H_2-receptor blockers to reduce stomach acid secretion, but we have little experience with its use in patients with CRF. It can be considered in patients in whom use of H_2-receptor blockers does not control vomiting. Sucralfate (Carafate) acts as a GI "bandage" that may be used to coat painful GI ulcers and promote food intake. We usually administer sucralfate to patients that have melena from GI bleeding.

Metoclopramide (Reglan) may be useful in animals with uremia that vomit or show signs of nausea (excessive licking of the lips, swallowing, drooling). The drug works partly by depressing the "vomiting center" in the brain and also by enhancing gastric emptying. We usually use this drug in patients in which H_2-receptor blockers have been ineffective, although some practitioners recommend metoclopramide as the first-line agent of choice. It can be given orally at 0.2 to 0.4 mg/kg tid to qid and may be most effective if given approximately 30 minutes before a meal.

When the animal is feeling better and has returned home, it can be offered food orally. Sick animals are more likely to eat familiar foods than novel foods. For this reason, dietary histories must be accurate enough that the current food can be purchased, if necessary, at the clinic. Patients are most likely to develop an aversion to unfamiliar foods when ill. If animals do develop an aversion to a food, they may never eat that food again. We have achieved more success with acceptance of veterinary foods for patients with CRF by introduction of the foods at home when patients are feeling better.

Dietary modification and nutritional support have traditionally been considered cornerstones of therapy in dogs and cats with CRF. Many earlier recommendations were based on the results of studies of diets fed to healthy young dogs and cats after renal failure was induced by removal of 83% to 92% of the total kidney mass (remnant kidney model). More recently published clinical studies of dogs and cats with naturally occurring CRF have documented beneficial effects of veterinary foods designed to accommodate the disease-induced limitations imposed by renal failure. Currently available "kidney-friendly" veterinary foods generally are restricted in phosphorus, protein, calcium, and sodium. They may be supplemented with sources of alkali (e.g., potassium citrate) and may contain a lower ratio of omega-6/omega-3 fatty acids than most commercial diets do. Compared with foods designed for healthy pets, kidney-friendly veterinary foods contain 70% to 80% less phosphorus and 30% to 50% less protein on an energy basis, although substantial differences exist among the available products. (For a selection of low-phosphorous and low-protein diets for dogs and cats, see Appendixes H and I). The canned forms of the diets generally are more restricted in phosphorus than their dry counterparts, and the dry (but not canned) forms of diets designed for cats are supplemented with potassium at approximately twice the level of foods for healthy cats, apparently in an effort to avoid kaliopenic nephropathy.

Restriction of phosphorus intake can have beneficial effects on renal function and mortality in dogs and cats with CRF. These effects are independent of protein restriction (i.e., protein restriction is not necessary for benefits to be achieved with phosphorus restriction). How phosphorus restriction exerts these beneficial effects is not precisely known, but they may be related to reduced renal mineralization and inhibition of secondary hyperparathyroidism. Decreased renal mineralization may result from lowered concentration and actions of parathyroid hormone (PTH) and possibly from a direct lowering of serum phosphorus concentration, which reduces the calcium x phosphorus concentration product.

Currently no veterinary foods that are both replete in protein and restricted in phosphorus are commercially available. It is theoretically possible to produce such foods, but the process is difficult in commercial formulations. Diets are restricted in phosphorus largely through limitation of their protein content, because phosphates often are associated with proteins in food. In addition, the source of dietary protein influences the amount of phosphate in the diet. The amounts of calcium and phosphorus added to the diet, as well as the form of the added phosphorus, influence the degree of phosphorus absorption. Considerable variability exists in the amount of phosphorus (measured in mg/100 kcal) in veterinary foods that contain similar amounts of protein, which provides the opportunity of matching the degree of phosphorus restriction with the patient's food intake without unnecessarily compromising protein intake.

In patients with early kidney failure, intestinal phosphorus binders (aluminum hydroxide, calcium carbonate, calcium acetate) may provide phosphorus restriction without the necessity of changing the diet. Conventionally, intestinal phosphorus binders are administered only when the serum phosphorus level is elevated, but reason may exist to administer them to patients with CRF before the serum phosphorus concentration rises. Phosphorus intake should be slowly reduced to approximately 60 mg/kg/day as GFR falls with disease progression.

Aluminum hydroxide and carbonate have been used extensively as intestinal phosphorus binders. Chronic aluminum ingestion has been demonstrated to be toxic in people with CRF (who usually are on dialysis), but toxicity in dogs and cats has not yet been identified. Calcium carbonate is an alternative intestinal phosphorus binder; the final dose may be as high as 100 mg/kg divided twice daily with meals. We usually start with half this dose, adjusting as necessary to maintain serum phosphorus concentration within the normal range. Although the potential aluminum toxicity is avoided, hypercalcemia can occur, especially if the patient simultaneously receives calcitriol supplementation. Calcium acetate recently has been approved for humans as an intestinal phosphorus binder, replacing aluminum salts and calcium carbonate. Sevelamer hydrochloride (Renagel) has been recently approved for use in humans as a phosphate binder that contains no calcium or aluminum. Calcium acetate binds phosphorus in the intestinal lumen better than calcium carbonate does and also reduces the risk of development of hypercalcemia. Intestinal phosphate binders work best when given with food or within a few hours of food ingestion, but have been shown to reduce serum phosphorus concentrations even when given to anorectic patients.

Achievement of normal serum phosphorus or PTH concentrations can be difficult in some patients despite a combination of dietary phosphate restriction and intestinal phosphate binders. In these cases, provision of a veterinary food with more severe phosphate restriction may be useful. Some diets with similar phosphate contents per 100 kcal of intake may exert different effects on the serum phosphorus concentration because of differences in biologic availability of the phosphorus for absorption. Increasing the dose of the intestinal phosphate binder to maximal recommended levels may also be needed to decrease the serum phosphorus. Uncontrolled metabolic acidosis and renal secondary hyperparathyroidism may contribute to hyperphosphatemia by accelerating bone dissolution. It sometimes becomes impossible to achieve normal serum phosphorus concentrations regardless of therapy in patients with very severe renal failure.

Although dietary phosphorus restriction can lower serum PTH concentrations in some dogs and cats with chronic renal disease or early renal failure, patients with greater loss of renal function require the addition of a phosphorus binder to the food to provide phosphorus restriction proportionate to the loss of renal mass. Return of serum phosphorus levels to normal does not guarantee the return of serum PTH levels to normal, because phosphorus restriction alone is successful only in patients with sufficient remaining calcitriol synthetic capacity once the inhibitory effects of excess phosphorus on calcitriol synthesis are removed.

Calcitriol, the biologically active form of vitamin D, may need to be provided daily to dogs and cats with severe CRF for the rest of their lives. Small daily oral doses of calcitriol effectively return the serum PTH level to one that is either normal or below the toxic threshold. Months of therapy with a dose of 2.5 to 3.5 ng/kg once daily may be required before the full beneficial effect is obtained. Serum phosphorus concentrations must decline to less than 6 mg/dl before and during calcitriol therapy. Phosphorus reduction relieves the phosphate-mediated inhibition of the renal 1-hydroxylase enzyme that catalyzes the final step in the calcitriol synthesis pathway, which results in enhanced endogenous synthesis of calcitriol and subsequent inhibition of PTH synthesis. A second reason to institute phosphorus restriction is to reduce the likelihood of soft-tissue mineralization through reduction of the serum calcium x phosphorus concentration product. A third reason is to increase ionized calcium concentrations in the parathyroid gland nucleus. Calcium, with its associated transcription factor, must bind to its DNA binding site in the parathyroid cell nucleus to fully effect a calcitriol-mediated decrease in PTH synthesis. As serum phosphorus concentrations decline, calcium ionization increases. Serum phosphorus concentrations in excess of 7 or 8 mg/dl can decrease ionized calcium by approximately 0.1 mg/dl, enough to increase PTH secretion. Control of secondary hyperparathyroidism is almost certain to fail in patients in whom serum phosphorus levels are maintained much above the normal range. We find that the effectiveness of calcitriol in control of hyperparathyroidism increases in patients when serum phosphate concentrations return to the normal range.

In our experience, hypercalcemia is a rare side effect of low-dose oral calcitriol treatment. When noted, it usually is associated with the use of relatively high doses of calcium-containing intestinal phosphate binders, especially calcium carbonate. If necessary, calcitriol may be given at bedtime to a patient with an empty stomach to minimize hypercalcemia. When compared with calcitriol, so-called "noncalcemic" calcitriol analogs were calcemic at effective doses and showed no advantage over therapy with calcitriol. Pulse dose oral calcitriol protocols are available that further minimize the severity of hypercalcemia in those patients that do develop hypercalcemia.

Metabolic acidosis of varying severity often accompanies CRF. Anorexia, nausea, vomiting, and weight loss may in part be caused by this acidosis. Muscle weakness, lethargy, hypokalemia, skeletal demineralization, hyperphosphatemia, and hypercalciuria may be exacerbated by chronic metabolic acidosis. Accelerated progression of CRF attributed to increased tubular ammoniagenesis during chronic metabolic acidosis has been suggested. Diet influences the amount of acid end-products generated that must be excreted by the patient. Egg protein has traditionally been assumed to be the most biologically utilizable protein, but studies in dogs with CRF revealed that egg protein–containing diets, which are high in sulfur-containing amino acids (methionine and cysteine or cystine), may be more acidifying than vegetable protein–based diets. Lower-protein diets can result in less acid production, especially if they reduce sulfur-containing amino acid intake. Veterinary foods designed for the treatment of renal failure are usually designed to be mildly alkalinizing through the addition of salts that are metabolized to bicarbonate (potassium citrate). Because many commercial foods in the United States have been formulated to be acidifying in both dogs and cats, these diets should be discontinued in favor of veterinary foods, if possible, particularly if the alkalinizing potential of phosphate binders cannot provide adequate control of the acidosis. Acid-base balance should be reevaluated after dietary modification to determine whether supplemental alkali is needed. Sodium bicarbonate, potassium citrate, calcium carbonate, and calcium acetate are sources of alkali.

Hypokalemia occurs more commonly in cats with CRF than in dogs with CRF. Hypokalemia can result from CRF and can also create chronic renal disease or failure in some instances in cats. Correction of hypokalemia is essential in these instances. Appropriate potassium supplementation protocols for cats with CRF and normal serum potassium concentration remain controversial. A study at OSU could not find a beneficial effect of potassium gluconate supplementation over that of sodium gluconate in a population of cats with CRF and normal serum potassium. Veterinary foods designed for treatment of renal failure often contain additional potassium supplementation in the form of potassium citrate.

Systemic hypertension occurs commonly in dogs and cats with CRF when determined by methods that indirectly measure blood pressure. Unfortunately, administration of diuretics and dietary salt restriction are not effective treatment for severe hypertension. Appropriate procedures for documentation and treatment of hypertension in dogs and cats with CRF are available in the veterinary nephrologic literature.

Choice of a suitable diet is based on the patient's appetite and the composition and quality of the existing diet. Most patients with CRF are older, sedentary animals and consume fewer calories than young, healthy animals. If a patient eats only 20 to 30 kcal/kg/day, more care must be taken with the use of nutrient-restricted diets to avoid depletion of nutrients, particularly protein. Protein restriction may be instituted when the SUN exceeds 80 mg/dl. The minimum protein requirement of dogs is approximately 2 g/kg/day; cats require 3 g/kg/day. In pet foods, 2 g of protein contains approximately 7 kcal, so a dog that eats 70 kcal/kg/day needs 10% of those calories as protein (7 of 70). If the dog eats only 30 kcal/kg/day, 23% of the total calories are needed as protein if the minimum number of grams of protein per day are to be supplied. Protein restriction should not result in depletion of the patient's reserves—those bodily proteins that are required to support immune responses to infection and wound healing after trauma or surgery. In contrast to carbohydrate (glycogen) and fat reserves, protein reserves are functional rather than anatomic. The adequacy of protein reserves can be assessed during the physical examination, however. Depletion of protein reserves is suspected when the quality of skin and haircoat is poor or if muscle wasting is present based on the muscle condition scale. A sensitive indicator of reserves, particularly in cats, is the resistance encountered to insertion of a needle during blood sample collection. This resistance is provided by collagen, which is reduced in protein-depleted animals. Loss of protein reserves is one cause of decreased serum albumin concentrations.

The risks associated with protein depletion are balanced against the risks associated with the increase in SUN and the deterioration in condition of animals with CRF that consume excess amounts of dietary protein. The greater the daily energy intake, the lower the percentage of dietary protein required to maintain reserves while avoiding excessive intake.

Results of recent research are changing our recommendations for nutrient modification in dogs with early signs of CRF. Restriction of phosphorus intake to approximately 60 mg/kg/day as soon as polyuria is recognized and supplementation of potassium intake (with alkalinizing salts if acidosis is a concern) to maintain serum potassium within the normal range may suffice until patients develop severe disease. Dietary change or administration of phosphorus binders, such as aluminum hydroxide, calcium carbonate, and calcium acetate, may be used to restrict phosphorus absorption. Phosphate binders and potassium supplements can be added to the diet in small amounts initially, with the amounts increased as the patient's tolerance and condition permit.

Sodium restriction may be beneficial in animals with systemic hypertension, but should be introduced gradually. Animals with CRF have lost most of their renal reserve capacity and cannot quickly adapt to significant, abrupt changes in nutrient intake. Modification of the fatty-acid composition of diets to reduce the n-6/n-3 fatty acid ratio also may be beneficial, and studies to investigate this are currently in progress.

Recent findings in cats with induced renal insufficiency suggest that feeding diets restricted in protein may not be necessary in this species. Cats fed 9 g of protein per kilogram of body weight per day had no more severe kidney lesions or lower GFR than did cats fed 5.2 g/kg/day. Studies of dogs and cats with naturally occurring CRF, however, determined that the feeding of a veterinary food (food intake was not measured), when compared with the feeding of a commercial diet, increased the longevity of most patients.

We give clients samples of the dry and canned forms of the veterinary foods we stock for patients with CRF, to allow the pet to select one that it prefers when it feels better and has returned to a familiar environment. We have been unable to identify any consistent preference among the diets, but most patients consume adequate amounts of at least one of the choices offered. If clients cannot switch the diet of the pet with CRF to a veterinary food, it is beneficial if even part of the daily food intake is composed of the veterinary food. Moreover, permitting clients to provide some of the daily intake in the form of treats such as graham crackers or vanilla wafers may be enjoyable to the patients, and may increase their energy intake.

Clients should be trained to monitor food intake and to recognize the signs of wasting. In animals with severe CRF, maintenance of adequate food intake is difficult regardless of the food offered. Because the prognosis for these patients is poor, we usually encourage the owners of affected pets to let their animals eat whatever they choose. Eating a diet that may not seem optimal for the patient's condition is preferable to not eating a veterinary food, no matter how appropriately formulated it is, and seems to decrease the anxiety of the owner. We encourage owners to feed their pets at least twice a day and to carefully observe the food intake. A reduction in an animal's appetite should prompt the owner to return the pet for reevaluation, because this is often the first sign of deterioration in the animal's condition.

Flavorings (e.g., small amounts of bacon drippings, hamburger grease, chicken drippings, tuna juice, clam juice, baby food) may be added to protein-restricted foods to enhance their appeal and the animal's intake. Some patients increase their intake of a protein-restricted food if the food is prewarmed in a microwave oven or fried. Patients with CRF that refuse veterinary foods may consume homemade protein- and phosphorus-restricted diets or a mixture of the veterinary food and the usual food. Multiple, small-volume meals may help avoid the overdistension of the stomach, nausea, and vomiting that might be encountered in these patients.

Perspective regarding the goals for patients with CRF must be maintained. If treatment recommendations are so stringent that they threaten to disrupt the bond between the pet and its owner, careful consideration must be given to whether or not the treatment is worth the risk. Support of a client's efforts to provide the level of care with which he or she is most comfortable may be the best intervention in some cases.

General daily nutrient recommendations for patients with chronic kidney disease are presented in Table 5-20.

See Box 5-1 and Appendixes H and I for reduced-protein and reduced-phosphorous diets for dogs and cats.

See Appendix L for an exchange list of foods.

Table 5-20

General Daily Nutrient Recommendations for Patients with Chronic Kidney Disease

		Severity			
Nutrient	Normal	Mild (Polyuria, No Azotemia)	Moderate (Polyuria, Mild Azotemia)	Severe (Blood Urea Nitrogen >80 mg/dl)	Uremia (Azotemia Plus Clinical Signs)
Water		Free choice			
Energy		20-70 kcal/kg			
Protein—quantity		2 (dogs)-3 (cats) g/kg			Reduce?
Protein—quality	Average	High biologic value?			
Phosphorus	60 mg/kg	No change	Restrict toward 20 mg/kg		
Sodium	20 mg/kg	No change	Restrict if blood pressure increased		
Potassium	60 mg/kg	Supplement as necessary			

CLIENT COMMUNICATION TIPS: Kidney Disease

- Determine the total daily caloric intake and calculate protein intake to assess whether the animal is receiving the minimum requirement. This is especially important for older pets, whose daily food intake may vary.
- If a client does not know how much food the pet consumes in a given day or week, instruct the client regarding completion of a 5-day food diary. A piece of notebook paper can be used, with columns created for the date, time, type of food or treat offered, quantity or serving size, and initials of the person who offers the food. Anything consumed by the pet is recorded in the food diary. Follow up with clients after the food diary has been completed to identify factors that can potentially be modified (e.g., products, serving sizes, behaviors).
- Communicate clearly with clients about the type, dosage, and cost of any nutritional supplements that are recommended.
- Educate clients regarding the important benefits of meal-feeding older pets rather than feeding on a free-choice basis. Individual meals allow the owner to observe appetite and water consumption and identify potential problems.
- Teach clients how to monitor food intake each day and how to watch for signs of wasting.
- Give clients a "sample pack" of three or more veterinary renal products (in canned and dry form) to be offered to the animal at home.
- Recommend that any dietary change be made gradually over a period of several days or longer. If food aversions are to be avoided, dietary changes should not be made in the hospital setting, but in the home and after the pet is feeling better.
- Tell clients to call the veterinarian if they have problems or questions.
- Discuss with the staff the criteria for determining which renal diets the veterinarians in the practice recommend, as well as those they avoid recommending. Which foods are on the practice's "A list," and why. Which are on the practice's "B list," and why. Help staff identify clients who are receptive to learning more about dietary recommendations.

TECH TIPS: Kidney Disease

One of the many challenges in caring for a pet is the successful feeding of a diet that is "good" for the kidneys. Many of the waste products in uremic poisoning are related to protein. For this reason, a reduced-protein diet may be prescribed.

The following feeding tips may help to make the transition a little easier.

- Before recommending a change in diets, ensure that the pet is feeling better.
- Until the diet is changed, the pet should be fed two or three meals a day rather than on a free-choice basis. This allows the owner to monitor how much the pet is eating.
- The pet is introduced to the new diet as described in Appendix D. As the pet begins to eat the new food, the intake of the previous diet should be reduced as much as possible.
- A variety of foods are available. Owners should try a different food if the pet does not like the first choice.
- Small quantities of flavoring agents can be mixed with foods to make them more palatable; flavoring agents include low-salt meat drippings, tuna juice, clam juice, and garlic powder. If clients wish to try another flavor, they should discuss it with the clinic staff.
- Adding warm water to dry foods or warming the foods may be helpful.
- Food should be placed in a large bowl and offered in a quiet, warm environment.
- The client is given advice on the minimum amount of food the pet requires each day. It is important that clients ensure that at least this amount is eaten.
- If the pet refuses to eat for any reason, the client should call the clinic. Refusal to eat for more than 2 days may indicate that the disease is getting worse.

If clients enjoy sharing their own food with their pets or offering special treats, the owners should be reminded that too much protein can make a pet sick because of waste-product buildup (uremic poisoning). Treats should be chosen carefully.

Box 5-1

Reduced-Phosphorus, Reduced-Protein Diet for Dogs and Cats

Contents of Diet

$1^1/_2$ cups (6 servings*) cooked meat (e.g., beef, chicken, pork, eggs)
4 cups (8 servings) cooked starch (e.g., rice, pasta, potato)
1 teaspoon vegetable oil
2 500-mg Tums tablets
1 complete vitamin-mineral supplement designed for a 2- to 3-year-old child
For cats, add 1 500-mg tablet taurine

Approximate Nutritional Analysis

Calories	1200 kcal[†]
Protein	60 g
Calcium	600 mg
Phosphorus	400 mg
Sodium	140 mg
Potassium	500 mg

---

*Servings refer to items in Appendix L, from which a much greater variety of foods may be chosen. In addition, up to two servings (total) from any of the dessert, fat, fruit, vegetable, and caloric supplement lists may be provided to enhance palatability and intake of the diet.
[†]Kilocalories are distributed as 20% protein and 40% each carbohydrate and fat.

OBESITY

Obesity is the most common nutritional problem we confront in daily practice. Studies suggest that obesity may affect as many as 40% of dogs and 30% of cats. We recently published our experience with an obesity therapy program for dogs that included dietary changes, monthly weight checks, and structured maintenance portion control. Clients were able to reduce their pets' weights by an average of 15% and to decrease the BCS an average of 2/9 during 6 months of weight reduction; the reduced weight was maintained for the subsequent 18 months. To our knowledge, this method is the most successful documented approach to obesity therapy. Despite the positive overall result, individual results varied widely, and nearly 50% of clients dropped out during the course of the study.

Although understanding of the causes of obesity in companion animals remains a daunting challenge for veterinary nutritional scientists, veterinary hospitals that offer a structured obesity therapy program provide a valuable service for clients. Our program is primarily managed by technicians and is based broadly on the principles of the transtheoretic model of change described in Chapter 6 and those of the placebo response discussed in the sections on complementary and alternative medicine in Chapter 6. After the veterinarian identifies the problem and offers the solution, the client and patient are referred to the technician, who has more time to focus on the complex issues raised during obesity therapy.

For all breeds and species, obesity results when energy intake exceeds expenditure. This explanation of the problem is simple, but the problem itself is complex, because an animal's innate drives are toward food intake and away from unnecessary activity. In light of this, some factors have been identified that further increase the risk of development of obesity in pets. For example, some research has suggested that various genetic factors influence the risk of obesity, with 30% to 70% of the risk in dogs attributable to breed. Some breeds that have been found to have a higher risk of becoming obese include Labrador retrievers, cairn terriers, cocker spaniels, dachshunds, Shetland sheepdogs, basset hounds, beagles, and King Charles spaniels. Other behavioral factors that commonly increase the risk of obesity include stealing food from owners or other pets and leading a more sedentary life-style. Owner habits to be considered include supplying a high caloric intake after the animal has been neutered, overfeeding pet food, providing too many treats, and promoting a sedentary life-style.

Many misconceptions exist regarding obesity and disease. Although the problem of obesity is common in both veterinary and human medicine, obese animals are not at risk for developing the same range of health problems that threaten obese human beings. Some disease processes that are common to both humans and animals, and some of the health risks involved, are discussed in the sections that follow.

Obesity and Disease

Diabetes

Two types of diabetes mellitus occur. Type 1 diabetes (IDDM) has common features in both humans and animals, with the exception of the age of onset. In veterinary medicine the disease is usually diagnosed in middle-aged animals (>6 years of age), whereas in humans the age of onset is much younger. Type 1 diabetes in humans results from inadequate insulin production by the pancreas; autoimmune, viral, and genetic factors may play a role in this process. The onset of symptoms is abrupt, and they can be life threatening.

Type 2 diabetes (NIDDM) is characterized by resistance to the action of insulin. As with Type 1, differences in Type 2 diabetes exist between animals and humans. For example, 60% to 90% of human patients with NIDDM are obese, and in these patients the glucose intolerance improves with weight loss. In animals, NIDDM occurs much more frequently in obese cats than in dogs, and categorization is not straightforward because most animals with Type 2 diabetes retain some need for insulin therapy. In addition, only 40% of the animals diagnosed with NIDDM are obese.

Animals with NIDDM have glucose intolerance along with the usual signs of diabetes mellitus, which can include polyuria, polydipsia, and polyphagia. Although these are the most commonly reported mild signs of diabetes, they can also result from other conditions.

Osteoarthritis

Extra weight increases pressure on the joints, which can worsen an already existing arthritic condition in animals, just as it does in humans. Although obesity and osteoarthritis often are associated, no cause-effect relationship between the two has been proved. In some cases excess weight may damage joints, whereas in others obesity may result from the decreased activity that occurs in patients with joint disease. Regardless of the relationship, both problems can become worse unless some type of intervention occurs. Loss of weight can relieve pressure on the joints, especially knee and hip joints, and possibly help prevent cruciate muscle tears.

Cardiovascular Problems

In humans, an association exists between high blood pressure and obesity. High blood pressure can lead to elevated risk of heart disease and stroke. Increased hypertension and elevated blood lipids can lead to blocked arteries. In animals, to date no clinical evidence has suggested that obesity results in hypertension. One study showed an increased risk of undefined "circulatory problems," but only in grossly obese dogs. Also, animals rarely develop atherosclerosis, so blocked arteries resulting from high blood lipid levels are not a concern.

Cancer

Several types of cancer have been associated with obesity in humans. Obese women are at higher risk for developing uterine, cervical, and breast cancers, and obesity in men increases their risk of colon, rectal, and prostate cancers. Many of these cancers are not common in animals, with the exception of mammary cancer. The relationship between obesity and cancer is discussed further in the section on Cancer earlier in the chapter.

Skin Problems

One study showed that obese cats had more than two times the risk of developing nonallergic skin conditions, compared with cats of optimal body condition. Dry, flaky skin and feline acne accounted for more than 50% of the skin problems; the rest included skin alopecia of unknown origin, seborrhea, eosinophilic ulcers, and cysts. These conditions in obese cats may reflect difficulties with grooming.

Surgical Risk
Obesity has been associated with increased surgical risk because of the larger mass or depth of mass to be penetrated before access to the abdominal cavity is gained, increased risk of fat necrosis after surgery, and delayed wound healing.

Prevention

Because of the common occurrence of and many risks associated with obesity in animals, an obesity therapy program can be an important addition to the services included in the weight-management program of a veterinary clinic. This section describes the program we have used at OSU with some success.

We believe that the best way to prevent pets from developing a weight problem is to educate clients about proper feeding techniques and to teach them how to evaluate a pet's body condition before its weight becomes a problem. This education should occur during the first visit to the clinic, regardless of the life stage of the animal. The best time to provide this information, however, is when the pet is still a puppy or kitten; proper intervention at the start of life can ensure a lifetime of moderate body condition. We provide "go-home kits" that contain food samples, literature on proper feeding practices, a pet food measuring cup, and a body condition scoring sheet, so that the owner can monitor the pet's condition and adjust the amount of food offered as necessary. We show clients how to assess body condition according to the rib cage, abdominal tuck, and waist parameters, and have them practice in our presence to ensure that they understand the procedure.

When an animal is spayed or neutered, its energy needs decrease by approximately 25%. Clients are advised at the time of neutering or spaying to decrease the amount of food offered or to change the diet to one of lower caloric density. In dogs, it may be appropriate at this time to change the diet from a growth food to one designed for adults, particularly if the dog has completed the majority of its growth. For cats, we recommend continuing growth foods for 12 to 18 months, until skeletal development is finished, to avoid problems associated with the increased acidifying potential of diets designed for adult cats. Many people believe that neutered pets automatically become overweight; if the guidelines are followed, the pet's body condition is assessed, and food intake is adjusted as necessary, weight gain should not be a problem. See Appendixes A and B regarding recommendations for feeding puppies and kittens.

Obesity Therapy Program

The goal of obesity therapy is not weight loss, but rather maintenance of the lost weight. We have found that a structured approach to obesity therapy is the best way to ensure success. As mentioned, our program builds on collaboration between the veterinarian and technician to assure the most efficient use of time for both. The veterinary technician leads and maintains the program after referral from the veterinarian, with each consulting with the other as appropriate for client management and patient care. The features of the program are as follows.

Veterinarian's Tasks

Physical examination. Before the obesity therapy program is begun, the veterinarian performs a thorough physical examination. This examination includes evaluation of fecal samples for parasites and evaluation of blood and urine samples to rule out metabolic diseases that could affect the animal's weight, such as diabetes or hypothyroidism. The process of identification and treatment of these problems builds client trust and prepares the client for the cooperation necessary for obesity therapy, if obesity remains a problem after the metabolic disorder has been addressed.

Screening. Once the veterinarian has established that the animal is overweight and has ruled out or treated comorbid conditions, he or she conducts a screening conversation with the client. The goal of this conversation is to determine whether the client realizes the pet is overweight and whether the client is willing to make the changes necessary to reduce the animal's weight. Suggestions for conducting this conversation are provided in the Transtheoretic Model section of Chapter 6. Willing clients are then referred to the technician for an additional obesity workup.

Technician Tasks

Obtaining the dietary history. A thorough and accurate dietary history should be taken (see Appendix C). The history is very important, because it provides essential information about the food intake of the pet, as well as the food-related bond between the pet and the owner. For example, the food-related relationship between a pet and an owner who pours a cup of food into a bowl once a day is quite different from that between an owner and a pet that eats the owner's food with him or her. An accurate dietary history can take 30 to 60 minutes to collect and is most successful when the owner makes sudden discovery of a factor that contributes to the problem and can be changed. Following are some suggestions that help elicit all the information needed to accurately determine an animal's caloric intake.

1. When discussing the animal's current pet food, be sure to request the exact name of the product and its form (i.e., canned or dry). If the animal is fed canned products, ask what size can the owner typically purchases. Canned cat food products, for example, vary in size from 3 ounces to 14 ounces. If the animal is fed dry food, ask how many 8-ounce dry measuring cups of food it receives. Show the client a sample measuring cup. If the client does not have this information (and they likely will not), ask them to measure the amount fed each day, even if it requires waiting an extra day or so until the information is available. It is important to specify that amounts of food be measured in 8-ounce cups, because cups of many different sizes exist. A client who says the pet receives two cups of food may mean two 4-ounce teacups or two 16-ounce stadium cups; the pet may be receiving half or twice as much food as might be assumed if the size of the cup were not identified.

2. When asking about the brand and number of treats fed, we ask, "What treats do you feed?" rather than, "Do you feed treats?" Although the question is leading, it is also open ended. Clients often offer more information if they conclude that we already know what they are doing and are not judgmental. As with pet foods, the exact name and size of the treat must be determined.

3. If a significant (>35%) amount of the pet's food intake consists of table food, try to obtain a list of the amounts and types of food offered. Often this is not easy. This

situation suggests a strong food-related bond between the owner and pet, which can complicate therapy. Unfortunately, most clients supplement their pets' usual diet with treats and table foods, rather than reducing the amount of regular diet provided and replacing the eliminated calories with other foodstuffs. Occasionally, pointing out this habit is sufficient for a client to begin an obesity therapy program.

4. Identify all the different people who may be feeding the animal (children, spouse, neighbors, other visitors to the home), and determine whether the patient may have access to the food of any other animal in the home. In addition, it is important to determine whether the animal has a tendency to try to steal food or to get into the garbage.

5. Ask the client to list all medications, nutritional supplements, vitamins, or complementary and alternative treatments the pet receives. Be sure to also ask about the type and amount of food (e.g., meat, cheese) the owner uses to disguise any medicines before giving them (another leading question). Some people use a whole slice of bologna to cover a pill; others use ice cream or peanut butter. These are potential sources of excess calories that should be discussed.

6. It is essential that the technician remain nonjudgmental throughout the entire dietary history interview. If owners sense disapproval of any kind, they may refrain from revealing all the food they actually offer.

7. On rare occasions a client may be encountered who feeds the pet only human foods, directly from the table, and who does not measure the food given. In this situation the owner must complete a food diary for 5 to 7 days, so that an attempt can be made to quantify the types and volumes of foods being consumed. A sheet of notebook paper can be used, with columns created for the date and time of feeding, the initials of the person offering the food, the food item fed, and the approximate size of the food item. Give the client examples to use as references when discussing portion size, such as a level tablespoon of peanut butter, a piece of meat the size of the owner's palm, or a dab of salad dressing the size of a thumbnail.

Calculation of caloric intake. Once all the necessary information has been collected, the number of calories the animal is currently taking in can be estimated. It may be necessary to contact one or more pet food manufacturers by phone or e-mail to obtain the caloric content of foods. Ask the manufacturers to send current nutritional information on all their foods so a file can be started. Such files save time and provide a wealth of information on the pet foods encountered locally. For determination of the caloric content of human foods, we use *Bowes and Church's Food Values of Portions Commonly Used* and the "USDA National Nutrient Database for Standard Reference," available on the World Wide Web site of the United States Department of Agriculture (http://www.nal.usda.gov/fnic/foodcomp/Data/SR15/sr15.html). Many comparable resources exist.

Determination of weight goal and calories required. The objectives of obesity therapy are improved health and reduction of disease risk—factors related to quality of life rather than to aesthetics. In most cases a 20% weight loss will remove even grossly obese animals from the high-risk category for obesity-related diseases. In cases in which a large loss of weight is required, it is best to start slowly; we set an initial goal of 10%. This approach is intended to avoid overwhelming the client with the amount of weight the animal needs to lose and to prevent discouragement when initial losses total only 1% to 2%. A body condition chart or poster can be used to show the owner where the pet is starting and what its body condition will be if the recommended amount of weight is lost. Once the initial goal is met, the pet's improved appearance and health often motivate the owner to continue until the desired body condition is attained.

Several formulas are used to determine caloric needs of animals, which can be graphed to produce a chart similar to the one shown in Figures 5-1 and 5-2 and used to determine an initial estimate of the desired intake. The two formulas that we typically use include the following linear equation for patients between 2 kg and 50 kg.

$$\text{Energy needs in kcals/day} = 30 \times \text{Kilograms of body weight} + 70$$

We also use the following exponential equation for all patients.

$$\text{Energy needs in kcals/day} = 97(\text{Kilograms of body weight})^{0.665}$$

Alternatively, a "rule of thumb" is that 45 kcal per kilogram of body weight per day are required; following this guideline produces a weight loss of approximately 1% per week. Because of the many variables associated with food intake, metabolic rate, and activity level, we make clear to owners that we expect to adjust the initial estimate as needed to achieve the desired rate of weight loss of approximately 1% per week.

Completion of the dietary plan. The details of any dietary plan for obesity therapy vary widely and are the result of experience, which dictates realistic goals, and negotiation with the client. Once the calories actually given and those required for weight loss have been estimated, they can be compared to see if any adjustments are necessary. Three scenarios commonly arise: the caloric intake exceeds the calories needed; the caloric intake is adequate, but the physical activity needs to be increased; or the caloric intake is below the minimum caloric requirement. All three cases can result from varying combinations of errors in intake estimation, low metabolism, and inactivity. If the caloric intake exceeds the calories needed and a large volume of food is offered in addition to the pet food, the difference between "replacement" and "supplementation" is explained to the client. Sometimes all that is necessary is a reduction in treats, pet food, or table food. If the caloric intake is adequate but the physical activity needs to be increased, the activity guidelines in this section help in provision of recommendations. If the caloric intake is below the minimum required, it may be necessary to change the food to one that is lower in calories or higher in "filler"—fiber, water, or air. It also may be suggested that the dietary intake be decreased by 10 kcal per kilogram of body weight per day. In all cases it is crucial to determine the nutrient intake of the diet to ensure that changes will not result in malnutrition. When any recommendations regarding energy restrictions are made, the other nutrient needs of the animal must be kept in mind to ensure that they continue to be met. A check of the overall adequacy of the diet is to estimate the protein intake as described in the section on kidney disease; dogs should consume a minimum of 2 g of protein per kilogram of body weight per day, and cats should consume 3 g of protein per kilogram of body weight per day to avoid the risk of protein depletion. Patients whose intake is close to this level are observed closely for muscle wasting and other signs of protein depletion.

Follow-up. One of the critical keys to a successful obesity therapy program is to follow the progress of the patient. We tell clients what the follow-up schedule is and ask them to agree to a preferred method and time of contact. Our first contact with the client occurs

1 week after initial recommendations are made, followed by repeat "check-ins" at 6 weeks, 3 months, 6 months, and 1 year. This allows us to monitor the patient's BCS and weight progress, to make adjustments as needed, and to continue to support and motivate the client. Such follow-up also helps to determine when the owner is becoming frustrated or is having problems with the plan, so that encouragement or suggestions can be offered to help keep them on the plan.

Database maintenance. We maintain a separate filing system for our obesity program patients. Each file contains a copy of the therapeutic plan, copies of the laboratory evaluations, a progress sheet to keep track of the patient's weight, and a communication sheet to keep track of problems the animal may be having and of the owner's reported successes.

Photographs. We photograph each patient at the start of therapy and again after the animal has achieved its weight goal. A photograph of the client and the patient can be given as a gift at the end of the year. Electronic photos can be kept in the database, and paper prints of the pictures can be taped to the inside of the patient's file for easy access.

Activity

Before recommendations are made that a patient's activity be increased, the practitioner should ensure that both client and patient are physically capable of accomplishing this. Activity recommendations must also take into account the client's schedule to avoid setting unrealistic and unattainable goals.

Many pets lead sedentary lives because of their owners' work schedules. We sometimes suggest that owners adjust the animal's environment to increase its activity. These adjustments can include placement of bowls such that the animal has to climb or jump to obtain food and water. Baby gates or similar barriers can be placed in doorways so that the animal has to work to get into and out of various rooms throughout the house. Toys are available that dispense pieces of dry dog or cat food when the animal moves the toy; these toys can simulate (or stimulate) hunting as well as slow down food intake.

If a client is too busy or is physically unable to exercise a pet regularly, the animal's activity can be increased by means of playful interactions within the home. Playing fetch by throwing a toy up (or down) the staircase is a good means of exercise and a better way to offer a treat than simply handing it to the pet. A favorite suggestion is to have the dog do "doggie push-ups"—command the pet to "sit" and "lie down" four or five times in a row before a treat is given. A large variety of interactive toys for dogs and cats (e.g., laser lights, fishing poles with feathers) promote increased activity. A good way to begin a new exercise program is to set a goal to increase the pet's activity by 1 minute per day until a goal of 10 minutes per day is reached. Once this goal is achieved, the duration can be slowly increased until the pet's activity is at the desired level.

Cats also can be trained, especially with food rewards (the rule is replacement of calories, rather than supplementation). In fact, some cats exercise very effectively by chasing pieces of their daily dry ration that are thrown by the owner. In addition, unlikely as it may sound, some cats can be trained to walk with a harness and leash. Many excellent books on the subject of cats and exercise are available; one with a chapter specifically on overweight indoor cats is *Felinestein*, by Suzanne Delzio and Dr. Cindy Ribarich. A link to this book is available online at www.nssvet.org/ici.

Reduced-Energy Diets

One aspect of obesity therapy, along with portion control and psychologic support of the client, is provision of a diet with fewer calories than the one currently consumed or one with added fiber or water to "dilute" the calories contained in the food. Unfortunately, no studies describing successful obesity therapy, defined as maintenance of the weight loss for the life of the patient, are available. For a selection of reduced-energy diets for dogs and cats, refer to Appendixes H and I. These diets may be used to maintain moderate body condition in patients with low energy needs (less than approximately 30 kcal/kg/day).

Summary

Obesity is a major nutritional problem affecting pets. The risks associated with obesity warrant an offer of intervention, which can be achieved at veterinary clinics by instituting

CLIENT COMMUNICATION TIPS: Obesity

- For obesity prevention, review the importance of body condition scoring and regular exercise with each client at every healthy-pet visit.
- Review the dietary history of overweight pets carefully. If a client does not know how much food the pet consumes in a given day or week, instruct the client regarding completion of a 5-day food diary. A piece of notebook paper can be used, with columns created for the date, time, type of food or treat offered, quantity or serving size, and initials of the person who offers the food. Anything consumed by the pet is recorded in the food diary. Follow up with clients after the food diary has been completed to identify factors that can potentially be modified (e.g., products, serving sizes, behaviors).
- Determine the total daily caloric intake and calculate protein intake to assess whether the animal is receiving the minimum or maximum requirement. This is especially important for sick or older pets, whose daily food intake may vary.
- Educate clients regarding the important benefits of feeding multiple small meals to overweight pets. Small meals improve metabolism and allow the owner to observe appetite and water consumption and identify potential problems.
- If the client elects to offer commercial treats, provide a list of low-calorie products and discuss "replacing" calories from the food bowl, rather than "supplementing" them.
- Teach clients how to assign a BCS to the pet, how to monitor food intake each day, and how to watch for signs of protein depletion (wasting).
- Recommend that any dietary change be made gradually over a period of several days or longer.
- Plan to have a member of the health-care team follow up with the client. Tell clients to call the veterinarian if they have problems or questions.
- For veterinarians and clients interested in homemade diet evaluation, the MSU Diagnostic Center for Population and Animal Health (DCPAH) provides diagnostic feed testing. Proximate analysis, mineral analysis, fatty acid profiles, and some vitamin analysis are available. The Nutrition Section of the DCPAH can be contacted at (517) 353-9312 for sample submission guidelines and fee schedules.
- Discuss with the staff the criteria for determining which "reduced-calorie" diets the veterinarians in the practice recommend, as well as those they avoid recommending. Which foods are on the practice's "A list," and why. Which are on the practice's "B list," and why. Help the staff identify clients who are receptive to learning more about dietary recommendations.

both an effective client education program for prevention and a structured program that includes long-term follow-up and support for obesity therapy. Veterinary technicians are a valuable resource for institution and management of these programs, which serve to benefit the patients, the clients, and the veterinary clinic.

SKIN DISEASE

Diagnosis

Many nutrients are required to maintain normal structure and function of the skin and haircoat of dogs and cats. For example, energy is required to replace that lost as heat, and as much as 30% of the daily protein requirement provides amino acids for resynthesis of skin and hair that is shed. Maintenance of the normal structure and appearance of hair additionally requires significant amounts of the sulfur-containing amino acids methionine and cysteine. Dietary fat provides the EFAs (linoleic acid for dogs and linoleic and arachidonic acids for cats) that are required for maintenance of normal membrane function of epithelial tissues. Minerals and vitamins are also required for normal skin and haircoat; clinical problems related to zinc and vitamins A and E have been reported.

The goals in taking the nutritional history are to determine whether the skin problem is nutrition related and, if so, to localize the problem to the animal or the diet. Nutrient-sensitive skin problems include adverse reactions to foods, food intolerance or allergy, protein-energy malnutrition (PEM), and mineral or vitamin responsive disorders. Diet-induced skin problems include food intolerance, primary and secondary nutrient deficiencies, and nutrient toxicities.

Diagnosis and classification of nutrition-related skin problems are based on dietary history and food evaluation. Questions regarding food intake are asked to determine whether the animal eats enough to meet its physiologic needs and whether the owner feeds an unconventional or homemade diet. For example, biotin deficiency (which can result in skin lesions), although rare, has been reported to occur in dogs fed large amounts of raw egg white. Specific questions should be asked regarding the type, amount, and frequency of prescribed medications or nutritional supplements being fed, because these substances can affect nutritional status.

Nutrient-Sensitive Skin Problems

A history that reveals adequate intake of an acceptable diet suggests the presence of a nutrient-sensitive problem, such as occurs with GI, hepatic, or renal disease. Genetic disorders resulting in supernormal nutrient needs, such as "Syndrome I" zinc deficiency, should be considered only after all other abnormalities have been ruled out and the feeding of a well-formulated diet has failed to improve the animal's condition.

Adverse reactions to foods. Adverse reactions to foods are not common, but they may be difficult to diagnose and frustrating to treat. Two major types of adverse reactions to foods occur: food intolerance, an adverse reaction to some constituent of the diet, and food allergy.

Food intolerance. Food intolerance, or a non–immune-mediated reaction to a food, seems to result most commonly from idiosyncratic sensitivities to compounds that most animals tolerate. Contaminants in the diet, such as toxins, bacteria, food additives, vasoactive amines, and other dietary constituents, also occasionally cause idiosyncratic reactions. Nutrient-sensitive food intolerance affects the GI tract more commonly than the skin. In contrast, diet-induced food intolerance may affect any system, depending on the offending agent. In both cases the treatment is the same: switch the patient to a different diet that is known to be satisfactory based on clinical experience.

Food allergies. Food allergies are immune-mediated reactions to normal constituents of food. Both immediate (type 1) and delayed (type 4) food allergies have been reported in dogs and cats.

Food allergies occur because of a defect in an animal's immune system; they are not caused by a particular problem with the diet. Animals may become allergic to any protein (as well as some other constituents of the diet) that is part of the regular diet or intermittently consumed (e.g., in snacks or treats). Some factors that influence the likelihood of an allergic reaction to a food include the sensitivity of the animal's immune system, the number of proteins in the diet, the amount of protein, the availability of the protein in the intestinal tract to the immune system, and the immunogenicity of the protein.

Food allergy is one of three major causes of pruritus in animals; the other two are flea allergy dermatitis and atopic dermatitis. Fleas are a common cause of pruritus in animals. Atopic dermatitis occurs in approximately 10% to 15% of dogs, and food allergy seems to be somewhat less common than this. Recognition of these three causes of pruritus is a key to effective therapy, because treatment directed at any of the causes may reduce the animal's pruritus to below the clinical threshold, at least initially. For example, if fleas are eliminated and the pruritus subsides, flea allergy dermatitis might be assumed to have been the sole cause of signs, whereas if atopic dermatitis is treated with hyposensitization, or food allergy is treated with food elimination, these conditions can easily be assumed to have been the entire cause of the problem. It may be more useful to consider the relative role of each of these conditions and plan treatment accordingly, because signs may return if treatment of only one of the conditions fails or if one of the other causes of pruritus becomes more important.

Food allergy most commonly occurs in dogs between 1 and 3 years of age; nearly 50% of dogs with the disease develop signs during this time. Approximately one third of dogs develop signs at less than 1 year of age, and approximately 15% develop signs at 4 to 11 years of age. No sex or breed predilection has been reported for food allergy, and most patients (approximately two thirds) have been fed the same diet for at least 2 years before the onset of clinical signs. Because food allergy is not usually associated with a sudden change in diet, either food intolerance or a non–diet-related problem should be considered more likely than an allergy if an adverse reaction to a food occurs after a recent change in food.

Animals with food allergy most commonly have a nonseasonal pruritus, in contrast to the more seasonal pattern associated with flea allergy. The anatomic distribution may be similar to that seen in dogs with atopic dermatitis. The majority of animals with food allergy also have otitis externa. Patients with food allergy generally respond less favorably to glucocorticoid therapy than do dogs with flea allergy or atopic dermatitis.

If food allergy is suspected based on the history and physical examination, the diagnosis can be confirmed through a positive response to an elimination diet. Other diagnostic methods, such as intradermal or serologic tests, have not been found to correlate well with subsequent provocative food challenge and are not recommended for the diagnosis of food allergy. The diet during the period of an elimination trial should consist of *only* one novel protein source and, if necessary, a carbohydrate source. The diet should be made by the owner rather than purchased, to ensure that a minimum number of antigens are fed to the affected animal. No nutrient supplements are necessary for the short duration of the trial. If meat is used for the protein source, it must be ground in machinery that has been thoroughly cleaned to avoid contamination with an allergenic protein. Although maximum improvement in signs may require as long as 10 to 12 weeks of feeding the elimination diet, some improvement should occur within 6 weeks if the animal has a food allergy *and* if the owners have fed only the prescribed diet, avoiding treats, supplements, chewable vitamins and minerals, heartworm preventatives, rawhide chew treats, and any other potential source of allergens. If the pet is intensely pruritic when the elimination diet is initiated, short (3-day) courses of oral corticosteroids may be administered. Antibiotics must be administered for treatment of pyoderma, and specific antifungal agents for treatment of yeast *(Malassezia* sp.) infections, when these conditions are present.

Commercial novel protein diets also may be used for elimination trials, but lack of improvement of signs in patients fed these diets does not absolutely rule out (or rule in, for that matter) the presence of food allergy, which can be accomplished only through complete adherence to a single-source home-cooked diet. In addition to novel protein diets, hydrolyzed protein diets recently have become available based on the premise that the smaller resulting proteins are less allergenic. The use of hydrolyzed proteins for nutritional management of food allergy appears to have come from the practice of feeding hydrolyzed milk protein formulas to infants with bovine protein allergy. Although a considerable percentage of infants with allergy to bovine milk protein appear to tolerate hydrolyzed milk proteins, the response appears to range from 55% to 100%, depending on the product tested. Until the effectiveness of veterinary hydrolyzed protein diets has been demonstrated in controlled trials in patients with food allergies, their role in therapy remains uncertain.

Although confirmation of the diagnosis of food allergy requires challenge with the original protein to confirm the return of clinical signs, most clients decline this procedure. Once the diagnosis has been made, animals often can be gradually weaned onto a commercial hypoallergenic diet for long-term treatment. If the chosen commercial diet is not tolerated, the animal usually relapses within 14 days. In this case the homemade diet is again fed until clinical signs are under control, after which a different therapeutic diet may be tried. If the patient cannot tolerate any commercial diet, the homemade diet can be formulated for long-term use in both dogs and cats with minimal supplementation.

One of the more popular recently recommended treatments for atopic dermatitis is supplementation with omega (n)-6 and omega (n)-3 EFAs. Both dogs and cats require the omega (n)-6 EFA linoleic acid, abbreviated C18:2(n-6). Cats also require arachidonic acid, abbreviated C20:4(n-6). The abbreviations indicate the number of carbons (C; 18 or 20) and the number of double bonds (two or four). The n-6 designation indicates that the first double bond is six carbon atoms beyond the methyl, or n-6, end of the fatty acid (Figure 5-10). In dogs, arachidonic acid (Figure 5-11) is formed by desaturation of linoleic acid (addition of another double bond) to form gamma-linolenic acid, elongation of C18:3(n-6) to C20, and desaturation again to form the next double bond, which results in the C20:4 designation. Cats lack the desaturase enzyme necessary to form gamma-linolenic acid and

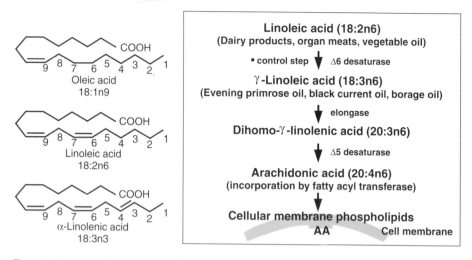

Figure 5-10 Family of polyunsaturated fatty acids.

Figure 5-11 Biosynthesis of arachidonic acid.

therefore require a dietary source of both arachidonic and linoleic acids. The minimum requirement for linoleic acid for dogs is somewhat greater than 2% of dietary energy. Cats require 2% of energy as linoleic acid and 0.04% as arachidonic acid.

In addition to the n-6 series of fatty acids, both n-3 and n-9 series fatty acids exist. The C18:3(n-3) fatty acid is called alpha-linolenic acid and can also be desaturated and elongated to form fatty acids with higher molecular weights. Although no requirement for n-3 fatty acids has been demonstrated in dogs or cats, these fatty acids may eventually be found useful as therapeutic agents. By competing with the n-6 series of fatty acids for the elongase and desaturase enzymes, these fatty acids may be used to block conversions of linoleic to arachidonic acid, the precursor of the prostaglandins. The n-9 series of fatty acids are not essential, because they can be made by the enzymes both dogs and cats have. There is also evidence that these types of dietary fats may increase the EFA requirement. Oleic acid, C18:1(n-9), a monounsaturated fatty acid found in many fats and oils, also competes for the desaturase and elongase enzymes, forming the triene (i.e., having three double bonds) 5,8,11-eicosapentaenoic acid. The ratio of this triene to the tetraene arachidonic acid in the plasma is used to diagnose EFA deficiency in humans; a ratio of greater than 0.2 indicates a deficiency. That the n-9 fatty acids can compete with the n-3 and n-6 fatty acids for elongation and desaturation enzymes may influence the response to treatment with supplemental fatty acids.

A variety of fatty-acid supplements, including plant-based and marine fish oils for oral administration, are available, and recently diets with altered fatty-acid compositions have been introduced. Studies of the response of the skin to modification of the amount and pattern of fatty-acid intake of patients with atopic dermatitis have yielded inconsistent results. Studies have not controlled the amount and type of fatty acid consumed, and the doses of fatty acids in veterinary supplements is less than 10% of those used in studies of human beings with skin disease. The content of veterinary diets marketed for skin disorders reportedly is higher. Additionally, nonspecific effects can affect the condition of patients with chronic inflammatory diseases, irrespective of diet.

The American College of Veterinary Dermatology recently concluded, based on review of more than 20 trials, that "[t]here is presently insufficient evidence to recommend for or against the use of EFA[s] to control clinical signs of atopic dermatitis."

Diet-induced EFA deficiency also can occur in dogs and cats. Diet-related causes of EFA deficiency are treated by changing the diet. Other causes of EFA deficiency may be treated by supplementation of the diet with a source of linoleic acid for dogs and with sources of both linoleic and arachidonic acid for cats.

The recommendation has been made that both animal and vegetable oils be provided to obviate the necessity for endogenous arachidonic acid synthesis. As shown in Table 5-22, marine (rather than terrestrial) animal fats are a more appropriate choice. Supplementation should not exceed 20% of total kilocalories as energy to avoid reducing intake of other essential nutrients in the diet (Table 5-23). Uncomplicated fatty-acid deficiency should respond to treatment in 3 weeks to 3 months.

Protein-energy malnutrition. Hair and skin abnormalities in veterinary patients commonly result from disease-induced decreases in food intake. Morphologic changes in the hair bulb and hair diameter are sensitive indicators of overall protein status, with hair-bulb atrophy and constriction and depigmentation of the hair shaft seen in humans after as little as 2 weeks of protein deprivation. The ratio of telogen to anagen hair increases with prolonged deficiency. Animals with PEM from any cause have dry, rough, thin haircoats. The hair is brittle and easily broken. The skin appears dry and thin and may appear to have increased or decreased pigmentation. PEM also may result in decubitus ulcers and impaired wound healing. A nutritional history helps determine whether the cause of the deficiency is decreased food intake or an inadequate diet. The minimum protein requirement of adult dogs at maintenance is quite low and should be adequately met by diets that contain more than 16% of energy as high-quality protein (~2 gm/kg body weight/day). Requirements for late gestation, lactation, and early growth are higher (approximately 25% to 30% of total calories). Adult cats should receive at least 20% of daily energy as protein (~3 gm/kg body weight/day), and 30% to 35% during late gestation, lactation, and early growth. In the absence of a dietary protein deficiency, other causes of protein loss should be investigated. These include malabsorption syndromes, nephropathies, pancreatic disease, and any chronic disease that inhibits normal food intake.

Mineral and vitamin deficiencies. Mineral and vitamin deficiencies in dogs and cats fed commercial diets are rare, so issues related to nutrient sensitive and diet-induced disorders are described together here.

Mineral deficiencies. Skin manifestations of mineral deficiency are seen most commonly with diet-induced primary (inadequate intake) or secondary (inadequate availability due to nutrient interaction) deficiencies of copper and zinc. Copper is required for melanin production and keratin synthesis. Copper deficiency has been reported to cause hypopigmentation and a dry, rough coat resulting from faulty keratinization of the hair and skin. An anemia similar to iron-deficiency anemia is expected because copper is required for iron transport to sites of heme synthesis. Because copper uptake is antagonized by excess dietary zinc, secondary deficiencies are also possible.

Table 5-22
Fatty Acid Content of Selected Lipid Sources

Oil	Fatty Acid (%)*					
	Linoleic Acid (C18:2[n-6])	Arachidonic Acid (C20:4[n-6])	Gamma-Linolenic Acid (C18:3[n-6])	Eicosapentaenoic Acid (C20:5[n-3])	Docosahexaenoic Acid (C22:6[n-3])	Alpha-Linolenic Acid (C18:3[n-3])
Safflower	70-80					0.5
Corn	50-55					1
Soybean	52-56	0.05				7.3
Tallow (beef)	2-4	0.0-0.2				0.5
Lard (pork)	10-20	0.3-1	0.1			0.5
Cod liver		25.4	0.4	6.9	0.9	1.2
Herring	13	20	0.4	6.3	0.6	1.2
Salmon	11.5	23.5	0.4	13	3	1.2

*Average values obtained from various sources.
Empty cells indicate the presence of <0.1% of fatty acid.

Table 5-23

Approximate Amount of Lipid to Add to Pet Foods to Increase Food Energy by 20%

Diet	Amount of Lipid (tsp)	Amount of Diet as Fed
Dry	1.5	1 cup
Soft or moist	1.5	1 cup
Canned, regular	2	13.2-oz can
Canned, gourmet	1	5.5-oz can

Two clinical syndromes of zinc deficiency have been described. Syndrome I occurs in Siberian huskies and occasionally in Alaskan malamutes. The lesions frequently occur with the onset of adulthood and during periods of stress. Both genders are affected, and appetite may or may not be depressed. Skin lesions include crusting and scaling with underlying suppuration around the mouth, chin, eyes, and ears. Thick crusts may also form on the skin overlying the points of the limb and on the vulva, scrotum, or prepuce. Hyperpigmentation of lesions occurs in some dogs. Affected animals are not usually pruritic unless lesions are excessively crusted. Parakeratosis and hyperkeratosis are usually evident in biopsy specimens. Treatment with 100 mg $ZnSO_4$ twice daily (10 mg/kg body weight/day) has been reported to be effective, as have low doses of oral glucocorticoids. Zinc therapy usually provides rapid resolution of the problem, but therapy may need to be continued indefinitely to prevent recurrence of signs.

Syndrome II is seen in rapidly growing pups of all breeds and is probably the result of a secondary zinc deficiency. Dietary zinc availability is reduced in high-calcium, high-phytate containing diets as a result of intestinal binding. When these diets (generally low-quality dry foods) are fed to animals with relatively high zinc needs, a deficiency may result. Skin lesions associated with this syndrome include extensive thickening and fissuring of the foot pads and nasal planum. Pups may be small for their ages, depressed, anorectic, and may have moderate lymphadenopathy, although lesions and clinical signs are quite variable. Response to zinc therapy is reported to be dramatic, with marked improvement occurring within 2 weeks. Syndrome II appears to result from ingestion of a nutritionally inadequate diet, which should be abandoned in favor of an excellent-quality diet designed for growing animals.

The National Research Council's recommendation for zinc intake is 1.94 mg per kilogram of body weight per day for growing puppies and 0.72 mg per kilogram per day for adults. Although supplementation may overcome the adverse effects of some diets, oversupplementation should be avoided. Adult men whose diet was supplemented with 300 mg of zinc sulfate per day (20 times the recommended daily intake) for 6 weeks demonstrated depressed lymphocyte and neutrophil function, and serum lipoprotein abnormalities. Excessive levels of dietary zinc also can inhibit absorption of copper and iron.

Vitamin deficiencies.

Fat-soluble vitamins. Vitamin A is required for maintenance of skin and epithelial tissue, but both excesses and deficiencies may result in cutaneous lesions. Dietary carotene is oxidatively cleaved to retinal and reduced to retinol in the intestinal mucosa of the dog. This cleavage does not occur in cats, which results in a dietary requirement for preformed vitamin A. Once formed, retinol is incorporated into chylomicrons and transported to the liver via the lymphatic systems. Retinol can serve all vitamin A–related functions, although it is often further metabolized in tissues to physiologically active forms. In the eye, retinol is oxidized to retinaldehyde, which participates in the visual cycle. Oxidation of retinol to retinoic acid results in the form of vitamin A that is active in epithelial differentiation. Vitamin A deficiency and toxicity result in hyperkeratinization and scaling of the skin, alopecia, poor haircoat, and increased susceptibility to microbial infection. Deficiency may result from dietary inadequacy and from diseases that decrease fat digestion, absorption, and transport. Kidney disease may result in increased vitamin A storage (because of reduced excretion), but the most common cause of vitamin A intoxication is oversupplementation with vitamin A, liver, or cod liver oil. In addition to cutaneous lesions, exostoses of both the axial and the appendicular skeleton may occur with vitamin A toxicity.

In addition to diseases related to dietary deficiency, vitamin A–responsive dermatoses have been reported in dogs fed an apparently adequate diet. Three cocker spaniels with idiopathic seborrhea characterized by generalized scaling, thick, focal, inflamed, crusty lesions of the thorax and ventral abdomen, and lack of response to a variety of antiseborrheic treatments were reported to respond to 10,000 IU of vitamin A per day in 5 to 8 weeks. The dogs were still normal after 1 to 4 years of therapy. Other practitioners have reported similar results. Because of the nonspecific nature of seborrhea and the real potential for vitamin A toxicity, allergic, endocrine, parasitic, and other causes of seborrhea should be ruled out before therapy is instituted. Biopsy evidence of follicular keratosis may support the diagnosis. Aquasol A has been recommended for treatment at 1000 to 2500 IU per kilogram of body weight per day. Bioavailability is enhanced if vitamin A is given with food. Lifetime therapy may be necessary, so the animal should be monitored for signs of vitamin A toxicity (dry, scaly skin, inappetence, bone and joint pain).

The synthetic retinoid 13-*cis*–retinoic acid (isotretinoin [Accutane]) has been used in humans to reduce skin inflammation and decrease sebaceous gland output. Its use in veterinary medicine has been reported, but its value in canine seborrhea appears to be limited. Etretinate is another synthetic retinoid used in human medicine and may be more efficacious than isotretinoin for treatment of disorders of keratinization. Further studies are needed to establish the appropriate role of these compounds in veterinary medicine.

Therapy with vitamin E (DL-alpha-tocopherol acetate) has been reported to be effective for some dermatologic problems. Deficiency of vitamin E may result when diets high in polyunsaturated fats are fed. Vitamin E is an antioxidant that may be depleted as the fats become oxidized. Vitamin E deficiency in dogs results in seborrhea, which resembles the effects of EFA deficiency and demodicosis. Vitamin E has been reported to be effective therapy for canine discoid lupus erythematosus and epidermolysis bullosa simplex (EBS) when given at 100 to 400 IU per dog per day. This dose is 20 to 80 times the daily requirement for a 10-kilogram dog. Although vitamin E is nontoxic, extremely high doses in humans (nearly 100 times the recommended dietary allowance) have resulted in transient nausea, flatulence, diarrhea, and, in one case, increased prothrombin time. The anticoagulant effects of vitamin E may be the result of antagonism of intestinal vitamin K transport or an effect at the level of prothrombin formation.

Water-soluble vitamins. Dietary deficiencies of biotin, riboflavin, and niacin have been reported in animals fed bizarre diets for prolonged periods. Signs of water-soluble vitamin deficiency are rather nonspecific and generally include dry, scaly skin and hair loss. Vitamin

Box 5-2
Homemade Diet and Treats

Homemade Diet
The following recipe will make enough food for a 10-20 pound pet for 3-6 days, and enough for a 50-pound dog for a day or two. It should be sufficient for long-term feeding of sedentary adult dogs. It should not be fed to pregnant, nursing, growing, or working dogs without veterinary supervision.

Ingredients
2 cups (8 servings) cooked meat (such as beef, chicken, pork, or egg)
4 cups (8 servings) cooked starch (such as rice, pasta, or potato)
Note: If the client wishes to substitute foods prepared in their home for the meats or starches listed above, refer to the exchange lists in Appendix L.

Homemade Treats
Novel protein treats can be made at home. Purchase a can of the food selected. Cut the food into thin slices, and place them on an ungreased cookie sheet. Bake at 250° for 1 hour or until crispy. Treats can be stored in the refrigerator.

C has been used as therapy for skin problems related to defective neutrophil function in humans, but reports of successful use of vitamin C in dogs and cats with similar problems are not available.

Novel Protein Diets
Novel protein diets are recommended when patients with allergies develop signs of skin or GI disease when exposed to antigens in food. The diets usually contain a single protein source not commonly used in commercial foods (recently, some diets that contain hydrolyzed proteins have become available). Both the provision of a novel protein source and a decrease in the amount of protein ingested may be beneficial. Because of the many proteins included in commercial pet foods, finding a single, novel protein the animal has not previously eaten may not be easy. Homemade diets may be prescribed (Box 5-2), especially for the diagnosis of allergies to foods, and are discussed in the section on Adverse Reactions to Foods.

See Appendixes H and I for a selection of novel protein diets for dogs and cats.

URINARY TRACT DISEASE

Stones
Urinary tract stones are a relatively common problem in dogs and cats. Most stones in dogs and cats have one major crystal component. Types of stones are presented in Table 5-24.

Urine is a complex solution of organic and inorganic ions. Many of these ions can remain in solution at higher concentrations in urine than in water because of the complex interactions that occur among the various constituents of urine. For several possible reasons (e.g., diet, decreased water intake, altered urine pH, relative lack of inhibitors of

CLIENT COMMUNICATION TIPS: Skin Disease

- Carefully review the dietary history with clients.
- If a client does not know how much food the pet consumes in a given day or week, instruct the client regarding completion of a 5-day food diary. A piece of notebook paper can be used, with columns created for the date, time, type of food or treat offered, quantity or serving size, and initials of the person who offers the food. Anything consumed by the pet is recorded in the food diary. Follow up with clients after the food diary has been completed to identify factors that can potentially be modified (e.g., products, serving sizes, behaviors).
- Determine the total daily caloric intake and calculate protein intake to assess whether the animal is receiving the minimum or maximum requirement. This is especially important for sick or older pets, whose daily food intake may vary.
- Educate clients regarding the important benefits of meal-feeding older pets rather than feeding on a free-choice basis. Individual meals allow the owner to observe appetite and water consumption and identify potential problems.
- Communicate clearly with clients regarding the type, dosage, and cost of any nutritional supplements you recommend.
- Teach clients how to monitor food intake each day.
- Recommend that any dietary change be made gradually over a period of several days or longer. If food aversions are to be avoided, dietary changes should not be made in the hospital setting, but in the home and after the pet is feeling better.
- Tell clients to call the veterinarian if they have problems or questions.
- If the client would like to feed a homemade diet, recommend the service provided at www.petdiets.com and ask that the client include the e-mail address of the practice, so that a report and updates are received.
- Discuss with the staff the criteria for determining which novel protein and "hypoallergenic" diets the veterinarians in the practice recommend, as well as which they avoid recommending. Which foods are on the practice's "A list," and why. Which are on the practice's "B list," and why. Help staff identify clients who are receptive to learning more about dietary recommendations.

TECH TIPS: Skin Disease

If an animal needs to be fed a diet that contains a protein to which it has not yet been exposed, compliance with the new diet often determines whether the outcome is successful or not. Getting accurate information and preparing the client ahead of time help ensure success. Following are some suggestions for enhancing compliance.

- Obtain a complete dietary history (see Appendix C) to determine if the complaint is caused or exacerbated by food choices.
- Supply the owner with samples of novel protein pet foods. Make sure that the samples are of foods that are available for the owner to purchase at a later time in the event that the pet likes the food.
- Give the owner written instructions on the proper way to make the transition to a new pet food (see Appendix D).
- Schedule a follow-up phone call after sufficient time has elapsed for the transition to the new food to ensure that no problems have occurred and to determine how effective the treatment has been.

Table 5-24
Prevalence of Selected Stone Types in Dogs and Cats*

Stone Type	Dogs	Cats
Struvite	55%	Approximately 45%
Calcium oxalate	27%	Approximately 45%
Urate	7%	7%
Cystine	1%	<1%
Silicate	1%	0%

From Lulich JP, Osborne CA, Bartges JW et al: Canine lower urinary tract disorders; and Osborne CA, Kruger JM, Lulich JP et al: Feline lower urinary tract disorders. In Ettinger SJ, Feldman EC: *Textbook of veterinary internal medicine,* Philadelphia, 1995, WB Saunders.
*Data from University of Minnesota Urolithiasis Laboratory and based on analysis of approximately 22,000 stones in dogs and 4800 stones in cats. Numbers do not total 100% because compound, mixed, and matrix stones are not included here.

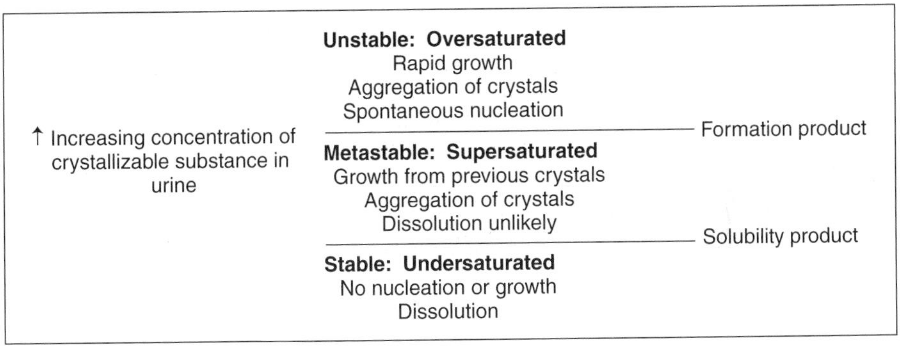

Figure 5-12 Factors involved in the growth of crystals in urine. (From Menon M, Resnick MJ: Urinary lithiasis: etiology, diagnosis, and medical management. In Walsh PC, Campbell MF, Retik AB et al, eds: *Campbell's urology,* ed 8, Philadelphia, 2002, WB Saunders.)

crystallization), the solubility product of a particular crystal may be exceeded, crystals may form, and these crystals may aggregate and grow. Because the urine is commonly supersaturated with a variety of ions, observation of crystals in the urine does not mean the patient is at risk for urolithiasis. Urine supersaturation depends on the amount of the ion ingested and excreted and the volume of urine produced. For this reason, ion concentration, urine volume, and frequency of urination are the most important factors influencing urinary stone formation. These relationships are shown in Figure 5-12.

Urine pH also affects crystal formation, as shown in Table 5-25. The urine pH can be affected by diet, intrinsic factors (e.g., renal tubular acidosis), and external stressors (e.g., hyperventilation syndrome).

Conditions and drugs (e.g., anticholinergic agents) that predispose to urine stasis can play an important role in stone formation, because crystals must reside in the urinary tract for a sufficient time for a urolith to form.

The common types of stones in dogs and cats are formed from struvite, calcium oxalate, and urate. Treatment of urinary stone disease may be divided into removal of identified

Table 5-25
Affect of pH on Crystal Formation

More soluble in acidic urine (pH less than approximately 6.8)	Struvite, calcium carbonate, calcium phosphate, urate
More soluble at intermediate pH (6-6.5)	Uric acid
More soluble in alkaline urine (pH greater than approximately 7)	Cystine
Minimal effect of urine pH	Calcium oxalate

stones and prevention of recurrence of stones. Relief of urinary tract obstruction, reestablishment of urine flow, and correction of fluid, electrolyte, and acid-base imbalances associated with obstruction and postrenal azotemia are the first steps in management of urolithiasis. Stones may be removed surgically, by hydropulsion, or through use of calculolytic diets, depending on the composition of the stone. A stone should be retrieved and submitted for quantitative analysis whenever possible.

Recurrence of stone formation may be prevented by changing the volume and composition of the urine. This can be achieved by increasing water intake and, if necessary, by feeding veterinary foods designed to reduce the risk of stone formation. The primary therapy for patients with urinary stone disease is to reduce the urine specific gravity (USG) and increase the frequency of urination. Patients that have formed a stone *should never be fed food dry.* This is not to say that they cannot be fed dry products, but at least 1 volume of water must be added to each volume of dry food before feeding, so that the food completely absorbs the moisture. In addition to canned products, water, other liquids, or salts may be added to the diet. The goal is to reduce the USG to <1.02 or to double urine output. Patients must be allowed frequent opportunities to urinate to prevent bladder distension. Salt should not be given to patients at risk for fluid retention or to dogs with oxalate and cystine urolithiasis because natriuresis may cause hypercalciuria and may increase urinary excretion of cystine. We recommend to clients that the urine of stone-forming pets be consistently clear, colorless, and odorless and that the pet should urinate often. In addition to these general recommendations, specific suggestions regarding the common stone types follow.

Struvite

The composition of struvite stones is $MgNH_4PO_4 \cdot 6H_2O$. Calcium phosphate (as carbonate apatite) often is present in these stones in small amounts (2% to 10%). The presence of three cations—Ca^{+2}, Mg^{+2}, and NH_4^+—detected by earlier qualitative methods was responsible for the name *triple phosphate* previously used to describe these stones. Struvite stones are spherical, ellipsoidal, or tetrahedral and may be present singly or in large numbers of varying sizes. In dogs and cats the bladder is the most common site of struvite stone formation, although struvite stones may occur at any site in the urinary tract. In dogs, struvite calculi tend to recur after surgical removal; the recurrence rate in one study was 21%.

Struvite stones in dogs usually are associated with urease-positive urinary tract infection (especially *Staphylococcus* and *Proteus* spp.), alkaline urine, struvite crystalluria, and a radiodense stone. Hydrolysis of urea by urease-positive bacteria liberates ammonia and carbon dioxide, which increases the pH of the urine and the availability of ammonium and phosphate ions for struvite formation. The solubility of struvite is markedly reduced in alkaline urine because of removal of protons from phosphate ions. The urine of all dogs with urolithiasis should be cultured. If urinary tract infection is present, appropriate antibiotic therapy and careful follow-up should be instituted to ensure elimination of the infection. Struvite solubility also is reduced in animals with persistently alkaline urine, even in the absence of urinary tract infection. In patients that form struvite stones in the absence of urinary tract infection, predisposing factors include a family history of struvite stones, a diet based on vegetable proteins, and distal renal tubular acidosis. Urinary tract infection usually is not present in cats with struvite stones.

Because of the primary role of urinary tract infection by urease-positive organisms in struvite urolithiasis of dogs, careful elimination of infection by appropriate antibiotic therapy and repeated patient follow-up to demonstrate eradication of infection are the most important aspects of medical management to prevent recurrence.

The use of urinary acidifiers to maintain urine pH in the range of 6 to 6.5 has been suggested in dogs because struvite and hydroxyapatite are most soluble in acidic urine. In most dogs with struvite urolithiasis, eradication of urinary tract infection returns urine pH to this range. Use of urinary acidifiers in the presence of infection with a urease-positive organism is futile. If urine pH remains alkaline after elimination of urinary tract infection, other potential causes of alkaline urine (e.g., dietary, familial, metabolic causes) should be investigated. In cats with struvite urolithiasis without urinary tract infection, urinary acidifiers once played a more important role, until most commercial cat foods were reformulated to reduce urine pH. Urine acidifiers should be given only to cats with urine pH consistently greater than 6.7 as measured by pH meter on urine collected at home, under free-choice feeding conditions, because travel to a veterinarian's office can cause hyperventilation, resulting in alkaline urine. Some concern exists that addition of acidifying compounds to cat foods may have contributed to the increasing incidence of calcium oxalate stones in cats. It seems more likely that it unmasked a population of susceptible individuals.

Calculolytic diets have been used successfully to induce dissolution of naturally occurring struvite calculi in dogs and cats. This type of veterinary diet is designed to promote undersaturation of the urine with the ions necessary for formation of struvite uroliths and to promote dissolution of existing struvite calculi. In dogs with struvite uroliths and urinary tract infection, dissolution is expected to take 2 or 3 months, and the diet is often recommended to be fed for 1 month after radiographic evidence of stone dissolution is obtained. Clinical findings in canine patients fed the Hill's s/d diet include polyuria-polydipsia and dilute urine, decreased blood urea nitrogen levels, increased alkaline phosphatase (hepatic isoenzyme), decreased serum phosphorus, and decreased serum albumin concentrations.

Certain precautions should be observed when use of calculolytic diets is considered for treatment of patients with struvite uroliths. Because of the low protein content, these diets should not be fed to growing puppies, pregnant or lactating bitches, or cats. Occasionally, nephroliths that have decreased in size after institution of the diet may pass into the ureter and cause ureteral obstruction and hydronephrosis.

Calcium Oxalate

Calcium oxalate stones are the most common type of kidney stones in people, and their incidence has been increasing in dogs and cats since the mid-1980s. These stones are composed of calcium oxalate monohydrate (whewellite) or calcium oxalate dihydrate (weddelite). Oxalate frequently is not detected on qualitative analysis, making quantitative analysis necessary. Calcium oxalate calculi usually are white in color and very hard; they often have sharp, jagged edges and may occur singly or in multiple numbers. They are found most often in the bladder and urethra, but they recently have been identified in the ureters and kidneys of cats with increasing frequency. The recurrence rate of calcium oxalate stones may be as high as 48%. When it occurs, urinary tract infection is thought to be a complicating (rather than a predisposing) factor to oxalate urolithiasis.

Oxalate is derived mainly from the diet, with small amounts produced endogenously from the metabolism of ascorbic acid (vitamin C) and the amino acid glycine. In human beings, increased dietary oxalate, increased colonic absorption of oxalate secondary to fat malabsorption, vitamin B_6 deficiency, and inherited defects of oxalate metabolism may predispose to the formation of calcium oxalate stones. The role of these and other diet-related factors in naturally occurring calcium oxalate urolithiasis in dogs and cats is poorly understood.

Altered calcium metabolism may play a role in development of oxalate urolithiasis. Increased urinary excretion of calcium (hypercalciuria) can result from increased absorption of calcium from the intestinal tract ("absorptive" hypercalciuria), from increased urinary loss of calcium ("renal leak" hypercalciuria), or from increased release of calcium from bone ("resorptive" hypercalciuria). In absorptive as compared with renal leak hypercalciuria, urinary calcium excretion is higher after feeding than during fasting. Chronic acidosis may be associated with increased urinary excretion of calcium resulting from increased calcium release from bone. Long-term feeding of an acidifying diet may contribute to this resorptive hypercalciuria.

In one study, miniature schnauzers had higher urinary calcium excretion during fasting than did beagles, and urinary calcium excretion increased threefold after feeding (i.e., hypercalciuria seemed to be absorptive). Dogs with hypercalcemia resulting from primary hyperparathyroidism may develop calcium oxalate (or calcium phosphate) stones because of PTH–mediated mobilization of calcium from bone (resorptive hypercalciuria).

Citrate forms a soluble complex with calcium and normally may be an inhibitor of calcium oxalate formation, at least in humans. Acidosis may be associated with de-creased urinary citrate excretion and, therefore, may predispose to calcium oxalate stone formation. The role of citrate in urinary stone formation in dogs and cats has not yet been reported.

Attempts to dissolve calcium oxalate stones in dogs and cats have so far been unsuccessful, and surgery is required to remove stones of this type. Postoperatively, the patient may be fed its presurgical diet (unless a specific contraindication is present) pending results of analysis of the stone. If the urine can be made clear, colorless, and odorless, with frequent urination, and if the urine contains no crystals, no further treatment may be necessary. If this cannot be accomplished, or if stone formation is recurrent, a veterinary food that has been demonstrated to reduce urinary supersaturation with respect to calcium oxalate in animals that form stones naturally should be fed. This recommendation is made because so many interacting variables determine urine supersaturation (some 100 simultaneous equations must be solved to obtain a single value for supersaturation) that a recommendation for altering the dietary content of one or more nutrients is futile. Phosphorus intake should not be restricted, because reduced phosphorus may result in increased activation of vitamin D_3 to calcitriol by 1-a-hydroxylase in the kidney and may cause increased intestinal absorption of calcium. In addition, urinary pyrophosphate may function as an inhibitor of calcium oxalate formation. Magnesium intake also should not be restricted because it may inhibit calcium oxalate formation. The diet should not be supplemented with sodium because natriuresis is associated with hypercalciuria. A diet with less animal protein may be beneficial, because a diet high in animal protein may be acidifying and could promote loss of calcium from the bones. Supplementation of the diet with citrate may be helpful, but no evidence supports or refutes this speculation. Administration of citrate as potassium citrate (Urocit-K) may be helpful, because urinary citrate may inhibit calcium oxalate formation and its alkalinizing effect may reduce release of calcium from the bones, although no data are available. Beyond this effect, therapeutic manipulation of urine pH is not known to be beneficial, because oxalate solubility is relatively unaffected by a wide range of urine pH. The recommended dosage of potassium citrate is 100 to 150 mg/kg/day, but it is unclear whether this dosage actually increases urinary citrate in dogs and cats. Sodium citrate should not be substituted because of the potentially adverse effects of the sodium on urinary excretion of calcium.

Avoidance of vitamin C has been recommended, because ascorbic acid is a metabolic precursor of oxalate, although it is not a documented cause of stone formation in animals. A number of commercial diets recently have become available that attempt to prevent recurrence of oxalate stones. Only the feeding of the Waltham S/O diet has been shown to result in urine that is undersaturated with both struvite and calcium oxalate.

Urate

Urate stones in dogs are composed of the monobasic ammonium salt of uric acid (ammonium acid urate). Calcium oxalate may be a secondary component of some urate stones, and urate stones found in dogs with portosystemic shunts often contain struvite in addition to urate. Urate stones are found most often in the dalmatian and English bulldog breeds, but other breeds also may be affected. Urate stones may be found in dogs with portosystemic shunts possibly because of reduced conversion of ammonia to urea and uric acid to allantoin. Urate stones do not occur commonly in cats, but some cases have been reported.

Urate stones are small, brittle, spherical stones with concentric laminations. They usually are multiple and light yellow, brown, or green. They are found most often in the bladder and urethra, and the recurrence rate may be as high as 50%. When it occurs, urinary tract infection appears to be a complication of urate urolithiasis rather than a predisposing cause.

A defect in uric acid metabolism in some male dalmatian dogs predisposes them to urate stone formation. This defect is merely a predisposing factor and not a primary cause of urolithiasis, because dalmatian dogs that do not develop stones excrete as much urate as stone-forming dalmatian dogs do, and because other breeds (e.g., English bulldog) also may develop urate urolithiasis.

Uric acid is derived from the metabolic degradation of purines. In all dogs but dalmatians, uric acid is converted to allantoin in the liver by the enzyme uricase. Dalmatian dogs have higher plasma uric acid concentrations and excrete much more uric acid in the urine than do dogs of other breeds. The defect in uric acid metabolism in the dalmatian is not caused by absence of hepatic uricase. The enzyme is present in the liver of dalmatians in amounts comparable to those found in other breeds. Impaired transport of uric acid into liver cells may reduce the rate of hepatic oxidation in dalmatians. The proximal renal tubules of dalmatian dogs also appear to reabsorb less and secrete more urate than do the kidneys of dogs of other breeds.

Dissolution and prevention protocols include some combination of urine dilution, low-purine diet, alkalinization of urine, and administration of allopurinol. Diets low in organ-derived meats reduce the ingested purine load. Feeding a low-protein, low-purine diet has been shown to reduce urinary excretion of urate in normal dogs. A purine-restricted, nonacidifying diet (e.g., Hill's u/d) has been recommended for dogs with urate urolithiasis, but no published clinical studies confirm its efficacy. If the dry form of the diet is fed, at least 1 volume of water per volume of food should be thoroughly mixed with the diet before feeding.

The usefulness of urine alkalinization in urate urolithiasis is uncertain. Canine urate calculi nearly always are composed of ammonium acid urate, and, whereas uric acid becomes more soluble in alkaline urine, urate becomes less soluble. Hydrogen and ammonium ions are thought to cause flocculation of ammonium urate in urine. Administration of $NaHCO_3$ or potassium citrate decreases urinary hydrogen and ammonium ion concentration. Administration of $NaHCO_3$ reduces renal tubular ammonia production, and the sodium load contributes to the induction of polyuria. Therefore, administration of $NaHCO_3$ at a dosage that keeps the urine pH at 7 to 7.5 has been recommended. The pKa of the following reaction is approximately 5.4.

$$Uric\ acid = Urate + H^+$$

However, the pKa of the following reaction is nearly 9.4.

$$NH_4^+ = NH_3 + H^+$$

As urine pH increases from 5.4 to 7.4, the amount of urate doubles, but the amount of ammonium decreases by only a negligible amount. Thus, alkalinization of the urine may be of limited benefit.

Allopurinol is a competitive inhibitor of the enzyme xanthine oxidase, which converts hypoxanthine to xanthine and xanthine to uric acid during purine metabolism. One of allopurinol's metabolites, oxypurinol, also is an inhibitor of xanthine oxidase. Allopurinol therapy reduces the amount of uric acid formed from hypoxanthine and is recommended for use in dogs with urate urolithiasis at a dosage of 30 mg/kg/day divided bid. A dosage of 30 mg/kg/day divided bid for 1 month, followed by 7 to 10 mg/kg/day, has been recommended for prevention of recurrence of urate stones. Xanthine stones may develop in some dogs receiving allopurinol at ≥30 mg/kg/day. Ideally, the dosage of allopurinol should be adjusted so that 24-hour urinary excretion of urate is approximately 300 mg. If the 24-hour urate excretion exceeds 300 mg, the allopurinol dosage should be increased; if it falls below 300 mg, the dosage should be decreased. The dosage of allopurinol should be reduced in the presence of renal failure because the kidneys excrete it. Allopurinol should be prescribed only after the desired increases in urine volume and frequency have been achieved to avoid formation of xanthine crystals or stones.

Idiopathic Cystitis in Cats

Lower urinary tract signs in cats often resolve spontaneously within 1 or 2 weeks regardless of treatment, which prevents accurate assessment of the success of treatments given during this time. Antibiotics, steroids, dietary change, and increased water intake are often prescribed initially to good effect, but none of these treatments is known to be effective in preventing subsequent recurrence of clinical signs.

Diet may play multiple roles in therapy for IC. In the presence of macroscopic crystalluria the changing of the diet to dilute the urine, as described in the section on urinary stone disease, without unnecessary alteration of the pH is indicated. Although most crystalluria usually is benign, severe crystalluria can aggravate an already-inflamed bladder. In a recent study, we found that nearly 60% of cats with IC ate 100% dry cat food; an additional 17% ate 75% of their total daily intake in the form of dry food. Compared with all cats, this is a disproportionate amount of total food intake as dry food. This does not mean that dry food consumption causes IC, but suggests that dry food consumption might unmask or aggravate the disorder in some susceptible cats (making IC a nutrient-sensitive rather than a diet-induced disease).

Consequently, we recommend that the client either add water to the dry food or change to canned foods, particularly if the patient is a male cat (because of the risk of urethral obstruction), if this change is feasible for the owner and the cat. Benefits of increased water intake include possible dilution of any noxious substances in urine, more frequent urination (which decreases bladder contact time with urine), and removal of any excess crystals. We also recommend that the same diet be fed for extended periods of time to reduce the stress that some cats seem to experience when the diet is changed. Suggestions for making dietary changes are provided in Appendix D.

We also treat our patients for pain and advise owners to attempt to modify the home environment to reduce stress. Therapeutic recommendations for pain relief are beyond the scope of this book and are presented elsewhere. Some comments concerning the effect of indoor housing on nutrition-related disease risk are appropriate, however, because it appears that stress responsiveness is very important in the development of flare-ups in cats with IC and may be important in precipitating the first episode of signs in susceptible animals. Additionally, stress responsiveness may play a role in other nutrition-related disorders, including urolithiasis, obesity, and diabetes mellitus. Unfortunately, stress responsiveness is difficult to quantify. Stress-responsive cats appear to be unusually threatened by seemingly minimal changes in the home environment, the weather, activity, use of the litter pan, food intake, owner work schedule, additions to or subtractions from the household population of humans and animals, and other factors. Regimens to reduce stress may prove essential in the management of cats with IC. In an attempt to reduce environmental stress, we recommend that the patient be provided places to hide, places to perch, and opportunities to express the natural predatory behavior of cats (e.g., climbing posts, toys that can be chased and caught). More information on this aspect of IC in cats is available on the World Wide Web site of the Indoor Cat Initiative (available at http://www.nssvet.org/ici).

CLIENT COMMUNICATION TIPS: Urinary Disease

- Review the dietary history carefully with the client.
- If a client does not know how much food the pet consumes in a given day or week, instruct the client regarding completion of a 5-day food diary. A piece of notebook paper can be used, with columns created for the date, time, type of food or treat offered, quantity or serving size, and initials of the person who offers the food. Anything consumed by the pet is recorded in the food diary. Follow up with clients after the food diary has been completed to identify factors that can potentially be modified (e.g., products, serving sizes, behaviors).
- Determine the total daily caloric intake and calculate protein intake to assess whether the animal is receiving the minimum requirement. This is especially important for sick or older pets, whose daily food intake may vary.
- Educate clients regarding the important benefits of meal-feeding older pets rather than feeding on a free-choice basis. Individual meals allow the owner to observe appetite and water consumption and identify potential problems.
- Teach clients how to monitor daily food intake and how to assign a BCS. Remind clients of the importance of regular exercise or play time every day.
- If prescription of a veterinary diet is necessary, allow clients to take home samples of several brands in both canned and dry forms. These products should be introduced in the home environment, and water should be added to dry products at each meal so that water intake is increased.
- Recommend that any dietary change be made gradually over a period of several days or longer. If food aversions are to be avoided, dietary changes should not be made in the hospital setting, but in the home and after the pet is feeling better.
- Tell clients to call the veterinarian if they have problems or questions.
- Discuss with the staff the criteria for determining which "urinary tract stone" diets the veterinarians in the practice recommend, as well as those they avoid recommending. Which foods are on the practice's "A list," and why. Which are on the practice's "B list," and why. Help staff identify clients who are receptive to learning more about dietary recommendations.

TECH TIPS: Urinary Disease

- Put together a "go-home" kit that includes handouts about cystitis and brochures for products that help increase water intake, such as the "pet water fountain."
- Prepare a list of brands and pHs of currently available commercial and veterinary foods that might be recommended, to aid clients in selection of a food that is appropriate for the pet.
- Give the client written instructions regarding the proper way to make the transition to a new pet food (see Appendix D).
- Schedule a follow-up phone call, to be made after sufficient time has elapsed for the dietary transition to have occurred, to ensure that no problems have developed.

SICK GERIATRIC CATS

Although old age is not a disease, the risk of development of many diseases increases as animals age. A 1996 survey revealed that the most common health problems of geriatric cats were oral disease (19.5%); CRF (2.4%); weight loss (2%); heart murmur (1.8%); hyperthyroidism (1.8%); tumor (1.7%); diabetes mellitus (1.4%); cat bite abscess (1.4%);

and vomiting (1.3%). Tentative dietary and feeding recommendations for cats with problems related to dietary sensitivities are provided in other sections of this chapter; readers should recognize that some of these recommendations are based on little more than clinical experience and that they should be adopted with caution.

Geriatric cats can be affected by many diseases that affect younger cats. In such cases dietary and feeding recommendations differ on the basis of increased concern for adequate nutrient intake in the face of decreased activity and appetite. Weight loss, heart murmur, and vomiting are signs of many problems, including some of those listed below. In such patients, nutritional advice depends on the underlying cause of the problem.

Oral Disease

Dental problems can inhibit food intake, depress appetite, and result in weight loss. A careful oral examination should be part of the physical examination of geriatric patients, and abnormalities should be treated appropriately. A change to a canned food may be necessary if dry foods can no longer be adequately chewed.

Chronic Renal Failure

Nutrients currently thought to be of concern in cats with CRF include phosphorus, protein, and potassium. Phosphorus restriction appears to be more important than protein restriction in retarding progression of chronic renal disease and its effects in dogs and rats. Because protein-containing ingredients are the primary source of dietary phosphate, a possible benefit of protein restriction is a reduction in dietary phosphorus. Dietary protein intake should be sufficient to maintain a BCS of 3/5, a goal generally achieved with the consumption of at least 3 g of high-biologic-value protein per kilogram of body weight per day. Dietary phosphate restriction may be helpful in cats with CRF, but clear benefits have not yet been documented. Unfortunately, the aversion of many cats to phosphate binders limits their use.

Protein intakes of 20 g per day did not have adverse effects on the kidneys of young cats with experimentally induced renal failure. In cats with naturally occurring disease (average initial SUN of 52 mg/dl and SCr of 3 mg/dl), one study found that provision of diets with 36% less protein and 52% less phosphorus than the reference diet for 24 weeks appeared to slow the rate of deterioration of the patients as perceived by the clinician and owner. On the other hand, inadequate protein intake can cause protein depletion and its consequences, even in healthy cats. There is no reason to restrict protein intake in cats with no clinical evidence of renal disease or with only mild azotemia.

Recommendations that dietary protein intake be restricted in patients with uremia are based on the premise that reduction of the intake of nonessential protein decreases the production of nitrogenous wastes, thereby ameliorating associated clinical signs, including anorexia, vomiting, uremic ulcers, lethargy, and weight loss. There is no compelling evidence that such effects occur in cats or that consumption of a restricted-protein diet slows the progression of renal disease.

Potassium depletion is common in geriatric cats, especially those with renal insufficiency. Potassium-replete, nonacidifying diets should be fed to help control hypokalemia. Although some practitioners have advocated oral potassium supplementation in all cats with CRF, not enough evidence exists at present to support such recommendations. However, oral potassium supplementation should be considered when serum potassium levels fall below 4 mEq/l. Potassium gluconate or potassium citrate can be used to correct hypokalemia and to correct or prevent its associated effects (e.g., hypokalemic myopathy, reduced renal function, and anorexia).

Metabolic acidosis is common in cats with CRF, so urine-acidifying diets should be avoided. Most diets intended for cats with renal failure are nonacidifying and therefore beneficial in this respect. Such diets are often restricted in phosphorus as well, which might help limit progression of renal disease, renal secondary hyperparathyroidism with resultant soft-tissue mineralization, and renal osteodystrophy. Potassium supplements have an alkalinizing effect and may limit progressive renal injury.

Cardiovascular Disease

Patients with CHF may be obese or cachexic, and energy requirements vary. Potassium depletion is a potential problem associated with the use of loop diuretics (e.g., furosemide) in patients with CHF. Magnesium deficiency may be more common in cats with CHF than is generally recognized because of the feeding of magnesium-restricted diets and magnesium wasting induced by diuretics, digitalis, and aldosterone. The feeding of urine-acidifying, magnesium-restricted diets to patients receiving diuretics or digitalis and to patients with hypertension or hypokalemia should be avoided. Hypertensive cats may benefit from sodium restriction, but dietary change alone is frequently insufficient to lower blood pressure.

Hyperthyroidism

Current nutritional recommendations are limited to assuring adequate intake of a satisfactorily nutrient-dense diet in an attempt to minimize weight loss. Ventriflexion of the head is occasionally seen in patients with hyperthyroidism. This sign may be a result of thiamin or potassium deficiency.

Cancer

Suggestions for nutritional support of cancer patients include the following.

Food intake should be monitored closely, and support provided before weight loss occurs. Easily digested, highly palatable diets that contain nutrients with high bioavailability may help the patient maintain nutrient reserves.

If invasive support is necessary, the enteral route is the preferred approach. Because of the slower healing response of most patients with cancer, gastrostomy and jejunostomy tubes should not be removed prematurely (i.e., before 2 weeks have elapsed), even if oral intake of food is resumed.

Provision of increased quantities of arginine, carotene, cystine, fiber, glutamine, omega-3 fatty acids, and taurine have been recommended, but no data currently support the benefit of such supplementation or validate any specific dosage.

Diabetes Mellitus

The primary goals of nutritional management for geriatric diabetic cats are similar to those for younger cats: to attain and maintain moderate body condition (3/5), to minimize postprandial fluctuations in blood glucose by feeding diets low in simple sugars, and to standardize the type of diet, quantity fed, and times of feeding to complement the effects of exogenously administered insulin or other therapy. Food intake should be monitored especially carefully in geriatric cats. The role of dietary fiber in the management of diabetes mellitus remains controversial.

Conclusions

The information discussed in the previous sections suggests that nutrition-related diseases are not common in primary care veterinary practice. The low frequency of occurrence of nutrition-related diseases may be the result of the high quality of pet foods.

Our clinical impression, not based on supporting data, is that more nutrition-related diseases are seen in tertiary care facilities. We are most commonly consulted regarding problems related to obesity, diseases of the kidney and lower urinary tract, inappetence, and growth. The frequency with which these problems are seen in our practices may reflect only our interests and those of our colleagues.

SICK GERIATRIC DOGS

Dietary therapy recommended for older dogs is similar to that for younger dogs. Avoidance of sudden dietary changes is particularly important in older dogs. Patients are rarely presented in such serious condition that abrupt modifications are necessary, and they may be less able to decrease rates of excretion quickly enough to avoid depletion if intake is suddenly reduced. Modifications to the diet should be made in increments over a period of a few days to a few weeks, depending on the severity of the problem, the appetite of the patient, and the wishes of the owner. No dietary change is effective if it is not instituted, and both the animal and the owner may resist drastic changes. If the owner is not convinced of the necessity of the change, it will not be made. A change is also less likely to be made if it is one of many changes in owner behavior recommended simultaneously.

A new diet should not be introduced until medical therapy has succeeded in improving the dog's condition. The dog then has a better appetite and is more likely to eat the new food. The dog is also less likely to associate the new diet with the illness and develop a learned aversion—a situation that occurs when a dog associates a food with the effects of illness and refuses to eat the food even though doing so does not result in a problem. Most of us have a learned aversion to a food that was eaten just before a bout of malaise. Such aversions may take years to overcome, despite the understanding that the food is blameless. Because learned aversions generally do not occur with foods that constitute a large portion of an individual's diet, an animal is more likely to eat familiar foods first. The poor acceptance of some veterinary therapeutic diets may be a consequence of trying to introduce them too early in the course of therapy.

Clinicians treating old dogs should be aware of the possibility of drug-nutrient interactions. Management of such chronic problems as CHF, renal failure, and cancer includes the prescription of drugs that may have nutritional side effects. This area of veterinary nutrition has not been thoroughly studied, but "digitalis cachexia," the magnesium and potassium wasting associated with thiazide diuretic use, and the antinutrient and food intake–depressant effects of cancer chemotherapeutic agents are examples of similar common problems in human geriatric medicine.

Dietary recommendations, as all the recommendations made to clients concerning their dogs, require consideration of the individual patient. Extreme care must be taken when attempting to extrapolate results of studies done in other species; it remains to be proved how similar old rats and old people are to old dogs. Normal aged dogs are not nutritional cripples. Keeping them lean, eating, and exercising goes a long way toward helping them reach their genetic life expectancy.

DIET-INDUCED PROBLEMS

Diet-induced problems result from nutrient deficiencies or excesses, the presence of toxins or antinutrients, and contamination or spoilage related to improper handling or storage. Such problems are rare and generally are caused by feeding errors committed by well-intentioned owners. The acquisition of knowledge about pet nutrition and its incorporation into satisfactory commercial diets has occurred relatively recently. Many inappropriate feeding practices were developed before high-quality proprietary pet foods were readily available and probably were based on uncritical observation of the effects of dietary manipulation on animal performance. Adult animals have relatively low nutrient requirements, and many survive ingestion of imbalanced diets literally for years. Poor feeding practices are often recognized only in lactating females, young growing animals, or high-performance athletes, because of their increased nutrient needs.

Oversupplementation with vitamins and minerals still is a relatively common practice. It is neither economic nor sensible to attempt to supplement a poor-quality food; if one deficiency is identified, others may be present but not clinically apparent. The food should be discarded in favor of a high-quality product that requires no supplementation. Another common error is the feeding of only one food item—generally meat. Feeding meat as the sole dietary item can cause metabolic bone disease in pets. In addition, some animals may become "addicted" to highly palatable, imbalanced diets, making it extremely difficult to switch them to a satisfactory diet. The feeding of large amounts of table scraps can be a problem. Table scraps are highly variable in nutrient content, are rarely nutritionally balanced, and, if fed in large quantities, may upset the balance of a satisfactory diet. Feeding dog food to cats can result in nutritional deficiencies if the dog food contains insufficient amounts of ingredients of animal origin. In addition to these general problems, a number of specific nutrient deficiencies and excesses may result in diet-induced disease, particularly in cats.

Vitamin A

One of the nutritional peculiarities of cats is their dietary requirement for preformed vitamin A. Neither orally nor intravenously administered β-carotene, the plant precursor of vitamin A, can be converted to vitamin A. Dogs and most other mammals possess an intestinal enzyme that cleaves dietary β-carotene to two molecules of vitamin A, which are absorbed. This enzyme is absent from the intestine of cats, which presumably meet their vitamin A requirement in the wild by consumption of animal tissue, especially liver. In the late 1950s and the 1960s vitamin A toxicity in cats fed diets of animal liver was reported from areas of South America and Australia, where animal byproducts were fed to cats as a primary nutrient source. The disorder was extensively studied after these reports, and although vitamin A toxicity currently is a minor veterinary problem, it still occasionally occurs in cats and dogs and in dogs fed large amounts of liver or cod liver oil for months to years.

The initial signs of vitamin A toxicity are cervical stiffness and forelimb lameness. The signs result from new periosteal bone production, which restricts joint movement and may pinch spinal nerves that exit from the vertebral foramina. Affected cats resist movement and resent handling. With an animal's continued exposure to excessive amounts of vitamin A, the bony changes may extend to the sternebrae, ribs, scapulae, long bones, and pelvis. Ankylosis of cervical vertebra and elbow joints may occur, and affected cats are typically unkempt because the movements of the head necessary for grooming become impossible. Switching the cat to a nutritionally satisfactory diet early in the course of the disease may result in resolution of the stiffness and discomfort if ankylosis has not yet occurred.

Vitamin E and Thiamin Deficiencies

Inadequately formulated diets that contain large amounts of fish have caused vitamin deficiencies in cats. The tissues of many fish contain a thiaminase enzyme that destroys thiamin. Improperly processed foods that contain fish have caused thiamin deficiency and even death in cats. Cooking destroys the enzyme, thereby protecting thiamin. Some processing techniques, especially canning, can also destroy large amounts of thiamin, so reputable manufacturers add excesses to the diet to ensure adequacy. Signs of thiamin deficiency include an initial period of decreased food intake and salivation, which may appear within 1 or 2 weeks of ingestion of a deficient diet and last for several days. A period of brief tonic convulsive seizures then occurs. During this period, ventriflexion of the head and loss of normal righting reflexes may occur. Retinal veins are dilated, and retinal hemorrhages may be seen. Abnormalities of the heart have also been reported during this stage, including sinus irregularity and bradycardia. Treatment during this period with thiamin, 5 mg orally or 1 mg parenterally, results in disappearance of all signs within 24 hours. Untreated cats develop extensor rigidity, subside into coma, and die within 48 hours of the appearance of these terminal signs.

Large quantities of fish in cat food have caused a deficiency of vitamin E. Fish contains high levels of polyunsaturated fatty acids that are easily oxidized, which may result in damage to cell membranes. A primary function of vitamin E is to prevent this oxidation, so manufacturers of all-fish diets must add sufficient amounts to ensure that a deficiency does not occur. Signs of vitamin E deficiency, so-called "steatitis" or "yellow fat disease," include depressed appetite and hypersensitivity to touch. A fever that does not respond to antibiotics usually is present. As the disease progresses, the subcutaneous fat becomes firm and nodular because of the accumulation of peroxidized polyunsaturated fats. Inflammation and necrosis are also present. Long-term treatment consists of a change in diet. Short-term treatment consists of enteral nutritional support via a feeding tube until the appetite returns.

Corticosteroids should be administered to decrease the inflammatory reaction. Vitamin E acetate, 100 mg per day, may be given for 1 or 2 weeks to replenish bodily stores.

Nutritional Secondary Hyperparathyroidism

The most common diet-induced disease of cats and dogs that is related to mineral nutrition is nutritional secondary hyperparathyroidism (NSHP). NSHP is a metabolic bone disease caused by consumption of homemade diets, usually all meat, which are deficient in calcium and imbalanced in calcium and phosphorus. The disease is most commonly seen in young, rapidly growing kittens, 10 to 20 weeks of age. Kittens with NSHP are usually presented with generalized stiffness, lameness (usually more prominent in the hind limbs), and joint pain on palpation. Constipation and abdominal distension may also be observed.

When animals are fed diets deficient in calcium, extracellular calcium levels decline, which causes the parathyroid glands to secrete PTH. PTH stimulates reabsorption of bone mineral calcium and phosphorus. PTH also acts on the kidneys to enhance phosphorus excretion and calcium retention, thereby returning extracellular fluid calcium levels to normal. Reabsorption of bone mineral in the growing kitten with calcium deficiency does not inhibit production of the organic bone matrix (thus the name *osteitis fibrosa*).

NSHP is diagnosed on the basis of nutritional history and radiographic signs. Bone demineralization results in progressively decreased skeletal radiodensity, bowing and folding of long bones, narrowing of the pelvic canal, and vertebral compression fractures in advanced cases. Serum biochemistry is of little value because of normal variation in plasma calcium, phosphorus, and alkaline phosphatase levels. NSHP is treated by provision of a nutritionally satisfactory diet for the animal's age. Supplemental calcium has been advocated, but is probably unnecessary. Dietary change results in rapid improvement of stiffness and pain, but constipation and bone abnormalities resolve more slowly and may be permanent.

NSHP is a disease better prevented than treated. Breeders and cattery owners should be interviewed about nutritional practices early in the physician-client relationship, and the hazards of inappropriate diets should be explained. Reliance on excellent-quality commercial cat foods without supplementation is the best insurance against NSHP during the critical nutritional period of early growth.

In addition to nutrient deficiencies, toxicities and imbalances, which are rare in our practices, formulation errors, and processing problems also can occasionally occur. With the advent of internet-based communications among veterinarians and veterinary nutritionists, these problems are more likely than ever to be recognized and the company informed. Postprocessing problems such as improper storage can result in stale, moldy, or infested foods. Clients usually are quick to notice changes in the smell or color, and the presence of nonfood materials in the diet they feed, so these problems usually do not affect the pet.

RECOMMENDED READINGS

Abood SK, Mauterer J, McLoughling M, Buffington CA: Nutritional support of hospitalized patients. In Slatter D, ed: *Textbook of small animal surgery,* ed 2, Philadelphia, 1993, WB Saunders.
Birchard SJ, Sherding RG: *Saunders manual of small animal practice,* Philadelphia, 2000, WB Saunders.

Borghi L, Meschi T, Schianchi T et al: Medical treatment of nephrolithiasis, *Endocrinol Metab Clin North Am* 31:1051, 2002.

Bunch SE: Pancreatitis. In Nelson RW, Couto CG, eds: *Small animal internal medicine*, ed 3, St Louis, 2003, Mosby.

Deli S, Ribarich C: *Felinestein*, New York, 1999, Harper Resource.

Edney A, Smith P: Study of obesity in dogs visiting veterinary practices in the United Kingdom, *Vet Rec* 118:391, 1986.

Elliott J, Rawlings JM, Markwell PJ, Barber PJ: Survival of cats with naturally occurring chronic renal failure: effect of dietary management, *J Small Anim Pract* 41:235, 2000.

Feldman EC: *Canine and feline endocrinology and reproduction*, Philadelphia, 1996, WB Saunders.

Freeman LM: Nutritional therapy of heart disease. Presented at: 26th annual Waltham Diets/OSU Symposium for the Treatment of Small Animal Diseases—Cardiology, October 19-20, 2002, Columbus, Ohio. Available at: http://www.vin.com/proceedings/Proceedings.plx?CID=WALTHAMOSU2002. Accessed December 2003.

Glickman L, Sonnenschein E, Glickman N et al: Pattern of diet and obesity in female adult pet dogs, *Vet Clin Nutr* 2:6, 1995.

Goodwin J-K, Strickland KN: The role of dietary modification and nondrug therapy in dogs and cats with congestive heart failure, *Vet Med* 93:919, 1998.

Grauer GF: Urinary tract disorders. In Nelson RW, Couto CG, eds: *Small animal internal medicine*, ed 3, St Louis, 2003, Mosby.

Guilford WG, Center SA, Strombeck DR et al: *Strombeck's small animal gastroenterology*, Philadelphia, 1996, WB Saunders.

Jacob F, Polzin DJ, Osborne CA et al: Clinical evaluation of dietary modification for treatment of spontaneous chronic renal failure in dogs, *J Am Vet Med Assoc* 220:1163, 2002.

Kittleson MD, Kienle RD, eds: *Small animal cardiovascular medicine*, St Louis, 1998, Mosby, Chapters 10 and 20.

Markwell PJ: Obesity. In Wills JM, ed: *The Waltham book of clinical nutrition of the dog and cat*, Tarryton, NY, 1994, Elsevier.

Mattheeuws D, Rottiers R, Kaneko JJ, Vermeulen A: Diabetes mellitus in dogs: relationship of obesity to glucose tolerance and insulin response, *Am J Vet Res* 45:98, 1984.

Mauldin GE, Davidson JR: Nutritional support of hospitalized cats and dogs. In Slatter DJ, ed: *Textbook of small animal surgery*, ed 3, Philadelphia, 2003, WB Saunders.

Meurs KM: Canine dilated cardiomyopathy—recognition and clinical management. Presented at: 26th annual Waltham Diets/OSU Symposium for the Treatment of Small Animal Diseases—Cardiology, October 19-20, 2002, Columbus, Ohio. Available at: http://www.vin.com/proceedings/Proceedings.plx?CID=WALTHAMOSU2002. Accessed 2002.

Miller AB: Dietary fat and the epidemiology of breast cancer. In Birt DF, ed: *Dietary fat and cancer*, New York, 1986, Liss.

Morris JG, Rogers QR, Pacioretty LM: Taurine: an essential nutrient for cats, *J Small Anim Pract* 31:502, 1990.

Nagode LA, Chew DJ, Podell M: Benefits of calcitriol therapy and serum phosphorus control in dogs and cats with chronic renal failure: both are essential to prevent or suppress toxic hyperparathyroidism, *Vet Clin North Am* 26(6):1293, 1996.

Osborne CA, Lulich JP, Bartges JW: *The ROCKet science of canine urolithiasis*, Philadelphia, 1999, WB Saunders.

Pennington JAT: *Bowes and Church's food values of portions commonly used*, ed 16, Philadelphia, 1994, JB Lippincott.

Remillard RL, Armstrong J, Davenport D: Assisted feeding in hospitalized patients: enteral and parenteral nutrition. In: Hand MS, Thatcher CD, Remillard RL, Roudebush P, eds: *Small animal clinical nutrition*, ed 4, Marceline, Mo, 2000, Mark Morris Institute.

Scarlett J, Donoghue S: Association between body condition and disease in cats, *J Am Vet Med Assoc* 212:1725, 1998.

6

Contemporary Issues in Clinical Nutrition

COMPLEMENTARY AND ALTERNATIVE VETERINARY MEDICINE

The history of medicine has never been a particularly attractive subject in medical education and one reason for this is that it is so unbelievably deplorable. . .bleeding, purging, cupping and the administration of infusions of every known plant, solutions of every known metal, every conceivable diet including total fasting, most of them based on the weirdest imaginings about the cause of disease, concocted out of nothing but thin air—this was the heritage of medicine until a little over a century ago.

Lewis Thomas, US physician, 1913-1993

As exemplified by Dr. Thomas' quotation, spectacular advances have been made in the science of medicine during the last 150 years or so. The discoveries of antibiotics, vaccines, and the principles of adequate nutrition and sanitation have demonstrated the value of the scientific approach to health problems. As a result, most education for health-care professionals focuses on the scientific aspects of treatment of disease. Disease, however, has both scientific and emotional aspects that can influence outcome. In addition to physiologic abnormalities, disease-induced fear and anxiety can affect outcome. Historical treatments were not intentionally deplorable, however. It is easy to understand why doctors would try anything when they had nothing to lose. Moreover, a few of the treatments for some disorders, admittedly very few, were better than no treatment at all.

Early physicians must have known that a patient's confidence in a physician's skill as a caregiver can play an important role in disease outcome. Throughout much of human history the arts of calming patients and instilling confidence in the expertise of the caregiver were the primary tools of the clinician. Few active drugs other than poppy sap and willow bark were available; the most common historical disease treatments, regardless of the malady, were application of feces and bloodletting. The scientific approach to the physiologic aspects of disease is a relatively recent historical development. Given its success, it is no wonder that the scientific approach to medicine has been embraced with the fervor expressed by Dr. Thomas.

The emotional aspects of disease have not disappeared, however. Humans are still fearful and anxious in the presence of disease, and medical scientists still have much to learn.

Practitioners of medicine have not yet gained the power over the emotional aspects of disease that they have over its scientific aspects, although clinical investigators acknowledge this aspect by using placebos in controlled clinical trials. Clinicians and clients also recognize differences in practitioners' "charisma" as well as their clinical skills.

Nutrition also has both scientific and emotional aspects. Animals require a relatively constant input of nutrients to construct and sustain them throughout life; our understanding of the mechanisms by which this occurs constitutes much of the science of nutrition. The emotional aspects of food are no less significant. All cultures and belief systems incorporate foods into their rituals, many foods are preferentially eaten in certain contexts, and many people consume "comfort foods" when confronted with stressful circumstances.

Knowledge of the existence and importance of the scientific and emotional aspects of disease, nutrition, and medicine can be used to enlighten the investigation of complementary and alternative veterinary medicine (CAVM). Complementary and alternative medical treatments have both scientific and emotional aspects, and consideration of both may aid in efforts to understand this area of patient care.

Complementary and alternative therapies are defined generally by the United States National Institutes of Health National Center for Complementary and Alternative Medicine (NCCAM) as "those treatments and healthcare practices not taught widely in medical schools, not generally used in hospitals, and not usually reimbursed by medical insurance companies." Another recently proposed definition for complementary medicine is "diagnosis, treatment, and/or prevention that complements mainstream medicine by contributing to a common whole, by satisfying a demand not met by orthodoxy, or by diversifying the conceptual frameworks of medicine."

Complementary and alternative therapies are not intrinsically better or worse than conventional treatments; they are merely different. Use of such therapies does not absolve the practitioner of the responsibility to be a thoughtful, informed clinician. One of the many challenges facing caregivers today is finding and interpreting information that will permit them to decide what role is appropriate for these approaches to treatment.

One form of CAVM is the use of nutrients in "supranutritional" quantities to achieve a pharmacologic effect. All nutrients are chemicals capable of producing a variety of physiologic effects on the body, of which their nutritional effects are only one. Nutrients used as "drugs" are referred to as *nutriceuticals*. The U.S. Food and Drug Administration's Dietary Supplement Health and Education Act of 1994 established a framework for labeling and providing information about nutrition-related products, herbs, and other botanicals. Under the act, labels can contain a statement describing how the product affects structure and function or general well-being in humans but specific health claims cannot be made. The label also must carry the disclaimer, "This statement has not been evaluated by the Food and Drug Administration. This product is not intended to diagnose, treat, cure, or prevent any disease."

Some of the interest in CAVM is scientific and has resulted from positive effects identified in human and veterinary patients during clinical trials. Some interest also may be emotional, arising from, for example, attraction to novel or exotic-sounding interventions, fear and anxiety, frustration with inadequate medical care (including emotional support), and occasionally superstitions and belief in miracles.

Unfortunately, if we as clinicians underrate the emotional significance of the desire for health and the fear of disease, we may unintentionally leave some people susceptible to quackery. Quackery is defined as "[p]romotion, for profit, of devices, services, plans, or products (including, but not limited to, diets and nutritional supplements) that do not work, or which are untested." (For more information, see http://www.quackwatch.org.) In a very real sense quackery appeals to the emotions; if we leave our clients vulnerable to such appeals by ignoring the power of emotion on health and disease, we may inadvertently empower the charlatans. The client who resorts to quack therapies may delay seeking care for a pet's problem and unwittingly expose the pet to dangerous treatments. In addition, quackery violates the "golden rule" of "do for others what you want done for you" and may delay legitimate research that seeks effective cures. We can avoid nutritional quackery by being wary of "experts" who, without credible supporting evidence, say such things as the following.

- "Diet causes disease." (This generalization is untrue, although all patients showed appetite before they became ill.)
- "Malnutrition is common." (This is true only if obesity is included as "malnutrition.")
- "Pet foods contain 'poisons'." (The increasing longevity of pets suggests otherwise.)
- "Natural vitamins and minerals are better than synthetic ones."
- "Our products [or techniques] can produce miracles." (Miracles by definition depend on belief.)
- "Supporters of traditional treatments are victims of a conspiracy."
- "We offer testimonials to support these claims." (The testimonials are always positive; even if the testimonials are true, however, without evidence it is impossible to distinguish whether the benefit was caused by the therapist or the therapy.)
- "The secret lies in buying our product." (Usually the product is sold at a handsome profit.)

Many in the medical establishment respond to quackery with emotionless appeals to science and logic rather than by combining their arguments with the emotional appeals that are used so successfully by the quacks. The weakness in this approach lies in the fact that logical arguments lack the strength of appeals to evolutionarily conserved instincts of belief and pack behavior that guide many actions on an unconscious level. Acknowledging both the emotional and scientific aspects of CAVM may help us identify the relative importance of each aspect of proposed treatments.

Information regarding safety and effectiveness of alternative and complementary therapies may be less readily available than information regarding those of conventional medical treatments. Research on these therapies is ongoing, and data are increasingly available. Information regarding a compendium of monographs, compiled by the German Federal Health Agency's Commission E, that describe the safety and efficacy of many common herbal treatments recently became available at the American Botanical Council's World Wide Web site (http://www.herbalgram.org).

One concern raised regarding supplements based on natural products is the consistency of the formulation. Companies may not have rigid quality-control standards to ensure the purity and reliability of the product. This may result in the presence of accidental contaminants, allergens, pollens, molds, and spores (as can occur in conventional products).

Contradictory pharmacologic effects have been reported for herbal preparations that contain different subspecies of the plant that is the primary ingredient, and the active principle may not be present at all stages of the plant's life cycle. For example, some herbs that are edible when immature are poisonous when mature. A new World Wide Web site called ConsumerLab (http://www.consumerlab.com) provides an evaluation of major herbal, mineral, vitamin, and other supplements.

One recent example of alternative nutrition in veterinary medicine has been raw-food diets for dogs and cats. The arguments in favor of provision of raw-food diets to pets include the fact that dogs and cats evolved as carnivores, eating raw foods, and the assertion that consumption of these diets results in improved coat and skin, improved "energy levels," and reduced incidence of disease (see http://www.barfworld.com). Other "facts" of evolution, including carnivores' short life expectancy in the wild, likely incidence of infectious disease, and the absence of evidence of any consistent benefits of raw-food diets, dilute the persuasive power of these arguments. Reports of adverse effects of feeding these diets also have appeared in the veterinary literature. Unfortunately, to our knowledge, no evidence-based evaluation of raw-food diets has occurred. This permits both proponents and detractors to continue to engage in largely emotional arguments, with little effort made to understand the appeal of preparing raw food for pets—a task abandoned by most pet owners generations ago.

Investigators in human medicine have attempted to understand the appeal of alternative therapies. Some researchers believe that medicine has lost its holistic perspective, with the result that patients seek help from caregivers who spend the time to get to know clients and listen to their concerns. Such practitioners may also treat the situation as a whole, rather than addressing only the patient's presenting symptoms—an approach that seems to be valued by some clients. Interest in raw foods may not truly reflect dissatisfaction with commercial diets, but rather may represent an increased satisfaction from a cultural perspective in preparing food for a pet that is considered a member of the family, as opposed to pouring dry chunks into a bowl.

Clients' sociologic needs can be met without putting their pets' nutritional welfare at risk. Clinicians can listen to the client's concerns, acknowledge that these concerns are valid for the client (even if they seem invalid to the practitioner), and try to help find a diet that appears to be as complete, balanced, and safe as possible. Many nutritional support services provide computer-based analyses for a fee to clients (one example can be found at http://www.petdiets.com). As long as none of the ingredients is contaminated, such a diet should be safe for adult animals for months or years. In our experience, clients appreciate this help and sometimes return to feeding commercial foods after a few months. More frequent checkups may be offered to provide more careful observation of the pet.

Clients can be provided care based on both evidence and emotion, and the combination may be more effective than either approach alone. Dr. Howard Brody has concluded from his experience with human patients that an encounter with a healer is most likely to result in a positive meaning (placebo) response when it changes the meaning of the illness experience for that individual in a positive direction. Such a positive change is most likely when the following three things happen.

- The individual is listened to and receives an explanation for the illness that makes sense.

Table 6-1
Owner Satisfaction with Care

	Strongly Agree	Agree	Neutral	Disagree	Strongly Disagree
1. I felt that my problem was carefully listened to.	5	4	3	2	1
2. I received an explanation for the problem that makes sense to me.	5	4	3	2	1
3. I feel that care and concern were expressed by the clinician.	5	4	3	2	1
4. I feel that care and concern were expressed by others in the hospital.	5	4	3	2	1
5. I feel more confident that I can gain some level of control over symptoms.	5	4	3	2	1

- The individual feels care and concern being expressed by the healer and others in the environment.
- The individual gains an enhanced sense of mastery or control over the illness or symptoms.

These factors may be equally important for parents of children and owners of veterinary patients, possibly because they reduce the perception of threat and the associated autonomic arousal. Discussion of a mechanism that explains this effect has recently been published by Bierhaus and associates. Our effectiveness can be checked using the scale shown in Table 6-1. Whether the evaluation is given to clients or performed mentally by the practitioner at the end of each client encounter, it may help improve "charisma" with clients.

EVALUATING INFORMATION ON THE WORLD WIDE WEB

An enormous amount of information related to nutrition has become available on the Internet in the last decade—a sometimes overwhelming amount. As Bill Rados, director of the U.S. Food and Drug Administration communications staff, has said, "My advice to consumers about information on the Internet is the same as it is for other media: you can't believe everything you see, whether it's in a newspaper, on TV, or on a computer screen. Since anyone—reputable scientist or quack—who has a computer, a modem, and the necessary software can publish a Web page, post information to a newsgroup, or proffer advice in an online chat room, you must protect yourself by carefully checking out the source of any information you obtain." Fortunately, the evidence-based medicine (EBM) model of grading evidence applies much more broadly than just to the scientific literature and can be used to grade any health-related information.

Information is available from a variety of sources on the Internet. For example, Internet groups such as Usenet groups permit people to post questions and read messages, much as they would on regular bulletin boards. Mailing lists permit messages to be exchanged by e-mail, with all messages sent to all group subscribers. Some services also provide "chat" areas in which users can communicate with each other in real time. By far the easiest source of information is the World Wide Web. Because the Web does not contain an index,

CLIENT COMMUNICATION TIPS: Raw-Food Diets

- Listen carefully and try to understand the owner's reasons for choosing this form of diet.
- Discuss with clients the importance of an accurate dietary history and use of body condition score and body weight to determine the most appropriate dietary plan for a pet.
- Review the current dietary history carefully. If a client does not know how much food the pet consumes in a given day or week, instruct the client regarding completion of a 5-day food diary. A piece of notebook paper can be used, with columns created for the date, time, type of food or treat offered, quantity or serving size, and initials of the person who offers the food. Anything consumed by the pet is recorded in the food diary. Follow up with clients after the food diary has been completed to identify factors that can potentially be modified (e.g., products, serving sizes, behaviors).
- Discuss issues of concern regarding raw-food diets, including the need for a complete and balanced diet and the increased risk of exposure to potential pathogens such as *Escherichia coli* and *Salmonella*.
- Teach clients about preparing raw foods using aseptic technique.
- Recommend that clients use a service such as the one provided at http://www.petdiets.com to formulate a complete and balanced diet for their pets. Initial fees start at $150.00, and reevaluation of the formula is possible after 6 or 12 months for a reduced cost of $50.00. If the client includes the veterinarian's e-mail address when paying for the dietary formulation, the veterinarian will also receive information pertaining to the homemade recipe.
- Educate clients regarding the important benefits of meal-feeding older pets rather than feeding on a free-choice basis. Individual meals allow the owner to observe appetite and water consumption and identify potential problems.
- Recommend that any dietary change be made gradually over a period of several days or longer.
- Tell clients to call the veterinarian if they have problems or questions.
- Help the staff identify clients who are receptive to learning more about dietary recommendations.

finding information requires a search engine. One popular search engine is Google (http://www.google.com). According to the University of California at Berkeley Library (http://www.lib.berkeley.edu/TeachingLib/Guides/Internet/Google.html), Google is distinguished by its ranking algorithm, which is based on how many other pages link to each page, along with other factors such as the proximity of search keywords or phrases in the documents. Google uses both the number of other pages that link to a page and the importance of the other links (measured by the links to each of them); the ranking of a particular page cannot be influenced or purchased. New users of Google who want help can simply type the words *Google tutorial* into the Google toolbar to find current tutorials.

Once potentially relevant information has been found, the National Institutes of Health and the National Cancer Institute suggest the following "10 Things to Know about Evaluating Medical Resources on the Web."

1. *Who runs the site?* A good health-related Web site makes it easy to learn who is responsible for the site and its information. On the National Center for Complementary and Alternative Medicine (NCCAM) Web site, for example, the name of the site is clearly marked on every major page, along with a link to the NCCAM home page.

2. *Who pays for the site?* It costs money to run a Web site. The source of a Web site's funding should be clearly stated or readily apparent. For example, the suffix ".gov" on a Web address denotes a federal government–sponsored site. Users should know how the site pays for its existence. Does it sell advertising? Is it sponsored by a drug company? The source of funding can affect what content is presented, how the content is presented, and what the site owners want to accomplish on the site.

3. *What is the purpose of the site?* This question is related to who runs and pays for the site. An "About This Site" link appears on many sites; if this link is present, use it. The purpose of the site should be clearly stated and should help users evaluate the trustworthiness of the information.

4. *From where does the information come?* Many health-related or medical sites post information collected from other Web sites or sources. If the person or organization in charge of the site did not create the information, the original sources should be clearly indicated.

5. *What is the basis of the information?* In addition to identifying the author of the material shown, the site should describe the evidence on which the material is based. Medical facts and figures should have references (e.g., to articles in medical journals). In addition, opinions or advice should be clearly set apart from information that is "evidence based" (i.e., based on research results).

6. *How is the information selected?* Is there an editorial board? Do people with excellent professional and scientific qualifications review the material before it is posted?

7. *How current is the information?* Web sites should be reviewed and updated on a regular basis. It is particularly important that medical information be current. The most recent update or review date should be clearly posted. Even if the information has not changed, it is important to know whether the site owners have reviewed it recently to ensure that it is still valid.

8. *How does the site choose links to other sites?* Web sites usually have a policy regarding links to other sites. Some medical sites take a conservative approach and do not link to any other sites. Some link to any site that asks or pays for a link. Others link only to sites that have met certain criteria.

9. *What information about users does the site collect, and why?* Web sites routinely track the paths visitors take through their sites to determine what pages are being used. However, many health-related Web sites ask users to "subscribe" or "become a member." In some cases they may do this in order to collect a user fee or to select information that is relevant to the user's concerns. In all cases this gives the site personal information about the user. Many credible health-related sites that request user information explain exactly what they will and will not do with the information. Many commercial sites sell "aggregate" (collected) data about their users to other companies—information such as what percentage of users are women with breast cancer, for example. In some cases they may collect and reuse information that is "personally identifiable," such as ZIP code, gender, and birth date. The user should be certain to read and understand any "privacy policy" or similarly worded disclaimer on the site, and not sign up for anything that is not fully understood.

10. *How does the site manage interactions with visitors?* The site should always contain directions for contacting the site owner in the event of problems or if a user has

---

Table 6-2

Recommended World Wide Web Sites

Academic

Many species	Cornell University	http://www.ansci.cornell.edu/
Horses	Ohio State University	http://ohioline.osu.edu/b762/
Dairy cattle	Pennsylvania State University, Michigan State University	http://www.das.psu.edu/dcn/ http://www.ans.msu.edu/community/facilities/dairy_farm.html http://www.dcpah.msu.edu/
Swine	Kansas State University	http://www.oznet.ksu.edu/library/lvstk2/MF2298.pdf
	Michigan State University	http://www.ans.msu.edu/community/facilities/swine_farm.html
	Ohio State University	http://ohioline.osu.edu/b869
	Purdue, Illinois	http://web.aces.uiuc.edu/faq/faq.pdl?project_id=12
Sheep	Virginia Polytechnic Institute	http://www.ext.vt.edu/pubs/sheep/410-853/410-853.html
Humans	Purdue	http://ag.ansc.purdue.edu/sheep/
Clinical nutrition	Tufts University	http://navigator.tufts.edu/
Diagnostics	Ohio State University	http://nssvet.org
	Michigan State University	http://www.dcpah.msu.edu/

Government

Many species	U.S. National Research Council	http://search.nap.edu/nap-cgi/naptitle.cgi?Search=nutrient+requirements
Humans	U.S. government	http://www.nutrition.gov/home/index.php3

(Continued)

questions or feedback. If the site hosts chat rooms or other online discussion areas, it should describe the terms of use for this service. Is the group moderated? If so, by whom and why? Spend time reading the discussion before joining in, in order to feel comfortable with the environment before becoming a participant.

Once satisfied with the credentials of the site, users can grade the evidence (or information) presented for its relevance and validity to the situation at hand and use it to refine the search.

Some of our favorite Web sites are listed in Table 6-2. The criteria used to evaluate these sites were similar to those listed previously and included the following.
- Ease of understanding
- Credibility of the source (e.g., university, individual expert, breed group, food company, zoo, veterinary hospital, individual [expert vs enthusiast])
- Identification of information sources
- Depth (technical level)
- Up-to-date information, evidence of regular revision
- Availability of contact information for further questions
- Presence and quality of links

Table 6-2
Recommended World Wide Web Sites—cont'd

Commercial		
Pet diet evaluation	PetDIETS	http://www.petdiets.com/
Dog and cat nutrition	Cycle Dog Food	http://www.cycledog.com/products.htm
	Friskies	http://www.friskies.com/
	Hill's	http://www.hillspet.com/index.asp?swf=1
	IAMS and Eukanuba	http://www.iams.com/splash /iams_splash_page.jhtml
	Nutro	http://www.nutroproducts.com/
	Pedigree	http://www. pedigree.com
	Purina	http://www.purina.com/home.asp
	Waltham	http://waltham.com/
Exotic pet and bird nutrition		http://zupreem.com
		http://exoticnutrition.com
		http://waltham.com (birds)
Journals		
	American Society for Nutritional Sciences	http://www.nutrition.org/
Organizations		
	Comparative Nutrition Society	http://www.cnsweb.org/
	American College of Veterinary Nutrition	http://www.acvn.org/
Other		
	Quackwatch	http://www.quackwatch.org/
	AltVetMed	http://www.altvetmed.com/
	American Botanical Council	http://herbalgram.org

As the amount of available information increases, continued improvement as wise consumers becomes more important; the ability to find credible information and evaluate its relevance and validity with regard to the needs at hand is a vital skill. Synthesizing information into usable knowledge continues to be a challenge.

EVIDENCE-BASED MEDICINE

The safety and efficacy of nutrients and veterinary foods can be experimentally tested. *Safe* means that the treatment does no harm and that the benefits outweigh the risks. *Efficacious* means that the treatment does what it claims to do—the likely benefit from the therapy when applied in an appropriate patient by a competent practitioner .

Safety and efficacy in patients may be assessed using the principles of evidence-based medicine (EBM). EBM is the conscientious, explicit, and judicious use of current best evidence in making decisions about the care of individual patients. The practice of EBM integrates an individual's clinical expertise with the best currently available clinical research evidence. *Clinical expertise* means the proficiency and judgment acquired through experience and practice (which leads to more effective and efficient diagnosis), and in more thoughtful and compassionate consideration of individual patients' predicaments, rights, and preferences when making clinical decisions about their care. *Current best evidence* means clinically relevant research, especially patient-centered clinical research that documents or examines the safety and efficacy of the treatment. Because new findings frequently become available, the emphasis on currentness helps practitioners avoid reliance on classic studies and evidence learned in school and promotes reliance on up-to-date information available from many electronic resources.

When new research is identified, it is examined to determine what was investigated—the associations between a treatment and an outcome, the efficacy of a treatment, or a therapy's effectiveness. Investigations of associations include uncontrolled observation of clinical phenomena and results of epidemiologic studies. By themselves, such studies cannot identify cause-effect relationships. For example, associations between smoking and lung cancer subsequently were confirmed in controlled studies, whereas those between β-carotene and cancer prevention were not supported when subjected to clinical trials. Efficacy trials are studies in which patients are recruited to determine whether a treatment works under *ideal* circumstances, often a controlled clinical trial. Effectiveness studies are designed to determine whether a treatment works when it is offered to clients that are free to accept or reject it as they might ordinarily do in a primary-care setting.

EBM provides veterinarians a mechanism for systematic and thoughtful evaluation of current research before it is applied in clinical practice. Critical thinking is fostered by comparing and contrasting new information with the generally accepted current standard. The systematic approach identifies pertinent questions regarding the validity, relevance, and strength of the research and helps determine when facts have become outdated (or that they were never really true).

The crucial question posed according to EBM is, "In *my* patients with [the problem of interest], does [the proposed therapy], when compared with standard therapy alone, truly lead to an improved outcome (i.e., is [this therapy] safer or more effective)?" This question contains many important points for consideration. It contains a reminder to ensure that the patient population studied is comparable to the patients seen in the clinician's practice. This may not be the case for university-based studies, results from countries in which feeding practices are different, or animals of different breeds or ages. The question requires comparison of the new therapy with current therapies, which can raise complex issues. For example, if the disorder studied is not a serious problem, and the standard therapy is cheap, safe, and effective, a practitioner might be reluctant to try a new treatment, whereas if the disease is lethal and no standard therapy is available, the inclination to try a proposed treatment might be much greater. This is particularly important in evaluation of treatments for chronic disorders with signs that wax and wane. Because an affected patient usually is presented for care when signs are at their worst, the patient's condition is likely to improve even if nothing is done. This effect is called *regression to the mean* and must be differentiated from any effect of treatment. For some disorders, a clinically significant increase in the time between flare-ups of signs may be more useful than the time required for a flare-up to remit. Caution must be used in interpretation of the statement, "no significant difference occurred." Technically, this statement means, "We did not find a difference, and we are 80%

(or some other percentage) confident that, if a difference truly exists, we would have found it." Unfortunately, the statement often is made when an insufficient number of animals have been studied or because too much variability was present in the animals that were studied. This error, called a *type II error*, can result in mistaken rejection of effective therapies. When investigators report the absence of a significant difference, they also should report their level of confidence that a difference would have been found if it had been present.

Finally, the question focuses attention on outcome rather than on process variables. A treatment that changes a "surrogate" physiologic measurement (e.g., blood urea nitrogen in dogs with kidney disease) without influencing an important clinical outcome such as quality of life, survival time, or cost of care may be of little value, whereas an important clinical outcome may be of interest regardless of its effects on surrogate variables.

When abstracts are read, the following questions may be asked. Application of the EBM criteria may be helpful in evaluation of articles about new nutritional (or other) therapies.

- *Can the results be applied to my patients?* Species, breed, age, sex, and specific disease problems are considered.
- *Are all of the clinically relevant outcomes considered?* Outcome as well as process variables are discussed.
- *Are the likely benefits worth the potential risks and costs?*

If the answer to any of these questions is "no," it may be preferable to spend time reading a more relevant article. If all questions are answered with a "yes," the following additional questions may be asked.

Are the results of the study valid?

- Was the assignment of patients to treatments randomized?
- Were all patients that entered the trial properly accounted for and attributed at its conclusion?
- Was follow-up complete?
- Were patients analyzed in the groups to which they were randomized?
- Were patients, health-care workers, and study personnel "blind" to treatment?
- Were the groups similar at the start of the trial?
- Aside from the experimental intervention, were the groups treated similarly?

What were the results?

- How extensive was the treatment effect?
- How precise was the estimate of the treatment effect?

These criteria, from the 1996 British Medical Journal article entitled "Evidence Based Medicine: What It Is and What It Isn't," are applicable to any proposed treatment, whether complementary or conventional.

In addition to the strength of evidence presented in published articles, information in books or on Web sites can be rated according to the scale presented in Table 6-3.

The grading approach avoids the temptation to reject or embrace a particular result without thoughtful consideration. The fact that a study does not receive an "A" grade does not mean the study is useless; rather, it suggests that more caution be applied if a decision is made to implement the recommendations, more vigilance exercised with regard to different outcomes in treated patients, and more consideration given to new evidence when it becomes available.

Table 6-3
Grading Evidence from Research Studies

Grade	Source of Evidence
A	Metaanalysis of randomized controlled trials
A–	At least one randomized controlled trial
B	Well-designed controlled study without randomization
B–	Other type of well-designed study
C	Nonexperimental study such as comparative, correlational, or case studies
C–	Opinion of experienced expert
D	Unbiased testimonial
F	Manufacturer-provided testimonials, "back-of-magazine" ads, and television "infomercials"

Throughout this book, clinical studies have been cited that were conducted in client-owned animals and the results of which were published in the peer-reviewed medical literature. Reports of such studies are increasing, and the quality of the reports is improving continually. One veterinary serial, *The Veterinary Journal*, and with others expected to follow, subscribes to the Consolidated Standards of Reporting Trials (CONSORT, available at http://www.consort-statement.org), which offers an evidence-based checklist and flow diagram to help improve the quality of reports of randomized controlled trials and proposes a standard method for researchers to report trials. The checklist includes items, based on evidence, that must be addressed in the report; the flow diagram provides readers with a clear picture of the progress of all participants in the trial, from the time they are randomized until the end of their involvement. The intent is to make the clinical research more transparent, so that a user of the data, whether the data are flawed or not, can more appropriately evaluate their validity with regard to the user's purposes.

The EBM approach can enhance the emotional aspects of the practice of medicine. These aspects include practitioners' confidence in their abilities, their compassion and empathy for clients, and their humility with regard to the vast complexity of nature. The questions listed previously for the screening of articles also can be used to assess the "emotional efficacy" of a treatment.

- *Can the results be applied to my patients?* The practitioner's confidence in his or her skills and attitudes, and those of the clients, are taken into consideration.
- *Are all of the clinically relevant outcomes considered?* Ease of use and impact on the quality of life of client and patient are taken into account.
- *Are the likely benefits worth the potential risks and costs?* Whether clients are being asked to do something they really cannot do should be examined.

There are, of course, alternatives to EBM; discussions of some of these have recently been published. Some of the suggested alternatives are presented in the following list. It is interesting to note that these alternatives are based on emotional response rather than evidence.

- Eminence based—the fame, age, and experience of the clinician are substituted for evidence; given the effect of this approach on practitioners, its effect on clients may be substantial

- Vehemence based—"might makes right," or volume does so
- Eloquence based—sartorial elegance and verbal eloquence are powerful substitutes for evidence
- Diffidence based—doing nothing because of a sense of despair may be better than doing something merely because inaction hurts the physician's pride
- Nervousness based—the physician orders as many tests as possible
- Confidence based—an approach restricted to surgeons

Credible veterinary information may be found in scientific research literature obtained through public libraries, university libraries, medical libraries, and online computer services and databases such as Medline. Controlled clinical trials usually provide the best information about the scientific effectiveness of a therapy and should be sought whenever possible. Problems still arise, however, because of the difficulties associated with experimentation, such as biologic variability, small sample size, researcher bias, careless interpretation, and use of anecdotal evidence. To guard against these risks, the following criteria should be considered before any scientific conclusion is accepted.

1. The *strength* of the effect—Was the result obviously clinically relevant or merely "statistically significant"?
2. The *consistency* of the effect—Did the outcome occur in all patients, in a particular group of subjects, or in subjects at a particular stage of disease?
3. The *specificity* of the effect—Was the outcome specific to the disease or more generalized and nonspecific?
4. The *temporality* of the effect—Which came first? This is particularly problematic in studies in which regression to the mean is likely.
5. The *dose-response relationship* of the effect—In nutrition (and other disciplines) dose-response effects may be not linear but more like an inverted U (also called a hormetic response), with improvement occurring when the initially inadequate dose is increased, followed by a plateau range at which no effect of increasing dose is observable, then deterioration as the dose becomes excessive. The shape of this curve is influenced by many factors, particularly species and age.
6. The *biologic plausibility* of the effect—All other things being equal (although they seldom are), the effect should conform to recognized biologic principles, or the principle to which the effect is attributed should be clearly explained.

Because of the importance of the compassionate belief in the value of the therapy on the part of the caregiver and the effect of the placebo response of the patient on the outcome of the treatment, the preferred method of testing a treatment is the prospective, blinded, placebo-controlled trial. Use of this method is particularly important for evaluation of treatments (even for such ubiquitous processes as inflammation) with potentially extensive emotional effects to separate the influence of the therapist from the effect of the therapy; this method has been applied to surgical and chiropractic procedures and to acupuncture.

Used thoughtfully, the EBM approach appears to permit useful refinement of veterinary medicine. It frees practitioners from reliance on outdated information, provides a systematic approach to the daunting "explosion" of information, and offers a grading system for prioritization of that information. It also provides clinicians the opportunity to reflect on and update their practices by providing external criteria for improvement. However, even when this method is used, the results must be evaluated with care. Physicians must remember the adage, "Only half the information in science is correct; unfortunately, no one knows which half."

Through careful consideration of all new treatments with regard to both the scientific and the emotional aspects of clinical medicine, the best possible overall care may be provided to patients.

THE TRANSTHEORETICAL MODEL OF BEHAVIORAL CHANGE AND ITS ROLE IN OBESITY THERAPY

The transtheoretical model (TTM) of behavioral change was developed by James Prochaska and his colleagues to help explain the process by which humans change their behavior. According to Prochaska, the name *transtheoretical* was chosen because the approach was developed from a synthesis of the comparative analysis of 18 major theories of psychotherapy and behavioral change. We have begun to apply TTM to our efforts in obesity therapy. Because obesity therapy is based on changing client behavior, use of this model has helped us to better understand the change process and has provided us with some useful strategies for helping clients. TTM has been used to promote changes in a wide variety of behaviors, as shown in Table 6-4.

The TTM approach is used by the Centers for Disease Control in the United States and by the British health-care system as part of health-promotion efforts. Although not a panacea, the approach provides a useful perspective for consideration of behavioral change.

Table 6-4
Behaviors Changed through Use of the Transtheoretical Model

Behavior or Condition Changed	Desired Change
Alcoholism	Abstinence
Dental hygiene—poor	Brush twice per day and floss each tooth
Delinquency	Acceptable social behavior
Depression	No more than 2 consecutive days of "feeling blue"
Drug abuse	Abstinence
Fat intake	≤30% of kcal/day
Gambling	Abstinence
High-risk sex	Condoms always used
Inactivity	Physical activity for at least 20 minutes three times a week
Mammography screening avoidance	National Cancer Institute guidelines met
Obesity (human)	Less than 20% overweight
Panic attacks	None in any normal situation
Physical abuse	Never hit or be hit by anyone
Physicians' practices	Assist change efforts
Procrastination	Never defer anything that hurts you or others
Radon gas exposure	Test for presence
Smoking	Abstinence
Sun exposure	Sunscreen used

Modified from Prochaska JO, Crawley B: *Changing for good,* New York, 1995, Avon Books.

The TTM describes six stages of change and nine processes that occur as a person passes through the stages. The stages are as follows.

1. Precontemplation (PC)—The person has no intention of adopting (and may not even be thinking about adopting) the recommended behavioral change.
2. Contemplation (C)—The person has formed either an immediate or a long-term intention to make the behavioral change but has not yet begun to make it.
3. Preparation (P)—The person has formed a firm intention to change the behavior in the immediate future and has made some attempt to change it.
4. Action (A)—The person consistently performs the changed behavior, but for less than 6 months.
5. Maintenance (M)—The person enters a period that begins 6 months after a successful behavioral change has occurred and continues to work to prevent relapse.
6. Termination (T)—The person's former behavior has been extinguished and no longer holds appeal.

The nine processes of change that occur during the journey of "stages-of-change" include the following.

1. Consciousness-raising—Learning more about the consequences of the behavior.
2. Helping relationships—Facilitating the process of change and increasing the probability of success.
3. Social liberation—Making changes in the environment to help the client begin and sustain change efforts.
4. Emotional arousal—Experiencing the sudden realization that change is both necessary and possible.
5. Self-reevaluation—Appraising the problem and assessing the situation that may exist once the behavior has been changed.
6. Commitment—Accepting responsibility for change; an acknowledgment by the client that only he or she can take appropriate action; commitment made first privately, then publicly.
7. Rewards—Providing reinforcement during the action stage of the change process.
8. Countering—Substituting healthy responses for unhealthy ones.
9. Environmental control—Remodeling the environment to assist in the change process.

The relationship between the stages and processes of change is illustrated in Figure 6-1.

The stages-of-change perspective recognizes that people are at different levels of readiness for change and may be receptive to different types of interventional messages. A different strategy is called for when helping someone who has no intention of changing a behavior than when helping someone who intends to change but has been unable to act on that intention. Similarly, someone who is trying to change but has not been able to consistently perform the desired behavior requires a different message or strategy than someone who is consistently performing the behavior. The stages-of-change model suggests that behavior is not an "all-or-nothing" phenomenon, that behavioral change can be viewed in terms of a sequence of steps, and that interventions can be tailored to the stage at which an individual is when contact is made with the practitioner.

Although a variety of instruments have been devised to determine the stage of change at which the client is when he or she is encountered in the clinic, the simple tool presented in

Precontemplation	Contemplation	Preparation	Action	Maintenance
Consciousness raising ⟶				
Helping relationships ⟶				
Social liberation ⟶				
	Emotional arousal ⟶			
	Self-reevaluation ⟶			
	Commitment ⟶			
			Reward ⟶	
			Countering ⟶	
			Environmental control ⟶	

Figure 6-1 The relationship between the stages and processes of change.

Table 6-5, which identifies the stage from the answers to a few questions, is usually adequate for our purposes.

Clients in precontemplation about a pet's weight problem may offer a variety of excuses for their lack of concern, which also may help identify this stage (Table 6-6).

These clients are not ready to make the desired change. Research has found that people are more likely to move into contemplation if the benefits of the change are described; focusing on the dangers of not changing and being judgmental about the necessity for change are more likely to create defensiveness, which is counterproductive.

When clients enter the contemplation stage, both the "pros" and the "cons" of changing often increase. This can result in procrastination—"I know I need to change, but. . . ." The risks associated with not changing, as well as the benefits associated with making the change, are explained at this time. The "pros" of change, rather than the "cons," are promoted in order to foster excitement about commitment to the change process.

Miller and Rollnick have described a process called *motivational interviewing*, which helps avoid the process of presenting good arguments for change only to find that clients are in disagreement. Many clients do not ask for help with weight problems; they either are not ready to change (PC stage) or are unsure about changing (C stage). Motivational interviewing is specifically geared toward preparing such people for change. For example, when a problem behavior such as obesity is mentioned, the avoidance of labeling, confrontation, and giving advice reduces the risk of creating defensiveness in the client. Ultimately, clients decide what is best for them and their pets.

The goal for the initial encounter is to encourage clients to explore the pet's problem and possible reasons for concern, at their own pace.

Table 6-5
Stages of Change for Clients

	PC	C	P	A	M	T
No intention to act	✓					
Intention to act within 6 months		✓				
Intention to act within 1 month			✓			
Taking action				✓		
Took action within last 6 months					✓	
Solved problem more than 6 months ago						✓

A, Action; *C*, contemplation; *M*, maintenance; *PC*, precontemplation; *P*, preparation; *T*, termination.

Table 6-6
Excuses for Pet's Obesity

Excuses	Examples
Ignorance	"I didn't realize my pet was fat."
Denial and minimization	"My pet isn't fat."
Rationalization	"Being fat isn't a problem for my pet."
Projection and displacement	"My neighbor is feeding her."
Internalization (demoralization)	"It's hopeless, I can't do anything."

Broaching the subject of a pet's obesity is an important first step. Two simple strategies are to establish rapport and to ask open-ended questions about the pet, at which time the subject of weight can be broached. For example, "Your dog weighs 50 pounds today. Do you recall how much he weighed last time?"

Once the subject has been raised, the goal is to help clients discuss their views regarding the pet's weight and any concerns they have about it. Following is a menu of strategies for attaining this goal, from the least-threatening (PC) to the most-threatening (late C) stage.

1. Ask about the pet's diet and activity in detail.
2. Ask about a typical day.
3. Ask about life-style and stresses. For example, "You say that feeding your pet is a way you relax and unwind; do you find yourself in this situation often?"
4. If the client expresses concerns about the pet's health, ask about the role the client perceives weight may play in these concerns.
5. When a concern is expressed, ask how much that concern bothers the client.
6. Ask about current and past feeding regimens.
7. Provide information, and then ask, "What do you think? Would it be useful to spend a few minutes looking at this whole question of what is the right body condition to maintain?"
8. Ask about concerns directly. This is effective only when the client is ready and willing to talk about the problem. Use an open-ended question such as, "What concerns do you have about your pet's weight?" rather than a closed question such as, "Are you concerned about your pet's weight?"
9. Ask about the next step. "Where do you want to go from here?"

Table 6-7
Decision Results

Aspect of Decision	"Pros"	"Cons"
Consequences to client	Save money on veterinary bills	Begging by pet
	Opportunity to engage in more play and activity with pet	Need to find other pet-related activities
Consequences to pet	Improved health	Food restriction
	Decreased risk of disease	Loss of owner-related activity
Reactions of client	I'll feel better about myself as a pet owner	See myself as stricter with my pet
		I'll be frustrated if I fail
	Proud of healthy pet	I'm not really sure my pet's weight is a health problem

This approach permits the client to engage in some self-evaluation regarding the conditions that have led to the increase in the pet's weight and to consider what it would be like if the pet were returned to its former condition.

Studies have found that for an individual to proceed from precontemplation to contemplation of change, the "pros" of the change must increase, and to proceed from contemplation of to preparation for change, the "cons" of the change must decrease. An example is presented in Table 6-7.

Once the client passes into the preparation phase, the strategy to solve the problem in the action stage must be identified using the following steps.

1. Create a plan of action. Do not let the client leap into action without a plan. The plan itemizes the steps to be taken and sets a date on which the plan will begin. Family, friends, and neighbors are informed of the plan, if appropriate.
2. Encourage continuing self-reevaluation to reaffirm the decision and envision the changed future.
3. Help clients turn away from the behaviors to be changed and make change a top priority.
4. Anticipate anxiety; for some clients, behavioral changes are as stressful as facing a major operation.
5. Confirm the client's commitment (willingness to act and belief in the ability to change).

The client's commitment may be evaluated using the quick self-assessment questionnaire shown in Box 6-1.

The action stage consists of the approximately 6-month period of concerted effort that is required to institute any desired change. During this time a system of rewards may be used to celebrate successes. Countering techniques, such as active diversion, exercise, relaxation, and counter-thinking ("My pet isn't begging for food—he wants attention"), can be used to sustain the effort. Environmental control can also be used to provide positive cues and reminders to the client and individuals in supportive roles.

It has been determined that people can make an effort at sustained change for approximately 6 months. The amount of change (weight loss) that has occurred at the end

Box 6-1
Client Self-Assessment Questionnaire

Fill in the appropriate score. (1, never; 2, seldom; 3, occasionally; 4, often; 5, repeatedly.)
1. ___ I tell myself that if I try hard enough I can change my pet's weight.
2. ___ I make commitments against giving in to my pet's begging.
3. ___ I use willpower to keep from overfeeding my pet.
4. ___ I tell myself I can choose to change or not.
Total the scores. A total greater than 14 suggests a readiness to act; a total less than 14 suggests that more preparation is needed.

of this time may be all the client is capable of (for the present, at least) before entering the maintenance stage. Sustaining the change achieved depends on avoiding (when possible) or planning for "tough times"—holidays, anniversaries, visits from friends or relatives, and other times of stress. Having the client make a list of such times and helping the client evaluate his or her ability to resist temptation under stressful conditions can help in identification of situations for which more planning is needed. Reviewing the reasons for change can help, as can renewing the client's commitment, offering congratulations when accomplishments are made, and exploring new ways of interaction with the pet.

The TTM approach acknowledges that clients often return to problem behaviors; only approximately 20% of people permanently conquer long-standing problems on the first try. They usually do not regress all the way to precontemplation, however, but to contemplation or preparation, from which they can be encouraged to continue efforts at change with the knowledge that this time it will be easier. Some reasons for relapse include the following.

- The costs of change are higher than anticipated in terms of personal time, psychic energy, and so on.
- Insufficient preparation is made for complications and potentially stressful situations.

It is important to reassure clients that a lapse is not a relapse. When they express dismay that they "gave a treat," we reframe the admission as a sign of success (the behavior has been recognized and "nipped in the bud") rather than a sign of failure ("this will never work").

The termination stage signifies loss of attachment to the problem behavior. Time will tell how many clients can be helped to this stage.

Is this model useful in all patients? As appealing as the TTM approach is (to us, at least) for treatment of obesity, prevention still seems a crucial part of health maintenance. For example, clients are taught to feed whatever amount is necessary to maintain a moderate body condition, regardless of the feeding directions on the package label. If the amount becomes distressingly small, a less energy-dense food or a smaller bowl can be recommended; also, dogs should be trained, and cats should be provided opportunities for nondestructive activity.

Success with clients who want (or need) to change is measured in the TTM approach by determining how far along the continuum of change the client has moved. A helpful way of concluding an interview with clients during the change process is to summarize the progress made so far, using personalized comments (e.g., "You've made a lot of progress in the past several weeks"), and reiterating the client's concerns and the changes the client has elected to make. Freedom of choice should be emphasized, as should the practitioner's willingness to provide whatever additional help is desired.

RECOMMENDED READINGS

Bierhaus A, Wolf J, Andrassy M et al: A mechanism converting psychosocial stress into mononuclear cell activation, *Proc Natl Acad Sci U S A* 100:1920, 2003.

Brody H: The placebo response: recent research and implications for family medicine, *J Fam Pract* 49:649, 2000.

Cockcroft P, Holmes M: *Handbook of evidence based veterinary medicine*, Oxford, UK, 2003, Blackwell.

Isaacs D, Fitzgerald D: Seven alternatives to evidence based medicine, *BMJ* 319:1618, 1999.

Miller WR, Rollnick S, Conforti K: *Motivational interviewing: preparing people for change*, ed 2, New York, 2002, Guilford.

Patterson K, Grenny J, McMillan R et al: *Crucial conversations: tools for talking when stakes are high*, New York, 2002, McGraw-Hill.

Prochaska JO, Crawley B: *Changing for good*, New York, 1995, Avon.

Sackett DL, Rosenberg WM, Gray JA et al: Evidence based medicine: what it is and what it isn't, *BMJ* 312:71, 1996.

Sackett DL, Straus SE, Richardson WS et al: *Evidence-based medicine: how to practice and teach EBM*, ed 2, London, 2000, Churchill Livingstone.

Nutrition for Exotic Pets

The basic principals of clinical nutrition presented in this book apply to exotic pets as well as to dogs and cats. With regard to diagnostic and therapeutic interventions, factors related to the animal, to the diet, and to feeding management are as pertinent in exotic pets as they are in more conventional companion animals. The animal-specific factors of species, breed, age, physiologic status, food intake, activity, and body and muscle condition scores can be applied to animals of any species, although the biologic database for many of the exotic species is smaller than that for dogs and cats.

A satisfactory diet for exotic pets must be complete, balanced, digestible, palatable, and safe. Our preference is that prepared complete and balanced foods from reputable manufacturers be used whenever possible, because these foods provide the greatest likelihood that an animal's nutrient needs will be met. Manufactured foods are not the only ones that these pets may be fed, but manufactured diets are associated with a higher probability of success than are diets consisting of homemade recipes, with which fewer people have expertise and experience. Foods for exotic pets are not overseen by the Association of American Feed Control Officials (AAFCO) at the levels that dog and cat foods are; we therefore generally recommend manufacturers with long-term commitment to the business, because such manufacturers seem more likely to conduct research and incorporate the experiences of their customers into their products.

Proper feeding practices for exotic pets depend on the natural history of the species and can be quite variable. We generally prefer that exotic species not be fed on a free-choice basis, because we have found that this type of feeding is more commonly associated with problems. For example, birds fed seed diets (which we do not generally recommend) may sort through the mixture and pick out only a few seeds and may leave seed hulls in the food container, which leads some owners to believe that more food is available than is actually the case.

In the absence of extensive experience with most commercial diets marketed for exotic pets we rely on consultation with colleagues who specialize in the care and treatment of exotic species (e.g., veterinarians or nutritionists in private practice, zoos, teaching hospitals, universities) and others who are credible sources of information.

General criteria for evaluating nutrition-related information on the Internet are presented in Chapter 6 and should be applied to any World Wide Web search conducted on exotic pet husbandry. We believe that a reliable Web site states the information source's credentials, is easy to understand, lists sources of information, is updated with some regularity, provides contact information in the event that additional questions arise, and

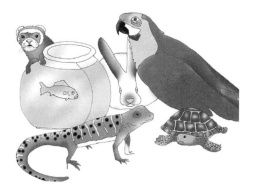

supplies relevant links to other resources. We recently asked veterinary students in our clinical nutrition classes to use these criteria to evaluate some of the more prominent Web sites related to exotic pet nutrition. The critiques provided by these veterinary students are included in Table 7-1, because they are useful examples of Web site evaluations.

Because of the lack of governmental regulation of commercially manufactured diets and nutritional supplements for exotic pets, no standardized criteria are currently available to critically evaluate commercial products. General knowledge of the biology and ethology of the species of interest, combined with consultation with knowledgeable breeders, enthusiasts, or veterinarians specializing in the care of exotic animals, is valuable in differentiating products that may be harmful from those that are helpful for clients and their pets.

Table 7-1

Sample Reviews of World Wide Web Sites Related to Nutrition of Exotic Pets

Site	Comments
General	
www.exoticpetvet.net	This site is maintained by two exotic pet experts, one of them a diplomate of the American Board of Veterinary Practitioners (ABVP) with a specialty in Avian Practice. The site has quite a bit of information on avian, primate, reptile, small animal, and pocket pet health, including nutrition. The experts also provide biographies and describe their practice.
	I chose this site because it contains veterinary information on many species (e.g., primates, avians, pocket pets) and also has links to other pertinent sites. I enjoy the fact that there is a place on this Web site established primarily "for vets to vets." This Web site was established by Dr. Margaret Wissman, a board-certified avian practitioner. She has written books (listed on the site) about iguanas, writes a monthly column in *Bird Talk* magazine, and has written sections for a new avian textbook and a new VCA textbook regarding exotic nutrition.
	This site is dedicated to many issues concerning the raising of exotic animals such as birds, primates, and pocket pets. Although the site does not have the most detailed nutritional information, it does have a lot of useful information regarding the raising of exotic animals. I like the page because it has a detailed description of the authors (one is a diplomate of the ABVP, Avian Practice). My main problems with the site include the facts that few links to further information are available and that no documentation that describes where the authors obtained their information is referenced.
	This Web site is not only very informative, with subject matter that includes nutrition, breeding, and common diseases, but it is also easy to understand. It contains information on birds, primates, reptiles, small animals, and pocket pets, as well as providing a search engine for its site and others like it. The information comes from two credible sources—an avian veterinarian who has written many books and magazine articles on the subject, and a zoologist with 30 years' experience. Anyone may contact them with specific questions, and they add new articles to the site often. All in all, I think this Web site would be a great reference tool for any exotic pet needs.
	This site has easy-to-understand information about how to feed a variety of exotic species. Its owner is a veterinarian. The site is maintained by a Webmaster who may be contacted

(Continued)

Table 7-1

Sample Reviews of World Wide Web Sites Related to Nutrition of Exotic Pets—cont'd

Site	Comments
General—cont'd	for more information. Each section lists the origin of its information as well as additional resources. The main site was the date the site was last updated, and it has several links to other sites.
http://www.exoticnutrition.com/	This site fulfills nearly all the criteria. It is well organized, has an adequate depth of information (with credible links for more in-depth information), is from a reliable source (an exotic pet food company), and lists contact e-mail addresses and telephone numbers. It is easy to use and seems to have pertinent nutritional as well as husbandry information about hedgehogs, prairie dogs, sugar gliders, and other exotic pets.
	I chose this Web site because it contains information on several popular species seen in a small animal practice. As its source is a pet food company, I think it is more reliable than a personal Web site. Also, there are links to other nutritional sites that give information on other species.
	This site is very good because, in addition to giving ideas on food sources, it also gives facts about each animal for which the company makes a product. In addition to feed, the company also has other products for the animals, and if we want to know about a species we need all the facts that we can get regarding the animal's life cycle.
	This Web site sells food for sugar gliders, prairie dogs, hedgehogs, and chinchillas. I chose it because it met the criteria we set in class: it is easy to understand and navigate; the source of information is a pet food manufacturer; and the depth of information is considerable. It has a frequently-asked-questions (FAQ) page for each species and goes into detail regarding the animals' natural diets and what they should be fed as household pets. Each page that describes the food that could be purchased lists the ingredients and the minimum and maximum quantities of nutrients and also describes why certain ingredients are important in the diet. The Web site lists an e-mail and telephone contact and the date of the most recent update.
	The only reservations I have about this Web site are that it may be biased, because the site's sponsor is trying to sell a product, and that if it is listed as a link on a nutritional Web site, people may believe that the nutritional site endorses this brand of food.
http://www.healthypet.com/ index.html	This site has several links, covers the nutritional needs of several species, is easy to understand, and is supported by the American Animal Hospital Association.

http://www.veterinarypartner.com/	This is a general site from the Veterinary Information Network and seems a good starting point. It contains many specific links. It has a current copyright, a general contact, and a contact address for the author of the specific article. There are also message boards and chat rooms, which allow contact with others who have the same interest.
http://www.zupreem.com/	This site features information and diets for zoo animals and a variety of other exotic animals. ZuPreem is a commercial manufacturer of food and is an extension of the Morris Animal Foundation, which in my opinion makes ZuPreem a credible source. The page offers links to other sites and seems to be easily navigable. Also, it lists both a contact phone number and address and welcomes questions from people visiting the site. It looked pretty good to me.
http://www.zeiglerfeed.com/default.asp	This is a great Web site. It is the Web page for Zeigler Brothers, Inc., a company that makes all kinds of foods for zoo animals, pocket pets, and laboratory animals. The site provides a list of all of the food products the company offers, along with information on what animal the diet is best for; the site also provides the protein, fat, and fiber content of the diets. Ways to contact the company are provided, as well as a feedback page for customers.

Birds and Fish

| http://www.waltham.com/ | This site has some very good information concerning birds. It discusses the components of a balanced bird diet, feeding birds in captivity, problems with obesity, and special need feeding (e.g., nesting, growing, molting, aging), and it includes a list of publications for further reading. The information is easy to understand and up-to-date. The site is from a reputable pet food company and includes links and contact information. |

Chinchillas

| http://exoticpets.about.com/cs/chinchillamed/ | I found this site to be the most useful and easiest to navigate. It is managed by a group of private individuals who are experienced in the care and management of chinchillas. They have written a book—*The Joy of Chinchillas*—which is outlined on the site. Some of my reasons for choosing this Web site are the following.
• The authors are experienced, and their opinions pertaining to different methods of feeding and care seem unbiased.
• The site lists common health problems of which chinchilla owners should be aware.
• The site contains a link to private veterinarians (on a state-by-state basis) who have had experience with and are knowledgeable regarding chinchilla care. This list allows owners or other veterinarians to contact or visit a chinchilla-experienced veterinarian in their area. |

(Continued)

Table 7-1

Sample Reviews of World Wide Web Sites Related to Nutrition of Exotic Pets—cont'd

Site	Comments
Chinchillas—cont'd	• The site contains information on how to feed a sick chinchilla, how to mix food, how to switch foods, and how to store food and extensive information on supplements that may be necessary for chinchilla health. • The site contains links to suppliers and vendors.
Ferrets www.texasferret.org/news/ 199607.shtml	This site has regularly updated articles on nutrition, resources, contacts, veterinarians, shelters, legal issues, health, and other topics.
Finches http://www.finchinfo.com/	This Web site on avian nutrition is wonderful. I am interested in finches, so I selected a Web site that has up-to-date, credible, and easy-to-understand information about the nutritional needs of pet finches. I was drawn to the Web site because it offers a variety of information about finches, including information on housing, health, breeding, egg laying, and different species. The nutritional information is very complete. The site contains information about vitamins and minerals (with each listed individually, along with signs of excess and deficiency), meal worms, seeds, fruits, and vegetables. Before I found this site, I had a difficult time finding information specifically about finch nutrition. I thought this site was very informative and fun.
Hedgehogs http://www.gohogwild.net/ghw98/ nutrition.htm	This is a great site for nutritional and feeding information for African pygmy hedgehogs *(Aterlerix albiventris)*. Even though I own a hedgehog, I learned some new things. The main problem I found is the visual display; the site is set up in outline form with some graphs at the end. The site contains a great deal of information, but it was tedious to scroll through it. Otherwise, the site meets most of the criteria: it is from a reliable source (the Wildlife Conservation Society); it contains a date and contact information (although there are no references); it contains a thorough list of what hedgehogs eat in the wild versus what they are fed in captivity and information on captive environments and obesity management. Hedgehogs are hindgut fermenters. They usually are insectivorous in the wild but may also eat some plants. In captivity they are usually fed commercial cat foods or commercial hedgehog food. Their diet should be supplemented with insects three or four times a week for fiber, and the site describes homemade diets with ingredients

that include cottage cheese, fruits, and vegetables. Insects should be given as treats as they can be high in fat.

The site suggests that hedgehogs receive only 70 to 100 kcal/day for basal energy needs. This site does not list the average normal weight for hedgehogs, but I have been told that 500 to 600 g is normal. These animals should be fed on a meal rather than a free-choice basis to prevent obesity, which is a common problem in captivity. This site is one of the more complete sites I found.

Ostriches

http://www.ostrichesonline.com/

This site has a wealth of information about ostriches, including an ostrich "dictionary." The site is a commercial one, and it appears to be run by an ostrich feed company. It allows users to buy many types of feed online, and gives information about each. The site is most likely biased in favor of the site owner's products.

Rabbits

http://carrotcafe.com/

"Pros" of site: Easy-to-understand format; depth of information very good; content includes daily requirements, appropriate diets for different life stages, diets for sick rabbits, description of various forms of food available. The site's source is an enthusiast, with help from a veterinary nutritionist. Contact availability, links to other sources, and FAQ are present, along with information regarding when to see the veterinarian.

"Cons" of site: Number of sources and links is limited. There is no date to indicate how up-to-date the site is.

This site offers a wide range of information, from technical (life-stage nutrient needs) to very basic (definitions of nutrients). It is easy to read. The major flaws are the lack of research articles and date of last update; however, this site is referenced by many other rabbit-related sites for its nutritional content.

Sugar Gliders

http://www.sugarglider.net/

This site has been updated in the last 3 months; has links and sources of information; and is easy to understand. It contains links to scientific articles regarding all aspects of sugar glider husbandry and nutrition. The site also contains an interactive chat room, a list of breeders, and a list of available veterinarians.

Turtles

http://www.healthypet.com/
Library/petcare-47.htm

This site is maintained by the American Animal Hospital Association, and the nutritional information is taken from a reptile-care textbook published by the Association in 1998.

RECOMMENDED READING

Fowler ME, Miller RE, eds: *Zoo and wild animal medicine: current therapy,* Philadelphia, 1999, WB Saunders.

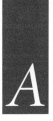

Nutrient Comparison Tables for Commercial Dog Foods

Table A-1
Gestation and Lactation

Diet	Mfg*	Weight (g)	Energy (kcal per can [canned diets] or per cup [dry diets])	Protein (g)	Fat (g)	CHO (g)	Fiber (g)	Ca (mg)	P (mg)	Na (mg)	K (mg)	Mg (mg)	Cl (mg)
Canned													
a/d	HIL	156	197	9.1	6.1	2.9	0.3	209	209	156	191	22	152
p/d	HIL	418	411	6.4	5.9	6.8	0.2	297	240	99	127	27	155
Puppy	HIL	418	519	7.1	5.6	9	0.3	338	234	97	193	32	185
Eukanuba MaxCal	IAM	170	340	7.5	7.1	1.3	0.3	190	150	55	180	13	135
Puppy	IAM	397	600	8.7	6	2.3	1	328	287	130	260	21	260
Dry													
p/d	HIL	99	411	7	5.1	7.7	0.6	398	280	79	161	31	115
Puppy Large Breed	HIL	99	336	8.1	2.9	13.8	0.7	287	229	106	220	29	196
Puppy	HIL	99	375	7.2	4.7	9.9	0.6	355	297	126	176	36	195
Eukanuba MaxCal	IAM	136	634	7.7	5.6	4.4	0.4	258	204	84	295	NA	237
Puppy Large Breed	IAM	90	368	7.5	4.1	10.4	1.5	227	180	92	188	26	201
Puppy	IAM	99	428	6.5	4	NA	0.9	NA	NA	NA	NA	NA	NA
Puppy Lamb and Rice	IAM	97	396	6.3	3.9	NA	1.2	NA	NA	NA	NA	NA	NA
Puppy Chow	PUR	NA	424	7	3.6	10	0.4	300	230	80	140	NA	NA
Puppy Chow Large Breed	PUR	NA	396	7.8	3.6	11.5	0.6	330	260	90	150	NA	NA

Amount per 100 kcal

*Diets listed alphabetically by manufacturer.

CHO, Carbohydrate; HIL, Hill's; IAM, Iams; Mfg, manufacturer; NA, not available; PUR, Purina.

Table A-2
Neonate Milk Replacers

Diet*	Mfg†	Weight (g)	Energy (kcal)	Protein (g)	Fat (g)	CHO (g)	Fiber (g)	Amount per 100 kcal					
								Ca (mg)	P (mg)	Na (mg)	K (mg)	Mg (mg)	Cl (mg)
Just Born Puppy													
Powder	FARNAM	NA	100	6.4	6.7	6	0.1	309	276	98	209	11.3	NA
Nurturall Powder	FARNAM	NA	100	6.3	6.7	5.9	0.06	293	257	101	238	10.7	NA
Mother's Helper													
Liquid	LAMBERT KAY	NA	100	6.1	7.7	3.7	0.4	176	139	59	164	21.4	NA
Mother's Helper													
Powder	LAMBERT KAY	NA	100	6.7	7.8	2.9	0.1	115	151	67	201	9.6	NA
Esbilac Liquid	PETAG	NA	100	6.9	7	4.8	0.3	191	150	86	204	19	NA
Esbilac Powder	PETAG	NA	100	6.6	7.7	3.4	0.06	250	207	55	209	7.4	NA
Milk Substitute	WALTHAM	NA	100	5.9	7	3.1	0	198	162	72	126	14.5	NA

*Feeding directions: Follow package instructions.
†Diets listed alphabetically by manufacturer.
CHO, Carbohydrate; Mfg, manufacturer; NA, not available.

Table A-3
Growing Dogs

Diet*	Mfgt	Weight (g)	Energy (kcal per can [canned diets] or per cup [dry diets])	Amount per 100 kcal									
				Protein (g)	Fat (g)	CHO (g)	Fiber (g)	Ca (mg)	P (mg)	Na (mg)	K (mg)	Mg (mg)	Cl (mg)
Canned													
Science Diet Puppy	HIL	418	519	7.1	5.6	9	0.3	338	234	97	193	32	185
Puppy Formula	IAM	396	600	8.6	6	NA	1	NA	NA	NA	NA	NA	NA
Eukanuba Puppy Growth Formula	IAM	283	418	8.8	6.1	NA	1	NA	NA	NA	NA	NA	NA
Dry													
Cycle Puppy	HEI	99	375	8.1	4.7	9	0.5	421	283	93	270	29	261
Science Diet Puppy	HIL	99	375	7.2	4.7	9.9	0.6	355	297	126	176	36	195
Science Diet Puppy Lamb and Rice	HIL	99	397	6.6	4.6	9.4	0.5	389	268	90	163	22	228
Eukanuba Puppy Weaning Diet	IAM	108	485	7.1	4.7	NA	0.9	NA	NA	NA	NA	NA	NA
Eukanuba Puppy Small Breed	IAM	108	485	7.1	4.7	NA	0.9	NA	NA	NA	NA	NA	NA
Eukanuba Puppy Medium Breed	IAM	108	485	6.8	4.2	NA	0.9	NA	NA	NA	NA	NA	NA
Eukanuba Puppy Lamb and Rice	IAM	94	387	6.6	4.6	NA	1	NA	NA	NA	NA	NA	NA
Original Puppy	IAM	100	428	6.5	4	NA	0.9	NA	NA	NA	NA	NA	NA
Puppy Lamb and Rice	IAM	97	396	6.4	4	NA	1.2	NA	NA	NA	NA	NA	NA

	Mfg												
Puppy Chow	PUR	108	424	7	3.6	10	0.4	300	230	80	140	NA	NA
Puppy Chow Healthy Morsels	PUR	96	346	7.9	3.9	10	0.5	340	340	100	150	NA	NA
ONE Puppy	PUR	96	414	6.7	4.4	8.6	0.4	410	287	93	105	NA	NA
Pro Plan Puppy Chicken and Rice	PUR	111	473	6.8	4.6	9	0.4	326	239	91	119	NA	NA
Pro Plan Puppy Lamb and Rice	PUR	105	444	6.8	4.7	8.5	0.4	317	243	74	124	NA	NA
Pro Plan Puppy Beef and Rice	PUR	108	447	6.9	4.6	8.4	0.4	288	247	85	123	NA	NA
Pro Plan Small Breed Puppy	PUR	112	468	8.9	5.9	8.1	0.4	347	316	108	158	NA	NA

*Feeding directions: Depends on appetite and activity of the puppy and the wishes of the owner.
†Diets listed alphabetically by manufacturer.
CHO, Carbohydrate; HEI, Heinz; HIL, Hill's; IAM, Iams; Mfg, manufacturer; NA, not available; PUR, Purina.

Table A-4
Adult Dogs—Commercial Diets

Diet*	Mfg†	Weight (g)	Energy (kcal per can [canned diets] or per cup [dry diets])	Protein (g)	Fat (g)	CHO (g)	Fiber (g)	Amount per 100 kcal					
								Ca (mg)	P (mg)	Na (mg)	K (mg)	Mg (mg)	Cl (mg)
Canned													
Skippy Chunks in Gravy	HEI	374	299	10.7	4.4	7.1	1	316	246	146	289	44	232
Skippy Select Cuts	HEI	288	374	11.6	3.7	8	0.6	454	318	164	347	39	352
Skippy Tender Strips	HEI	265	373	12	3.7	7.4	1	332	267	168	271	42	267
Science Diet Adult	HIL	418	435	6.2	4.1	13.6	0.2	164	164	72	215	30	206
Eukanuba Adult Maintenance	IAM	284	366	7	4.6	NA	0.8	NA	NA	NA	NA	NA	NA
Eukanuba Adult Large Breed	IAM	284	329	6	4.3	NA	0.9	NA	NA	NA	NA	NA	NA
Eukanuba Adult Lamb and Rice	IAM	284	372	6.9	4.6	NA	0.8	NA	NA	NA	NA	NA	NA
Beef and Rice	IAM	397	506	7.1	4.7	5	0.8	203	170	NA	170	NA	NA
Chicken and Rice	IAM	397	524	6.8	4.5	4.4	0.8	328	250	109	203	NA	NA
Lamb and Rice	IAM	397	521	6.9	4.6	NA	0.8	NA	NA	NA	NA	NA	NA
Turkey and Rice	IAM	397	510	7	4.7	4.9	0.8	257	217	129	225	NA	NA
Liver and Chicken	IAM	397	564	6.3	4.2	4	0.7	189	145	58	124	NA	NA
Dry													
Cycle Adult	HEI	96	338	6.3	3.4	14	0.7	261	173	82	263	39	193
Science Diet Adult	HIL	99	380	5.9	3.8	12.8	0.3	173	159	76	184	30	120
Adult Large Breed	HIL	99	365	6.2	3.8	13.2	0.4	192	165	70	170	33	108
Science Diet Beef and Rice	HIL	91	337	5.8	3.7	13.7	0.4	164	154	73	173	27	112
Science Diet Chicken and Rice	HIL	91	337	5.8	3.7	13.8	0.5	167	148	89	159	28	111

	Mfg												
Science Diet Lamb and Rice	HIL	99	364	5.7	3.9	13.3	0.6	257	184	70	157	26	187
Eukanuba Adult Maintenance Small Bite Formula	IAM	94	405	5.8	3.7	NA	1.2	NA	NA	NA	NA	NA	NA
Eukanuba Adult Maintenance	IAM	94	405	5.8	3.7	9.6	1.2	254	196	127	189	NA	NA
Eukanuba Adult Lamb and Rice	IAM	94	386	5.6	3.4	10.9	1	292	231	143	209	NA	NA
Eukanuba Adult Large Breed	IAM	88	344	5.9	4.1	11.3	1.3	227	202	109	235	NA	NA
Chunks and Mini Chunks	IAM	94	381	6.4	3.7	NA	1	NA	NA	NA	NA	NA	NA
Adult Large Breed	IAM	90	363	5.7	4	11.7	1.2	468	396	165	256	NA	NA
Adult Lamb and Rice	IAM	91	330	6.1	3.3	NA	1.4	NA	NA	NA	NA	NA	NA
Dog Chow	PUR	109	400	5.8	3.2	13	0.5	300	240	70	150	NA	NA
Dog Chow Lamb and Rice	PUR	103	407	5.6	4	11	0.5	250	220	80	140	NA	NA
Dog Chow Little Bites	PUR	108	373	5.9	3.2	13.8	0.6	310	250	80	190	NA	NA
Beneful	PUR	97	341	7.3	3.5	11.5	0.5	340	300	100	150	NA	NA
ONE Beef and Rice	PUR	105	441	6.6	4.4	8.9	0.4	302	216	77	122	NA	NA
ONE Chicken and Rice	PUR	105	449	6.9	4.2	8.9	0.4	287	205	78	122	NA	NA
ONE Lamb and Rice	PUR	105	451	6.5	4.3	9	0.4	315	235	113	115	NA	NA
Pro Plan Chicken and Rice	PUR	105	441	6.3	4.5	10	0.5	302	221	94	125	NA	NA
Pro Plan Turkey and Barley	PUR	99	388	6.5	4.3	10	0.5	268	245	71	130	NA	NA
Pro Plan Lamb and Rice	PUR	98	401	6.5	4.3	11.7	0.6	238	197	90	129	NA	NA
Pro Plan Beef and Rice	PUR	98	390	7	4.3	9.8	0.5	303	230	88	155	NA	NA

*Feeding directions: Amount and frequency should be adjusted as necessary for maintenance of a moderate body condition and normal muscle condition score.

†Diets listed alphabetically by manufacturer.

CHO, Carbohydrate; *HEI*, Heinz; *HIL*, Hill's; *IAM*, Iams; *Mfg*, manufacturer; *NA*, not available; *PUR*, Purina.

Table A-5
Performance Dogs

Diet (all dry)*	Mfg†	Weight (g)	Energy (kcal/cup)	Protein (g)	Fat (g)	CHO (g)	Fiber (g)	Amount per 100 kcal					
								Ca (mg)	P (mg)	Na (mg)	K (mg)	Mg (mg)	Cl (mg)
Active Adult	HIL	122	560	6.1	5.5	7	0.4	188	154	6.9	165	21	177
Eukanuba Adult Premium Performance Formula	IAM	96	430	6.6	4.4	7.1	0.9	264	202	121	176	22	132
Hi Pro	PUR	116	441	6.9	4.1	9.9	0.4	410	260	100	120	28	151
Pro Plan Performance Formula	PUR	108	477	7.2	4.9	7.4	0.3	274	202	86	118	18	189

*Feeding directions: Feed to moderate body condition.
†Diets listed alphabetically by manufacturer.
CHO, Carbohydrate; HIL, Hill's; IAM, Iams; Mfg, manufacturer; PUR, Purina.

Table A-6
Geriatric Dogs

Diet*	Mfg†	Weight (g)	Energy (kcal per can [canned diets] or kcal per cup [dry diets])	Amount per 100 kcal									
				Protein (g)	Fat (g)	CHO (g)	Fiber (g)	Ca (mg)	P (mg)	Na (mg)	K (mg)	Mg (mg)	Cl (mg)
Canned													
Science Diet Senior	HIL	418	415	5.1	3.7	15.9	0.5	191	170	43	202	29	181
Eukanuba Senior Maintenance	IAM	284	320	8	3.1	NA	0.9	NA	NA	NA	NA	NA	NA
Active Maturity Chicken and Rice	IAM	397	459	7.8	3	NA	0.9	NA	NA	NA	NA	NA	NA
Active Maturity Beef and Rice	IAM	397	473	7.6	3	NA	0.8	NA	NA	NA	NA	NA	NA
Dry													
Cycle Senior	HEI	104	350	5.1	2.8	16.6	0.7	299	249	21	382	36	231
Science Diet Senior	HIL	99	363	4.9	3.9	14.4	0.8	171	144	46	149	28	117
Eukanuba Senior Maintenance	IAM	85	341	6.8	3	NA	1	NA	NA	NA	NA	NA	NA
Eukanuba Senior Large Breed	IAM	86	336	6.6	2.6	NA	1	NA	NA	NA	NA	NA	NA
Active Maturity	IAM	85	331	6.2	3.2	NA	1.3	NA	NA	NA	NA	NA	NA
Dog Chow Senior 7+	PUR	105	351	7.7	3.1	12.5	1.5	350	270	90	190	NA	NA
Pro Plan Senior	PUR	103	385	7.7	3.6	10	0.5	292	233	70	153	NA	NA

*Feeding directions: Animals should be meal-fed, and intake observed. Goal is maintenance of moderate body condition without loss of muscle mass.
†Diets listed alphabetically by manufacturer.
CHO, Carbohydrate; HEI, Heinz; HIL, Hill's; IAM, Iams; Mfg, manufacturer; NA, not available; PUR, Purina.

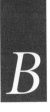

Nutrient Comparison Tables for Commercial Cat Foods

Table B-1

Neonate Milk Replacers

| | | | | | | | Fiber | Amount per 100 kcal | | | | | |
Diet*	Mfg†	Weight (g)	Energy (kcal)	Protein (g)	Fat (g)	CHO (g)	(g)	Ca (mg)	P (mg)	Na (mg)	K (mg)	Mg (mg)	Cl (mg)
Just Born Kitten Powder	FARNAM	NA	100	8.4	4.9	8.3	NA	216	233	115	293	29	NA
Just Born Kitten Liquid	FARNAM	NA	100	8.2	5.5	7	NA	216	233	115	293	29	NA
Whiskas Cat Milk	PEDIGREE	NA	100	6.4	5	10	NA	186	186	138	258	22	NA
Feline Milk Substitute Powder	WALTHAM	NA	100	8.2	5.2	4.4	NA	217	177	98	138	16	NA

*Feeding directions: Follow package instructions.
†Diets listed alphabetically by manufacturer.
CHO, Carbohydrate; *Mfg*, manufacturer; *NA*, not available.

Table B-2
Growing Cats

Diet*	Mfg†	Weight (g)	Energy (kcal per can [canned diets] or per cup [dry diets])	Protein (g)	Fat (g)	CHO (g)	Fiber (g)	Amount per 100 kcal					
								Ca (mg)	P (mg)	Na (mg)	K (mg)	Mg (mg)	Cl (mg)
Canned													
p/d	HIL	156	219	10.1	6.5	2.3	0.1	228	185	107	185	18	185
Kitten Science Diet	HIL	156	230	10.6	7.3	1.6	0.1	298	251	129	183	24	217
Kitten Savory Cuts	HIL	156	207	8	6	2.2	0.3	196	166	98	128	17	136
Kitten	IAM	170	280	8.8	6.4	NA	0.6	NA	NA	NA	NA	20	NA
Dry													
p/d	HIL	122	498	8.1	5.4	7.3	0.2	277	227	92	185	18	212
Kitten Science Diet	HIL	122	510	8.2	5.8	6.3	0.3	269	231	81	166	20	143
Eukanuba Kitten Chicken and Rice	IAM	121	568	7.7	4.7	NA	0.5	NA	NA	NA	NA	20	NA
Kitten	IAM	102	468	7.4	4.8	NA	0.6	NA	NA	NA	NA	21	NA
Kitten Chow	PUR	105	415	10.3	3.8	0.4	6.8	310	280	80	210	30	NA
ONE Kitten Formula	PUR	117	512	9.5	4.4	0.2	5.3	277	249	82	204	27	NA
Pro Plan Kitten Chicken Rice Formula	PUR	99	460	7.7	4.8	0.2	6.1	272	255	82	158	22	NA

*Feeding directions: Feed to moderate body condition.
†Diets listed alphabetically by manufacturer.
CHO, Carbohydrate; HIL, Hill's; IAM, Iams; Mfg, manufacturer; NA, not available; PUR, Purina.

Table B-3
Adult Cats—Commercial Diets

Diet*	Mfg	Weight (g)	Energy (kcal per can [canned diets] or per cup [dry diets])	Protein (g)	Fat (g)	CHO (g)	Fiber (g)	Amount per 100 kcal					
								Ca (mg)	P (mg)	Na (mg)	K (mg)	Mg (mg)	Cl (mg)
Canned													
Science Diet	HIL	156	174	10.3	5.6	5.4	0.6	215	159	94	196	18	196
Adult Savory Cuts	HIL	156	170	9.6	6.2	4.9	0.7	208	180	101	193	14	199
Salmon Formula	IAM	170	219	7.8	5	NA	0.6	NA	NA	NA	NA	20	NA
Turkey and Giblets	IAM	170	234	7.3	4.7	NA	0.6	NA	NA	NA	NA	20	NA
Ocean Fish Formula	IAM	170	232	7.3	4.8	NA	0.6	NA	NA	NA	NA	20	NA
Beef Formula	IAM	170	234	7.3	4.7	NA	0.6	NA	NA	NA	NA	20	NA
Catfish Formula	IAM	170	236	7.2	4.7	NA	0.6	NA	NA	NA	NA	20	NA
Chicken Formula	IAM	170	241	7	4.6	NA	0.6	NA	NA	NA	NA	20	NA
Lamb and Rice	IAM	170	248	6.7	4.5	NA	0.5	NA	NA	NA	NA	20	NA
Dry													
ONE Salmon and Tuna	PUR	102	381	9.1	3.4	7.8	0.4	374	291	121	222	30	NA
Cat Chow	PUR	102	394	8.3	3.3	9.6	0.4	310	320	70	190	30	NA
Meow Mix	PUR	95	360	8.1	2.1	9.6	0.2	320	290	100	210	30	210
Pro Plan Turkey and Barley	PUR	106	431	8	4.4	8.8	0.2	400	344	44	174	27	NA
Adult Recipes Science Diet	HIL	122	496	7.8	5.2	8.5	0.3	209	167	71	156	15	162
Pro Plan Salmon and Rice	PUR	96	406	7.7	3.6	8.5	0.3	245	238	57	165	19	NA
Pro Plan Beef and Rice	PUR	96	405	7.4	4	8.1	0.3	288	253	54	168	19	NA
Eukanuba Lamb and Rice	IAM	114	533	7.3	4.5	NA	0.5	NA	NA	NA	NA	20	NA

	Mfg												
Eukanuba Chicken and Rice	IAM	114	536	7.2	4.5	NA	0.5	NA	NA	NA	21	NA	NA
Original Adult	IAM	97	433	7.1	4.7	NA	0.7	NA	NA	NA	20	NA	NA
Ocean Fish and Rice	IAM	102	459	7.1	4.7	NA	0.7	NA	NA	NA	20	NA	NA
Lamb and Rice	IAM	102	461	7.1	4.7	NA	0.7	NA	NA	NA	20	NA	NA

*Feeding directions: Feed to moderate body condition. Diets listed in decreasing order of grams of protein per 100 kcal.
CHO, Carbohydrate; *HIL*, Hill's; *IAM*, Iams; *Mfg*, manufacturer; *NA*, not available; *PUR*, Purina.

Table B-4
Geriatric Cats

Diet*	Mfg†	Weight (g)	Energy (kcal per can [canned diets] or per cup [dry diets])	Protein (g)	Fat (g)	CHO (g)	Fiber (g)	Amount per 100 kcal					
								Ca (mg)	P (mg)	Na (mg)	K (mg)	Mg (mg)	Cl (mg)
Canned													
Science Diet Senior	HIL	156	162	9.7	4.9	7.4	1.1	183	144	87	183	18	154
Senior Savory Cuts	HIL	156	150	9.6	5.8	5.4	1.1	219	177	115	198	17	198
Active Maturity Chicken and Rice	IAM	170	204	9.2	6.3	NA	0.8	NA	NA	NA	NA	20	NA
Active Maturity Fish and Rice	IAM	170	196	9.6	6.5	NA	0.9	NA	NA	NA	NA	20	NA
Dry													
Science Diet Senior	HIL	99	386	8.1	4.7	8.8	0.5	207	164	72	210	19	197
Active Maturity	IAM	91	373	7.8	4	NA	0.7	NA	NA	NA	NA	20	NA
Active Maturity Hairball	IAM	95	365	8.3	4.3	NA	1.7	NA	NA	NA	NA	30	NA
Senior Cat Chow	PUR	110	400	9.9	2.5	10.7	0.5	346	292	88	240	30	NA
Pro Plan Senior Cat Formula	PUR	108	464	8.4	3.8	6.5	0.3	298	282	93	186	NA	NA

*Feeding directions: Feed to moderate body condition.
†Diets listed alphabetically by manufacturer.
CHO, Carbohydrate; HIL, Hill's; IAM, Iams; Mfg, manufacturer; NA, not available; PUR, Purina.

Diet History Sheet

DIETARY HISTORY EVALUATION FORM

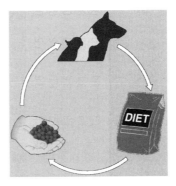

Date: _____   Reason for today's visit: _____
Weight (lb): _____   Body condition score (1-5)_____
Current_____ Usual_____
History taken by: _____

I. Pet Information
Pet name: _____   Species:_____
Breed: _____   Age: _____   Sex: _____
Spayed or neutered? _____
Pet's activity level (type, duration, frequency): _____
_____
Current or past diseases or problems: _____
_____
Current medications: _____
_____
Most recent thyroid level check: _____
How is pet's appetite? _____
Estimated energy needs (see chart): _____

187

II. Diet Information

The following descriptions should be sufficiently specific that a member of the practice could go to a store and purchase the food described.

Food Fed (Brand Name; Dry or Canned?)	How Much Is Fed? (What Is the Size of the Cup or Can Used?)	How Often Is the Food Fed? (Is It Fed on a Free-Choice Basis? How Many Meals per Day?)	Calories per Day
Usual			
Recent (since when?)			
			Total calories per day: _____

What Type of Treats or Table Food Is Fed Each Day? What Is Brand Name of Treat or Special Food?	How Much?	How Often?	Calories Per Day
Pet treats: Size S, M, L, XL			
Rawhides, pig ears, etc.			
Table food (be specific):			
Breakfast			
Lunch			
Dinner			
Between meals			
Food covering medication			
Additives to pet food for flavoring (e.g., gravy, broth)			
Vitamins or supplements			
			Total calories per day: _____

III. Owner and Environmental Information

Who feeds the animal? _____

On average, how many hours a day is the pet home alone? _____

How many adults and children in the household? _____

How many pets in the household? _____

What types of pets? _____

Where is the pet fed? _____

Does the animal have access to other pets' food? _____

Is there competition for food? _____

Is more than one animal fed out of each feeding dish? _____

Is the animal prone to getting into the trash? _____

Is the animal contained in a yard or does it have access to the neighborhood? _____

_____

How frequently is the animal boarded or in the care of someone else? _____

IV. Current Protein Intake

Minimum requirements

Dogs: 2 g per kilogram (lean body mass)

Cats: 4 g per kilogram (lean body mass)

Protein evaluation

1. Calculate protein needs of animal by multiplying minimum protein requirement by the animal's lean body mass.

2. Using information in dietary history, calculate how much protein the animal is currently taking in per day (most food product keys give protein content in grams per 100 kcal).

3. Evaluate protein status and consider a diet with more protein if needed.

    Pet's minimum protein requirement: _____ g/day

    Current protein intake: _____ g/day

    Action taken: _____

_____

    Comments: _____

_____

_____

_____

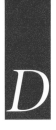

Food Transition Sheet

Making a change to a new pet food may not seem easy or convenient at first, but it can often improve a pet's health and quality of life. To help owners and pets through this process, we offer the following suggestions, collected from clients who have successfully made the change.

ADVICE CONCERNING THE PET

1. Before the pet's diet is changed, the pet should be at home, feeling better, and eating its usual diet normally. If the pet has food available all the time and refuses the new diet, the feeding schedule may be changed to meal-feeding, with food left out for only 1 hour at each feeding time.
2. A simple way to begin making the change is to offer the new food in the pet's usual feeding bowl, which is placed next to another bowl that contains the old diet. If the foods are put in similar bowls, the change may be easier. If the pet eats the new diet readily, then the old food is removed. If the pet does not eat the new diet after an hour, it is removed until the next feeding time. At the next feeding time the process is repeated; fresh new food is always provided. Once the new diet has become familiar to the pet (usually in 1 or 2 days), the animal should start eating it readily. When this occurs, the amount of the old diet offered is decreased by a small amount (approximately 25%) each day until the change is complete. If this strategy is used, the change should be completed over a period of 1 to 2 weeks.
3. If necessary, small quantities (less than a tablespoon per cup or can) of the pet's favorite food or meat or fish juice can be mixed with the new food initially to make it more appealing. Owners who want to try other flavors should check with the veterinarian first.
4. The pet should be fed in a quiet environment where it will not be distracted.
5. The veterinarian will provide advice regarding the minimum amount of food the pet should eat each day. If the pet does not eat all its food every day, this may be normal. A weight loss of up to 10% of the pet's body weight is not a cause for concern during the period of transition.
6. A variety of foods are available that may help the pet. Owners should not hesitate to ask the veterinarian to recommend a different food if the pet will not eat after the previous steps have been taken.

ADVICE CONCERNING THE OWNER

1. The change process should be started when the owner has as few "outside distractions" as possible so that the owner can monitor the process.

2. Owners should plan where the new food will be bought (the veterinary team can help), where in the house it will be stored, how the empty cans will be discarded, and so on, before the change process is initiated. A few minutes of thoughtful planning of the new routine may save hours of frustration later.

3. If the owner enjoys interacting with the pet during feeding time, the veterinary team can suggest some alternative activities, such as play, teaching tricks, and walking. Such activities also can be used to distract the pet if it seems to beg for food. When pets beg, often what they really want is the owner's attention, and they would be just as satisfied with other forms of interaction as with food.

4. The importance of the dietary change should be explained to other members of the household; the veterinarian can help the owner with this.

Detailed Feeding Directions for Prevention of Nutrition-Related Developmental Orthopedic Disease

1. The diet fed (brand name, form [canned, dry, semimoist], product name) and the daily amount consumed by the dog are determined.
2. A body condition score (BCS) is assigned using a 1 to 5 scale, where 1 is cachexic, 3 is moderate, and 5 is obese.
3. If the BCS is greater than 3, daily food intake is reduced by approximately 10%, and this amount is fed until the dog has reached a BCS of 2 or 3.
4. Once the desired body condition of 2 or 3 is attained, food intake is increased only enough to sustain this body condition until the patient is completely grown. If the amount fed declines to a level that concerns the owner, a food of lower caloric density that is complete and balanced for growth (or all life stages), based on feeding trials conducted according to protocols approved by the Association of American Feed Control Officials, may be substituted on an equal-energy basis.
5. Manufacturers' feeding recommendations are used as a starting point if the animal already has a BCS of 2, but the amount fed should be decreased as described in step 3 as needed. Because of the variability in growth rates and activity levels among dogs, they should be fed whatever amount is necessary to maintain a BCS of 2 during the growth period. After adult stature is achieved, the BCS may be allowed to rise to 3 if the owner so desires.
6. A feeding frequency that is appropriate for the circumstances of the owner, from feeding once daily to feeding on a free-choice basis, should be suggested.
7. If these guidelines are followed, supplementation of any kind in excess of that already present in pet foods is unnecessary.
8. Fresh, clean water must be available at all times.
9. The puppy may be switched to a recommended adult food at 6 months of age (or earlier depending on the nutritional claim), or at suture removal for animals that undergo neutering procedures after 3 months of age.
10. Following these recommendations should minimize the risk of nutrition-related developmental orthopedic disease. Clients should be aware that genetic peculiarities and trauma can also cause developmental orthopedic disease.

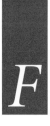

Protein Calculation Sheet

CURRENT PROTEIN INTAKE

Minimum Requirements

Dogs: 2 g of protein per kilogram (lean body mass)
Cats: 4 g of protein per kilogram (lean body mass)

PROTEIN EVALUATION

1. Calculate protein needs of an animal by multiplying minimum protein requirement by the animal's lean body mass.
2. Using information in the dietary history, calculate how much protein the animal is currently taking in per day (most food product keys give protein content in grams per 100 kcal).
3. Evaluate protein status and consider a diet with more protein if needed.
   a. Pet's minimum protein requirement: _____ grams per day
   b. Current protein intake: _____ grams per day
   c. Action taken: _____

Enrichment Recommendations for Indoor Cats

In 2001 the Executive Board of the American Veterinary Medical Association (AVMA) announced that the AVMA "strongly encourages owners of domestic cats in urban and suburban areas to keep them indoors." The Board concluded that "[f]ree-roaming cats are in danger of injury or death caused by vehicles, attacks by other animals, human cruelty, poisons, traps, and disease. They also have increased potential to transmit or serve as reservoirs for some zoonoses." Indoor cats also appear to be at increased risk for some disorders, including behavioral problems, dental disease, endocrine disease, idiopathic cystitis, and urolithiasis. Because these diseases can be influenced by the cat's perception of threat, reduction of perception of threat by environmental enrichment seems appropriate as adjunctive therapy for many of the common feline disorders. As zoo veterinarians have experienced, efforts to enrich the indoor environment of cats should yield important health benefits to cats.

A recently published list of requirements for overall welfare includes availability of food, water, and rest areas; opportunity for social contact, reproduction, locomotion, play and stretching, exploration, body care (grooming, thermoregulation, comfort seeking, evacuation, and territorialism); and reactivity (predictability and controllability, self-protection, ability to avoid danger and aggression). The consensus of experts in cat behavior seems to be that cats benefit from appropriate access to resources, control of interactions with owners, and a tolerable intensity of conflict. The environment of indoor pet cats might be improved through an assessment of their circumstances and improvement of conditions found wanting. "Opportunities for reproduction" was omitted because many indoor-housed cats are neutered (this aspect could be considered for intact animals), and "reactivity" was incorporated under other headings.

For cats with a disease that might be aggravated by an enhanced perception of threat, consideration of many aspects of the environment seems preferable to confining the focus to the area most obviously related to the problem (e.g., the litter box of cats with a urinary problem or the diet of obese cats). We also have found it beneficial to institute environmental modifications slowly, one at a time, and in such a way that the cat can express its like or dislike for the change.

Based on their natural history, cats may prefer to eat, drink, and eliminate privately in a quiet location in which they will not be startled by other animals, sudden movement, or the activity of an air duct or appliance that may begin operation unexpectedly and from which they can perceive an escape route if threatened. When the type or presentation of food, water, or litter is changed, the offering of choices in separate, adjacent containers rather than replacement of the usual offering with a new one permits cats to express their preferences. Play and feeding behaviors mimic predatory activities for cats. These may be simulated by hiding small amounts of food around the house or by putting dry food in a container from which the cat has to extract individual pieces or that the cat must move for the food pieces to be released, if such interventions appear to appeal to the cat. Cats also seem to have preferences for water that can be investigated. Consideration may be given to freshness, taste, and movement (water fountains, dripping faucets, or water pumped into a bowl by an aquarium pump) and to the shape of container (some cats seem to resent having their vibrissae touch the sides of the container while they are drinking). Food and water bowls should be cleaned regularly unless individual preference suggests otherwise.

Cats interact with both the physical structures and the other animals, including humans, in their environment. The physical environment should include opportunities for climbing, scratching, hiding, and resting. Cats seem to prefer to monitor their surroundings from elevated vantage points; provision of climbing frames, hammocks, platforms, raised walkways, shelves, or window seats has been recommended. Playing a radio or television to habituate cats to sudden changes in sound and human voices also has been recommended, and videotapes that provide visual stimulation are available.

Some cats may prefer to be petted and groomed, whereas others may prefer play interactions with owners. The play interactions with cats may include lures, laser pointers, or teaching behaviors. Cats also may enjoy playing with toys, particularly those that are small, that move, and that mimic prey characteristics. These can be divided into those that mimic birds (feathered toys on strings), small mammals, or insects (some cats enjoy chasing tossed pellets of dry food). For cats that prefer novelty, a variety of toys should be provided and rotated or replaced regularly.

In multicat houses, cats interact with one another. Because cats housed in groups do not appear to develop the dominance hierarchies or pack communication strategies many other species do, they attempt to circumvent antagonistic encounters by avoiding others or decreasing their activity. Unrelated cats housed together in groups appear to spend less time interacting with cohabitants than related ones do. These cats may strongly prefer to have their own separate set of resources (food, water, litter box, and resting area) to avoid competition for resources and unwanted interactions. Published guidelines for introducing new cats into a home are available and may be recommended to clients who are adding cats to the household.

Preferences regarding litter type have been documented in individual cats, and cats with a history of lower urinary tract problems seem to prefer unscented, clumping litter. Litter box size and whether the box is open or covered also may be important to some cats. Some cats seem quite sensitive to dirty litter boxes.

Veterinary behaviorists report that indoor cats are overrepresented among cats presented to pet behavior counselors with behavioral problems, most of which are related to improper housing conditions. Moreover, epidemiologic evidence suggests that indoor housing is a risk factor for some common feline diseases. Risk factors, however, must be kept in perspective. Indoor housing is likely to interact in complex ways with other factors. These factors might include unidentified microorganisms or predispositions in some cats. What these predispositions might be remains to be determined, but the breed predispositions found in epidemiologic studies of some problems suggest they may be partially genetically determined. Cats have some basic needs that result from their heritage as solitary hunters of small prey. They seem to prefer to have their own space, to feel as though they are "in control" of their surroundings, and to have choices when changes are made. If these needs are not met, some cats may feel stressed. This may add to the stress caused by disease, making it harder for the cat's condition to return to normal. Unfortunately, for any particular cat we cannot predict what factors, if any, might affect the animal or which factors are the most important. To help identify the aspects of a cat's basic needs that might be improved, we have described what "ideal" housing might include. Most cats do not need such an environment to be happy, but making the house more "cat friendly" might help some cats cope with some kinds of disease problems. Owners may look over the following resource checklist, think about the home from the cat's point of view, and check off the items that accurately describe the cat's current housing circumstances.

	Yes	No
Food and Water Each cat has its own food and water bowl in a convenient location that provides some privacy while the cat eats or drinks, and an escape route.		
Bowls are situated such that another animal cannot sneak up on the cat while it eats.		
Bowls are situated away from appliances or air ducts that could come on unexpectedly while the cat eats or drinks.		
Food and water are kept fresh (daily).		
Bowls are washed regularly (at least weekly) with a mild detergent.		
The brand or type of food purchased is changed infrequently (less than monthly).		
If a new food is offered, it is put in a separate dish next to the familiar food so the cat can choose to eat it if it wants to.		
Rest Each cat has its own resting area in a convenient location that still provides some privacy.		
Resting areas are situated such that another animal cannot sneak up on the cat while it rests.		
Resting areas are situated away from appliances or air ducts that could come on unexpectedly while the cat rests.		
If a new bed is provided, it is placed next to the familiar bed so the cat can choose to use it if it wants to.		
Movement Each cat has the opportunity to move around the environment freely; explore, climb, stretch, and play if it chooses to.		

(Continued)

	Yes	No
Social Contact		
Each cat has the opportunity to engage in play with other animals or the owner if it chooses to.		
Body Care		
Scratching posts are provided.		
Each cat has the opportunity to move to a warmer or cooler area if it chooses to.		
Each cat has a hiding area where it can get away from threats if it chooses to.		
Each cat has its own space that it can use if it chooses to.		
Each cat has its own litter box in a convenient, well-ventilated location that gives the cat some privacy and an escape route.		
Boxes are located on more than one level in multilevel houses.		
Boxes are situated so another animal cannot sneak up on the cat while it uses them.		
Boxes are situated away from appliances or air ducts that could come on unexpectedly while the cat uses them.		
The litter is kept clean and is scooped as soon after use as possible (just as the toilet is flushed after each use), at least daily.		
Boxes are washed regularly (at least weekly) with a mild detergent (such as dishwashing liquid) rather than strongly scented cleaners.		
Unscented, clumping litter is used.		
The brand or type of litter purchased is changed infrequently (less than monthly).		
If a new type of litter is offered, it is put in a separate box so the cat can choose to use it if it wants to.		

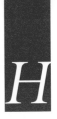

Veterinary Diets for Dogs

Table H-1
Novel Protein Diets

	Marketed for Use in Patients with	Avoid Feeding to Patients with	Nutrient Modifications	Commercial Substitutions
	Dermatitis caused by food allergy; inflammatory bowel disease		Protein to which the patient has not been exposed	Any containing a protein that is novel to the patient

| | | | Energy (kcal per can [canned diets] or per cup [dry diets]) | Amount per 100 kcal | | | | | | | | | |
Diet*	Mfg†	Weight (g)		Protein (g)	Fat (g)	CHO (g)	Fiber (g)	Ca (mg)	P (mg)	Na (mg)	K (mg)	Mg (mg)	Cl (mg)
Canned													
Average values‡				8.5	5.5	6.5	0.4	330	260	230	160	23	220
d/d—Lamb	HIL	418	582	3.2	5.7	10.3	0.8	108	65	72	115	9	180
d/d—Whitefish	HIL	418	582	3.9	4.5	14.8	1	163	90	90	172	12	271
Eukanuba Response Catfish and Potato	IAM	397	502	8	6.7	5.8	0.3	293	206	158	491	20	253
Eukanuba Adult Lamb and Rice	IAM	283	372	6.9	4.6	4.2	0.8	210	190	140	150	20	110
Lamb and Rice	IAM	397	521	6.9	4.6	4.2	0.8	220	160	90	180	10	110
Rabbit and Potato	IVD	397	389	7	5.2	9.3	0.6	392	384	213	264	19	NA
Whitefish and Potato	IVD	397	401	6.6	4.1	9.4	0.5	248	233	213	318	26	NA
Venison and Potato	IVD	397	536	5.3	5.5	8.8	0.2	244	170	119	141	22	NA
Duck and Potato	IVD	397	468	4.9	6.2	8.5	1	161	167	71	216	14	NA
Selected Protein—Lamb and Rice	WAL	374	371	9.1	5.7	8.9	0.7	404	333	44	182	40	303

Dry

	Mfg												
Average values‡				6.5	3.5	12	0.8	340	250	135	140	30	170
d/d—Duck, egg, or salmon (average)	HIL	99	375	4.1	3.6	15.2	0.4	155	105	71	163	15	235
z/d—Low allergen	HIL	99	363	5.1	3.9	13.4	1	160	133	100	309	22	171
z/d Ultra—Allergen Free	HIL	71	261	4.3	3.4	15	0.7	166	126	75	158	13	227
Eukanuba Response—Herring and Potato	IAM	74	301	5.5	3.1	11.6	0.5	238	216	127	370	30	255
Eukanuba Response—Kangaroo and Oats	IAM	91	381	4.9	3.6	12	0.7	161	133	118	153	40	240
Duck and Potato	IVD	98	312	7.1	3.4	15.5	0.7	357	305	104	312	29	NA
Rabbit and Potato	IVD	96	344	6.1	3.2	14.4	0.6	301	321	54	292	28	NA
Venison and Potato	IVD	98	343	6.5	3.1	13.8	0.9	311	321	72	352	34	NA
Whitefish and Potato	IVD	97	341	6.1	3.4	14.3	0.4	292	327	103	297	31	NA
HA Formula—Soy	PUR	83	302	5.3	2.6	14.8	0.4	350	260	60	170	30	170
ONE—Lamb and Rice	PUR	106	451	6.5	4.3	9	0.4	315	235	113	115	30	200
Pro Plan—Lamb and Rice	PUR	97	401	6.5	4.3	11.7	0.6	238	197	90	129	30	200
LA Formula—Salmon	PUR	100	394	7.1	4.2	11.3	0.5	450	270	60	180	40	160
Select Protein Catfish and Rice	WAL	81	266	7.2	2.8	14.3	1.3	582	379	124	215	30	364

*Feeding directions: Once a diagnosis of food allergy is made and a diet to which the patient has no reaction is found, it is important that the owner understand that the patient should not be given any foods, supplements, or treats that may contain provocative antigens.

†Diets listed alphabetically by manufacturer.

‡Average values for commercial diets of healthy pets.

CHO, Carbohydrate; HIL, Hill's; IAM, Iams; IVD, Heinz; Mfg, manufacturer; NA, not available; PUR, Purina; WAL, Waltham.

Table H-2
Nutrient-Dense Diets

	Marketed for Use in Patients with	Avoid Feeding to Patients with	Nutrient Modifications (Varies with Diet)	Commercial Substitutions
	Increased nutrient needs; gastric volume restriction; dogs with diarrhea	Decreased nutrient needs	Increased nutrient density	High-protein, high-fat canned dog foods; meat-containing baby foods

| | | | Energy (kcal per can [canned diets] or per cup [dry diets]) | Amount per 100 kcal | | | | | | | | | |
Diet*†	Mfg	Weight (g)		Protein (g)	Fat (g)	CHO (g)	Fiber (g)	Ca (mg)	P (mg)	Na (mg)	K (mg)	Mg (mg)	Cl (mg)
Canned													
Average values‡				8.5	5.5	6.5	0.4	330	260	230	160	23	220
p/d	HIL	418	591	6.4	5.9	6.8	0.2	297	240	99	127	27	155
Eukanuba Maximum Calorie	IAM	170	340	7.5	7.1	1.3	0.3	190	150	55	180	13	135
Clinicare	ABB	246	237	5.7	6.5	7.1	NA	177	135	58	177	13	104
CV Formula (Feline)	PUR	156	223	8.7	5.5	4.7	0.2	250	190	50	270	20	220
a/d	HIL	156	197	9.1	6.1	2.9	0.3	209	209	156	191	22	152
Chicken Baby Food	HEI	71	84	NA	NA	NA	NA	NA	NA	NA	NA	NA	NA
Dry													
Average values‡				6.5	3.5	12	0.8	340	250	135	140	30	170
Eukanuba Maximum Calorie	IAM	123	634	7.7	5.6	4.4	0.4	258	204	84	295	NA	237
p/d	HIL	122	411	7	5.1	7.7	0.6	398	280	79	161	31	115

*Feeding directions: Consider usual diet when choosing dry or canned form. Feed favorite foods if risk of learned aversion is present. Feed small, frequent meals if appetite is poor. Monitor food intake. If intake is less than recommended in "Energy needs of sedentary dogs and cats," see the discussion of treatment of inappetence in the Critical Care section of Chapter 5.
†Diets listed in order of decreasing energy.
‡Average values for commercial diets of healthy pets.
ABB, Abbot Laboratories; CHO, carbohydrate; HEI, Heinz ; HIL, Hill's; IAM, Iams; Mfg, manufacturer; NA, not available; PUR, Purina.

Table H-3
Dental Diets

Diet	Mfg	Weight (g)	Energy (kcal per cup)	Protein (g)	Fat (g)	CHO (g)	Fiber (g)	Ca (mg)	P (mg)	Na (mg)	K (mg)	Mg (mg)	Cl (mg)
												Amount per 100 kcal	
Canine t/d	HIL	68	257	4	3.9	12.9	2.5	135	98	50	154	18	151

CHO, Carbohydrate; *HIL*, Hill's; *Mfg*, manufacturer.

Table H-4

Modified Fiber Diets

Diet*†	Mfg	Weight (g)	Energy (kcal per can [canned diets] or per cup [dry diets])	Amount per 100 kcal									
				Protein (g)	Fat (g)	CH (g)	Fiber (g)	Ca (mg)	P (mg)	Na (mg)	K (mg)	Mg (mg)	Cl (mg)
Canned													
Average values‡				8.5	5.5	6.5	0.4	330	260	230	160	23	220
OM Formula	PUR	354	189	17.8	3.4	8.8	7.7	470	430	110	430	NA	210
r/d	HIL	404	292	8.5	2.8	12.7	7.3	221	180	83	277	47	166
w/d	HIL	418	330	5.3	3.8	15.3	3.6	180	157	79	180	25	213
Dry													
Average values‡				6.5	3.5	12	0.8	340	250	135	140	30	170
r/d	HIL	77	205	8.4	2.9	13	7.7	207	178	104	285	48	141
w/d	HIL	84	226	5.8	2.7	15.3	5.4	194	157	67	221	29	164
OM Formula	PUR	128	276	10.3	2.1	14	3.4	470	470	70	270	NA	100
DCO	PUR	133	320	6.9	3.4	13	2.1	330	250	90	190	30	220
High Fiber	WAL	NA	227	6.2	2.5	16.4	1.5	380	420	80	280	46	290
Eukanuba Optimum Weight Control	IAM	77	253	8.1	2.2	14.9	0.8	314	246	304	178	NA	369

*Feeding directions: Fiber can be purchased separately and added (gradually, until effective) to the patient's current diet; some examples are given in the table below. Recommended dosages vary widely; we recommend starting with 1 tablespoon per cup or can of food and increasing the dosage until the desired clinical effect is achieved. Clients should be told that the increase in fecal volume and frequency that results from increased consumption of bulking fiber is the intended effect.

†Diets listed by fiber content (grams per 100 kcal) in decreasing order.

‡Average values for commercial diets of healthy pets

CHO, Carbohydrate; EUK, Eukanuba; HIL, Hill's; Mfg, manufacturer; NA, not available; PUR, Purina; WAL, Waltham.

Food	Amount per Tablespoon (g)	Total Fiber	Insoluble	Soluble
Wheat bran	5.3	2.7	2.3	0.3
100% Bran cereal	6.4	1.8	1.6	0.2
All-Bran cereal	5	1.4	1.2	0.2
Oat bran	6.7	1	0.5	0.5
Metamucil	5.8	3.4	0.7	2.7
Canned pumpkin	0.6	5*	N/A	N/A

*5 g in each half cup; 4 servings per 16-ounce can of Libby's canned pumpkin (Nestlé).

Table H-5
Reduced-Fat Diets

Diet*	Mfg	Weight (g)	Energy (kcal per can [canned diets] or per cup [dry diets])	Amount per 100 kcal									
				Protein (g)	Fat (g)	CHO (g)	Fiber (g)	Ca (mg)	P (mg)	Na (mg)	K (mg)	Mg (mg)	Cl (mg)
Canned													
Average values†				8.5	5.5	6.5	0.4	330	260	230	160	23	220
Eukanuba Low-Residue	IAM	397	447	7.8	4.7	7	0.5	193	179	158	212	NA	215
Reduced Fat	IAM	283	338	5.9	4.6	6.5	0.8	230	190	130	260	30	240
EN	PUR	354	424	7.6	3.4	12.1	0.2	220	130	90	150	NA	190
i/d	HIL	418	548	5.8	3.1	11.7	0.2	221	183	99	206	19	275
Low Fat	WAL	385	375	9.1	1.7	15.8	0.4	470	350	200	270	25	300
Dry													
Average values†				6.5	3.5	12	0.8	340	250	135	140	30	170
Eukanuba Low Residue Puppy	IAM	85	435	6.7	4.5	7.2	0.4	241	188	84	157	NA	170
i/d	HIL	99	379	6.3	3.2	12.5	0.3	270	197	109	221	22	262
EN	PUR	122	397	6.1	2.8	13.1	0.3	330	210	90	140	NA	210
Reduced Fat	IAM	71	275	4.9	2.8	14.6	1	230	180	120	190	10	130
Reduced Fat Large Breed	IAM	71	275	4.9	2.8	14.6	1	230	180	120	190	10	130
Eukanuba Low Residue Adult	IAM	82	328	5.9	2.5	12.9	0.5	226	181	106	206	NA	261
Low Fat	WAL	NA	264	6.9	1.9	17.2	0.6	340	320	130	200	29	290

*Diets listed by fat content in decreasing order.
†Average values for commercial diets of healthy pets.
CHO, Carbohydrate; *HIL*, Hill's; *IAM*, Iams; *Mfg*, manufacturer; *NA*, not available; *PUR*, Purina; *WAL*, Waltham.

Table H-6
Reduced-Sodium Diets

Diet*†	Mfg	Weight (g)	Energy (kcal per can [canned diets] or per cup [dry diets])	Protein (g)	Fat (g)	CHO (g)	Fiber (g)	Amount per 100 kcal					
								Ca (mg)	P (mg)	Na (mg)	K (mg)	Mg (mg)	Cl (mg)
Canned													
Average values‡				8.5	5.5	6.5	0.4	330	260	230	160	23	220
CV	PUR	354	638	3.6	6.5	10.1	0.3	150	80	20	250	10	260
h/d	HIL	418	542	3.7	5.9	10.7	0.1	162	123	15	177	29	69
Dry													
Average values‡				6.5	3.5	12	0.8	340	250	135	140	30	170
Early Cardiac Support	WAL	85	319	6.4	4.3	12.3	1.2	200	195	68	205	21	210
h/d	HIL	99	387	4.2	4.6	13.1	0.4	188	127	15	181	36	79

*Feeding directions: Dry diets may be preferable to decrease obligatory water intake. Canned canine diets should be used with caution for the reasons mentioned previously. Dogs that consume 20 kcal per pound per day receive only approximately 4 mg of sodium per pound per day.

†Diets listed by sodium content (milligrams per 100 kcal) in decreasing order.

‡Average values for commercial diets of healthy pets.

CHO, Carbohydrate; *HIL*, Hill's; *Mfg*, manufacturer; *PUR*, Purina; *WAL*, Waltham.

Table H-7
Reduced-Energy Diets

Diet*		Marketed for Use in Patients with	Avoid Feeding to Patients with	Nutrient Modifications (Varies with Diet)	Commercial Substitutions								
		Obesity	Increased nutrient needs	Decreased fat, increased fiber or moisture	Reduced-calorie diets								
					Amount per 100 kcal								
Diet*	Mfg	Weight (g)	Energy (kcal per can [canned diets] or per cup [dry diets])	Protein (g)	Fat (g)	CHO (g)	Fiber (g)	Ca (mg)	P (mg)	Na (mg)	K (mg)	Mg (mg)	Cl (mg)
Canned													
Average values†				8.5	5.5	6.5	0.4	330	260	230	160	23	220
OM Formula	PUR	354	189	17.8	3.4	8.8	7.7	470	430	110	430	NA	210
Calorie Control	WAL	360	196	12.1	5.8	3.3	0.9	500	330	170	590	60	390
r/d	HIL	404	292	8.5	2.8	12.7	7.3	221	180	83	277	47	166
w/d	HIL	418	372	5.3	3.8	15.3	3.6	180	157	79	180	25	213
Eukanuba Restricted Calorie	IAM	397	445	8.2	4.2	7.6	0.5	205	196	98	161	NA	179
Dry													
Average values†				6.5	3.5	12	0.8	340	250	135	140	30	170
r/d	HIL	77	205	8.4	2.9	13	7.7	207	178	104	285	48	141
Calorie Control	WAL	NA	212	8.8	2.8	13.1	1	610	410	120	380	50	400
w/d	HIL	77	226	5.8	2.7	15.3	5.4	194	157	67	221	29	164
Eukanuba Restricted Calorie	IAM	65	238	6.2	1.8	15	0.5	263	211	55	211	NA	164
OM Formula	PUR	127	276	10.3	2.1	14	3.4	470	470	70	270	NA	100

CHO, Carbohydrate; HIL, Hill's; IAM, Iams; Mfg, manufacturer; NA, not available; PUR, Purina; WAL, Waltham.
*Diets listed by energy density in increasing order.
†Average values for commercial diets of healthy pets.

Table H-8
Urolithiasis Diets

Marketed for Use in Patients with	Avoid Feeding to Patients with	Nutrient Modifications	Commercial Substitutions
Urolithiasis	Increased nutrient needs	Reduced minerals	Depends on stone type
Struvite		Decreased phosphorus, magnesium, urine pH, protein?	Most dry cat foods
Oxalate		Decreased calcium; increased magnesium, citrate, urine pH; decreased protein?	
Urate		Decreased protein; increased urine pH	

Diet	Mfg*	Weight (g)	Energy (kcal per can [canned diets] or per cup [dry diets])	Protein (g)	Fat (g)	CHO (g)	Fiber (g)	Ca (mg)	P (mg)	Na (mg)	K (mg)	Mg (mg)	Cl (mg)	pH
								Amount per 100 kcal						
Average values†				8.5	5.5	6.5	0.8	330	260	230	160	23	220	NA
Canned														
Struvite														
c/d	HIL	418	439	6	6.2	12.1	0.2	162	124	76	143	16	162	6.2-6.4
s/d	HIL	418	573	1.8	5.7	12.5	0.5	58	22	270	95	5	504	5.9-6.1
S/O	WAL	385	575	3.7	6.7	NA	0.8	220	193	327	180	14	447	5.5-6
Oxalate														
k/d	HIL	418	554	3.1	5.4	11.2	0.2	174	45	38	83	28	98	6.8-7.2
S/O	WAL	385	575	3.7	6.7	NA	0.8	220	193	327	180	14	447	6.3-6.5

	Mfg													
Urate														
u/d	HIL	418	598	2.2	5.3	11.1	0.3	56	35	49	77	6	91	7.1-7.7
Dry														
Average Values†				6.5	3.5	12	0.8	340	250	135	140	30	170	NA
Struvite														
c/d	HIL	99	413	4.7	4.7	11.1	0.5	129	112	57	143	25	105	6.2-6.4
S/O	WAL	NA	434	3.4	3.7	NA	0.4	169	111	260	195	14	330	5.5-6
Oxalate														
k/d	HIL	99	396	3.3	4.4	14	0.3	184	55	52	152	21	159	6.8-7.2
S/O	WAL	NA	434	3.4	3.7	NA	0.4	169	111	260	195	14	330	6.3-6.5
Urate														
u/d	HIL	76	396	2.3	4.7	14.7	0.6	85	45	47	125	11	8.2	7.1-7.7

Add one cup of water per cup of dry food and let stand at least 5 minutes before serving.

*Diets listed alphabetically by manufacturer.

†Average values for commercial diets of healthy pets.

CHO, Carbohydrate; *HIL*, Hill's; *Mfg*, manufacturer; *NA*, not available; *WAL*, Waltham.

Table H-9
Reduced-Phosphorus–Reduced-Protein Diets

Marketed for Use in Patients with	Avoid Feeding to Patients with	Nutrient Modifications	Commercial Substitutions
Advanced kidney failure	Increased nutrient needs	Decreased phosphorus, protein	Some geriatric diets
Advanced liver failure	Increased nutrient needs	Decreased protein	Some geriatric diets
Hypertension	Increased nutrient needs	Decreased sodium	Some geriatric diets

Diet	Mfg	Weight (g)	Energy (kcal per can [canned diets] or per cup [dry diets])	Amount per 100 kcal									
				Protein (g)	Fat (g)	CHO (g)	Fiber (g)	Ca (mg)	P (mg)	Na (mg)	K (mg)	Mg (mg)	Cl (mg)
Canned													
Average values*				8.5	5.5	6.5	0.4	330	260	230	160	23	220
Medium Phosphorus and Protein	WAL	385	625	4.8	7.2	6.5	0.3	170	80	60	180	14	360
g/d	HIL	418	464	4.6	2.6	15.6	0.4	153	99	54	189	23	207
l/d (Liver)	HIL	418	534	4.2	5.7	11.9	0.5	196	149	47	211	20	164
Low Phosphorus and Protein	WAL	385	607	3.5	5.6	11.9	0.3	220	60	40	150	12	140
NF Formula	PUR	354	500	3.5	5.9	10.8	0.4	110	60	50	160	10	90
k/d	HIL	418	554	3.1	5.4	11.2	0.2	174	45	38	83	28	98
u/d	HIL	418	598	2.2	5.3	11.1	0.3	56	35	49	77	6	91
Dry													
Average values*				6.5	3.5	12	0.8	340	250	135	140	30	170
Eukanuba Early Stage	IAM	71	285	4.8	3.3	13.5	0.6	170	99	119	157	NA	274
g/d	HIL	99	358	4.7	2.8	16.6	0.2	154	105	47	160	15	165
Medium Phosphorus and Protein	WAL	NA	307	4.7	3.6	15.1	0.5	190	110	40	160	22	185

Low Phosphorus and Protein	WAL	NA	287	3.9	3.6	17.5	0.5	170	80	40	160	22	150
l/d (Liver)	HIL	99	437	3.7	5.0	10.5	0.5	164	128	43	189	18	162
NF Formula	PUR	110	459	3.6	3.6	14.0	0.2	170	70	50	190	20	130
Eukanuba Advanced Stage	IAM	71	293	3.4	3.1	13.8	0.4	132	56	105	126	NA	256
k/d	HIL	99	396	3.3	4.4	14.0	0.3	184	55	52	152	21	159

*Average values of commercial diets of healthy pets.
CHO, Carbohydrate; *HIL*, Hill's; *IAM*, Iams; *M/g*, manufacturer; *PUR*, Purina; *WAL*, Waltham.

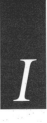

Veterinary Diets for Cats

Table 1-1
Novel Protein Diets

Marketed for Use in Patients with: Dermatitis caused by food allergy; inflammatory bowel disease

Avoid Feeding to Patients with: Protein to which the patient has not been exposed

Commercial Substitutions: Any food that contains a protein that is novel to the patient

Diet*	Mfg†	Weight (g)	Energy (kcal per can [canned diets] or per cup [dry diets])	Protein (g)	Fat (g)	CHO (g)	Fiber (g)	Ca (mg)	P (mg)	Na (mg)	K (mg)	Mg (mg)	Cl (mg)	pH
												Amount per 100 kcal		
Canned														
Average values‡				11	6	3	0.4	325	280	200	180	20	260	NA
d/d—Lamb	HIL	156	224	8	5.7	5.4	0.3	112	105	77	161	8	209	6.2-6.4
Eukanuba Response—Lamb	IAM	170	222	7.9	4.9	4.7	0.3	237	206	76	130	12	69	6-6.4
Lamb and Green Peas	IVD	167	215	7	7.4	3.4	0.6	116	123	80	138	13	94	6
Venison and Green Peas	IVD	156	215	8.3	7.4	2.6	0.4	130	138	109	130	12	80	6.4
Rabbit and Green Peas	IVD	167	190	8.9	6.7	3.4	0.5	551	308	75	103	21	112	6.8
Duck and Green Peas	IVD	156	190	8.1	7	3.4	0.5	221	197	90	107	20	123	6.5-6.6
Select Protein—Venison	WAL	165	152	11.1	4.3	7.7	0.7	340	270	260	330	20	NA	NA
Dry														
Average values‡				8.5	3.8	10	0.6	280	260	180	105	25	180	NA
z/d	HIL	77	396	9.6	3.9	9.3	0.3	172	147	88	180	18	221	6.2-6.4
Lamb and Green Peas	IVD	99	279	9.5	3.8	9.8	1.5	329	495	98	235	45	125	NA
Venison and Green Peas	IVD	99	261	9.4	3.8	10	1.5	543	503	70	200	43	100	7.2

Rabbit and Green Peas	IVD	99	288	9.2	3.7	10.4	1.8	287	222	86	243	38	96	6.8
Duck and Green Peas	IVD	99	290	9.1	3.7	10.5	1.5	409	321	97	259	39	141	NA
Select Protein—Duck	WAL	NA	264	9.3	3.5	10.8	1.3	520	370	190	210	23	410	NA

*Feeding directions: Once a diagnosis of food allergy is made and a diet to which the patient has no reaction is found, it is important that the owner understand that the patient should not be given any foods, supplements, or treats that may contain provocative antigens.

†Diets listed alphabetically by manufacturer.

‡Average values of healthy cat diets.

CHO, Carbohydrate; HIL, Hill's IVD, Heinz; IAM, Iams; NA, not available; WAL, Waltham.

Table 1-2
Nutrient-Dense Diets

Marketed for Use in Patients with	Avoid Feeding to Patients with	Nutrient Modifications (Varies with Diet)	Commercial Substitutions
Increased nutrient needs; gastric volume restriction; cats with diarrhea	Decreased nutrient needs	Increased nutrient density	High-protein, high-fat canned cat foods; meat-containing baby foods

			Energy (kcal per can [canned diets] or per cup [dry diets])	Amount per 100 kcal									
				Protein (g)	Fat (g)	CHO (g)	Fiber (g)	Ca (mg)	P (mg)	Na (mg)	K (mg)	Mg (mg)	Cl (mg)
Diet*	Mfg†	Weight (g)											
Canned													
Average values‡				11	6	3	0.4	325	280	200	180	20	260
Eukanuba Maximum Calorie	IAM	170	340	7.5	7.1	1.3	0.3	190	150	55	180	13	135
Clinicare	ABB	246	237	8.6	5.3	7.1	NA	152	126	53	157	11.4	115
CV Formula	PUR	156	223	8.7	5.5	4.7	0.2	250	190	50	270	20	220
p/d	HIL	156	219	10.1	6.5	2.3	0.1	228	185	107	185	18	185
a/d	HIL	156	185	9.1	6.1	2.9	0.3	209	209	156	191	22	152
Chicken Baby Food	HEI	71	84	9.8	7.2	0	0	64	120	40	135	NA	NA
Sheba—Beef	KAL	100	78	13	6.7	NA	0.3	420	250	237	220	24	NA

Dry

Average values‡			8.5	3.8	10	0.6	280	260	180	105	25	180
Eukanuba Maximum Calorie	IAM	123	602	8.2	5.5	3.5	0.3	248	199	101	168	17	195
p/d	HIL	122	498	8.1	5.4	7.3	0.2	277	227	92	185	18	212

*Feeding directions: Consider usual diet when choosing dry or canned form. Feed favorite foods if risk of learned aversion is present. Feed small, frequent meals if appetite is poor. Monitor food intake. If intake is less than recommended in "Energy needs of sedentary dogs and cats," see discussion of treatment of inappetence in the Critical Care section of Chapter 5.

†Listed in order of decreasing energy.

‡Average values of healthy cat diets.

ABB, Abbot Laboratories; *CHO*, carbohydrate; *HEI*, Heinz; *HIL*, Hill's; *IAM*, Iams; *KAL*, KalKan; *NA*, not available; *PUR*, Purina.

Table 1-3
Dental Diets

Diet	Mfg	Weight (g)	Energy (kcal per cup)	Protein (g)	Fat (g)	CHO (g)	Fiber (g)	Amount per 100 kcal						
								Ca (mg)	P (mg)	Na (mg)	K (mg)	Mg (mg)	Cl (mg)
Feline t/d	HIL	76	291	8.3	4	8.1	2.2	243	183	89	157	16	203
Dental Diet	FRI	57	226	2.6	3.1	12	1.5	508	432	183	204	32	210

CHO, Carbohydrate; *FRI*, Friskies; *HIL*, Hill's; *Mfg*, manufacturer.

Table I-4
Modified-Fiber Diets

Diet*	Mfg†	Weight (g)	Energy (kcal per can [canned diets] or per cup [dry diets])	Amount per 100 kcal									
				Protein (g)	Fat (g)	CHO (g)	Fiber (g)	Ca (mg)	P (mg)	Na (mg)	K (mg)	Mg (mg)	Cl (mg)
Canned													
Average values‡				11	6	3	0.4	325	280	200	180	20	260
r/d	HIL	156	116	11.4	2.8	10.1	5.5	215	202	94	228	27	242
w/d	HIL	156	148	11	4.4	6.5	2.9	169	158	116	232	21	285
OM	PUR	156	150	11.3	3.7	5.9	2.6	310	250	80	230	30	240
DM	PUR	156	194	11.9	5	1.09	0.8	240	230	80	170	20	160
Dry													
Average values‡				8.5	3.8	10	0.6	280	260	180	105	25	180
r/d	HIL	77	263	11.4	2.9	9.6	4.4	311	255	86	233	25	193
OM	PUR	122	326	11.2	2.5	11	2.3	370	340	80	200	30	260
w/d	HIL	77	281	11	2.8	10.4	2.2	319	251	74	232	23	189

| Eukanuba Optimum Weight Control | EUK | 93 | 357 | 9.8 | 3.2 | 9.1 | 0.5 | 310 | 256 | 104 | 203 | 23 | 175 |
| DM | PUR | 91 | 592 | 13.2 | 3.9 | 2.9 | 0.3 | 270 | 250 | 20 | 170 | 150 | 30 |

*Feeding directions: Fiber can be purchased separately and added (gradually, until effective) to the patient's current diet; some examples are given in the table below. Recommended dosages vary widely; we recommend starting with 1 tablespoon per cup or can of food and increasing the dosage until the desired clinical effect is achieved. Clients should be told that the increase in fecal volume and frequency that results from increased consumption of bulking fiber is the intended effect.

†Diets listed by fiber content (grams of fiber per 100 kcal) in decreasing order.

‡Average values of healthy cat diets.

CHO, Carbohydrate; EUK, Eukanuba; HIL, Hill's; Mfg, manufacturer; PUR, Purina.

Food	Amount per Tablespoon (g)	Total Fiber	Insoluble	Soluble
Wheat bran	5.3	2.7	2.3	0.3
100% Bran cereal	6.4	1.8	1.6	0.2
All-Bran cereal	5	1.4	1.2	0.2
Oat bran	6.7	1	0.5	0.5
Metamucil	5.8	3.4	0.7	2.7
Canned pumpkin	0.6	5*	N/A	N/A

*5 g in each half cup; 4 servings per 16-ounce can of Libby's canned pumpkin (Nestlé).

Table I-5
Reduced-Fat Diets

Diet*	Mfg	Weight (g)	Energy (kcal per can [canned diets]; per cup [dry diets]; or per pouch [semimoist diets])	Amount per 100 kcal									
				Protein (g)	Fat (g)	CHO (g)	Fiber (g)	Ca (mg)	P (mg)	Na (mg)	K (mg)	Mg (mg)	Cl (mg)
Canned													
Average values†				11	6	3	0.4	325	280	200	180	20	260
i/d	HIL	156	161	9.8	4.8	7.4	0.2	290	203	87	261	22	251
Eukanuba Low Residue	IAM	170	165	10.4	4.2	7.8	0.5	300	238	127	279	21	273
Dry													
Average values†				8.5	3.8	10	0.6	280	260	180	105	25	180
i/d	HIL	122	473	9.5	4.8	7.5	0.3	257	200	85	251	19	239
Eukanuba Low Residue	IAM	94	369	8.4	3.4	10	0.3	243	220	75	234	25	207
Semimoist													
EN	PUR	42	118	9.5	3.9	7.3	0.2	380	450	70	180	30	NA

*Diets listed by fat content in decreasing order.
†Average values of healthy cat diets.
CHO, Carbohydrate; HIL, Hill's; IAM, Iams; Mfg, manufacturer; NA, not available; PUR, Purina.

Table 1-6

Reduced-Sodium Diets

Diet*†	Mfg	Weight (g)	Energy (kcal/can)	Protein (g)	Fat (g)	CHO (g)	Fiber (g)	Ca (mg)	P (mg)	Na (mg)	K (mg)	Mg (mg)	Cl (mg)
								Amount per 100 kcal					
Canned													
Average values‡				11	6	3	0.4	325	280	200	180	20	260
h/d	HIL	156	197	11	6.8	5.5	0.4	205	197	79	229	17	182
CV Formula	PUR	156	223	8.7	5.5	4.7	0.2	250	190	50	270	20	220

*Feeding directions: Dry diets may be preferable to decrease obligatory water intake. Canned feline diets should be used with caution for the reasons mentioned previously. Cats that consume 20 kcal per pound per day receive only approximately 4 mg of sodium per pound per day.

†Diets listed by sodium content (milligrams per 100 kcal) in decreasing order.

‡Average values of healthy cat diets.

CHO, Carbohydrate; *HIL*, Hill's; *Mfg*, manufacturer; *PUR*, Purina.

Table I-7
Reduced-Energy Diets

	Marketed for Use in Patients with	Avoid Feeding to Patients with	Nutrient Modifications (Varies with Diet)	Commercial Substitutions
	Obesity	Increased nutrient needs	Decreased fat; increased fiber or moisture	Reduced calorie diets

				Amount per 100 kcal									
Diet*	Mfg	Weight (g)	Energy (kcal per can [canned diets] or per cup [dry diets])	Protein (g)	Fat (g)	CHO (g)	Fiber (g)	Ca (mg)	P (mg)	Na (mg)	K (mg)	Mg (mg)	Cl (mg)
Canned													
Average values†				11	6	3	0.4	325	280	200	180	20	260
Calorie control	WAL	165	111	12.4	5.7	2.9	0.6	410	340	400	370	23	410
r/d	HIL	156	116	11.4	2.8	10.1	5.5	215	202	94	228	27	242
w/d	HIL	156	148	11	4.4	6.5	2.9	169	158	116	232	21	285
OM Formula	PUR	156	150	11.3	3.7	5.9	0.2	310	250	80	230	30	240
Eukanuba Restricted Calorie	IAM	170	204	9.5	4.1	4.5	0.2	233	208	92	150	18	167
Dry													
Average values†				8.5	3.8	10	0.6	280	260	180	105	25	180
Calorie control	WAL	NA	211	12.9	2.4	9.8	1.2	670	400	200	280	24	510
w/d	HIL	76	245	11	2.8	10.4	2.2	319	251	74	232	23	189
r/d	HIL	76	263	11.4	2.9	9.6	4.4	311	255	86	233	25	193
Eukanuba Restricted Calorie	IAM	76	298	8.6	2.4	10.6	0.5	255	232	120	235	20	204
OM Formula	PUR	NA	326	11.2	2.5	11	0.2	370	340	80	200	30	260

*Diets listed by energy density in increasing order.
†Average values of healthy cat diets.
CHO, Carbohydrate; *HIL,* Hill's; *IAM,* Iams; *Mfg,* manufacturer; *NA,* not available; *PUR,* Purina; *WAL,* Waltham.

MANUAL OF VETERINARY DIETETICS

Table 1-8
Urolithiasis Diets

Marketed for Use in Patients with	Avoid Feeding to Patients with	Nutrient Modifications	Commercial Substitutions
Urolithiasis	Increased nutrient needs	Reduced minerals	Depends on stone type; most dry cat foods
Struvite		Decreased phosphorus, magnesium; urine pH, protein?	
Oxalate		Decreased calcium; increased magnesium, citrate, urine pH; decreased protein?	
Urate		Decreased protein; increased urine pH	

Diet*	Mfg	Weight (g)	Energy (kcal per can [canned diets]; per cup [dry diets]; or per pouch [semimoist diets])	Amount per 100 kcal										
				Protein (g)	Fat (g)	CHO (g)	Fiber (g)	Ca (mg)	P (mg)	Na (mg)	K (mg)	Mg (mg)	Cl (mg)	pH
Canned														
Average values†				11	6	3	0.4	325	280	200	180	20	260	NA
Struvite														
c/d	HIL	156	164	9.9	5	6	0.5	143	114	133	191	13	286	6.2-6.4
s/d	HIL	156	215	8.8	7.1	3.3	0.4	130	109	181	196	9	348	5.9-6.1
Eukanuba Low pH/S	IAM	170	198	9.5	6.2	3.5	0.2	242	190	95	181	21	138	5.9-6.3
UR formula	PUR	156	217	8.6	7.6	3.4	0.02	190	170	90	200	10	290	5.9-6.3
S/O Control pH	WAL	165	175	7.5	8	1.9	0.2	170	210	210	210	15	180	6.3-6.5

Oxalate													
x/d	HIL	156	162	9.5	4.5	7.4	0.2	154	125	67	202	20	115	6.6-6.8
Eukanuba Mod pH/O	IAM	170	198	9.1	5.9	3.2	0.2	233	173	99	267	21	147	6.3-6.9
S/O Control pH	WAL	165	175	7.5	8	1.9	0.2	170	210	210	210	15	180	6.3-6.5
Dry													
Average values†				8.5	3.8	10	0.6	280	260	180	105	25	180	NA
Struvite													
c/d	HIL	76	285	8.5	4.1	10.3	0.2	197	184	106	210	15	258	6.2-6.4
s/d	HIL	122	521	7.4	5.8	6.6	0.2	233	165	151	193	16	329	5.9-6.1
Eukanuba Low pH/S	IAM	102	441	7.8	3.9	8	0.4	236	203	112	198	18	191	5.9-6.3
UR Formula	PUR	227	366	8.3	2.7	10.7	0.3	260	200	60	200	20	260	5.9-6.3
S/O Control pH	WAL	NA	390	8.8	4.7	8.3	0.5	170	210	220	230	15	510	6.3-6.5
Oxalate													
x/d	HIL	76	286	8.5	4.1	10.2	0.3	196	162	85	209	20	244	6.6-6.8
Eukanuba Mod pH/O	IAM	105	451	7.6	3.9	8	0.4	238	205	104	305	19	151	6.3-6.9
S/O Control pH	WAL	NA	390	8.8	4.7	8.3	0.5	170	210	220	230	15	510	6.3-6.5
Semimoist													
Struvite													
UR Formula	PUR	42	120	9.7	3.7	6.5	0.3	370	400	60	190	30	130	5.8-6.2

*Diets listed alphabetically by manufacturer.

†Average values for healthy cat diets.

CHO, Carbohydrate; HIL, Hill's; IAM, Iams; M/g, manufacturer; NA, not available; PUR, Purina; WAL, Waltham.

Table 1-9

Reduced-Phosphorus–Reduced-Protein Diets

Marketed for Use in Patients with	Avoid Feeding to Patients with	Nutrient Modifications	Commercial Substitutions
Advanced kidney failure	Increased nutrient needs	Decreased phosphorus, protein	Some geriatric diets
Advanced liver failure	Increased nutrient needs	Decreased protein	Some geriatric diets

Diet	Mfg	Weight (g)	Energy (kcal per can [canned diets] or per cup [dry diets])	Protein (g)	Fat (g)	CHO (g)	Fiber (g)	Ca (mg)	P (mg)	Na (mg)	K (mg)	Mg (mg)	Cl (mg)
Canned													
Average values*				11	6.0	3	0.4	325	280	200	180	20	260
g/d	HIL	156	165	8.1	4.5	8.5	0.8	152	123	66	171	19	133
l/d	HIL	156	164	7.2	5.3	8.7	0.4	200	133	48	219	10	191
Eukanuba Multi-Stage Renal	IAM	170	205	6.6	5.4	7.2	0.5	174	158	116	191	18	158
Clinicare RF	ABB	244	237	6.3	6.7	6	NA	124	103	52	119	9	67
k/d	HIL	156	219	6	5.4	7.3	0.5	128	78	64	214	7	114
NF Formula	PUR	156	NA	6	5.7	5.9	0.5	200	100	30	190	20	90
Low Phosphorus and Protein	WAL	165	287	5.7	8.6	2.4	0.3	190	80	120	210	31	500
Dry													
Average values*				8.5	3.8	10	0.6	280	260	180	105	25	180
g/d	HIL	76	297	7.9	4.5	9.9	0.3	120	130	79	176	13	161
NF Formula	PUR	NA	NA	7.2	3	11.9	0.3	160	100	50	210	20	150
l/d	HIL	122	505	7.1	5.2	8.3	0.4	199	151	62	202	17	151

Amount per 100 kcal

k/d	HIL	122	477	6.7	5.2	10.3	0.2	178	114	56	175	14	142
Eukanuba Multi-Stage Renal	IAM	122	535	6.4	5.3	7.8	0.5	150	114	102	148	11	164
Low Phosphorus and Protein	WAL	NA	381	5.8	5.2	10.1	1.1	180	100	40	170	17	90

*Average values for healthy cat diets.

ABB, Abbot Laboratories; CHO, carbohydrate; HIL, Hill's; IAM, Iams; NA, not available; PUR, Purina; WAL, Waltham.

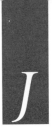

Basic Homemade Diet for Cats and Dogs

The following recipe is designed to nourish pets without making their diseases worse. The recipe makes enough food for a 10- to 20-pound pet for 3 to 6 days and enough for a 50-pound dog for 1 or 2 days. The veterinarian may be able to give the owner additional information regarding a specific pet's needs.

INGREDIENTS

2 cups cooked meat (beef, chicken, or pork)
4 cups cooked starch (rice, pasta, or potato)
1 teaspoon canola or vegetable oil
2 500-mg Tums tablets
1 complete vitamin-mineral supplement for a 2- to 3-year-old child
For cats, add one 500-mg taurine tablet

NUTRITIONAL INFORMATION

Calories: 1200 (distributed as 20% protein, 40% each carbohydrate and fat)

Nutrient	Diet	Requirement
Protein	60 g	62 g
Calcium	600 mg	2000 mg
Phosphorus	400 mg	1700 mg
Sodium	140 mg	200 mg
Potassium	500 mg	2000 mg

PREPARATION

- Cook meat according to type of meat and personal preference; the method is not important.

- Cook starch according to directions.
- Combine meat and starch with other ingredients and mix well (the vitamin supplement can be given separately to dogs if they will accept it).

INCREASING VARIETY IN A PET'S DIET

If an owner would like to substitute other foods prepared in the home for the meats or starches used in the recipe, the exchange lists in Appendix L may be followed. These lists are called *exchange lists* because the foods within a group may be substituted for one another. In the recipe, $1^1/_2$ cups of meat is equal to 6 exchanges, and 4 cups of cooked starch is equal to 8 exchanges. If, for example, the owner wants to use cheese rather than meat as a protein source, then six $^1/_4$-cup servings ($1^1/_2$ cups total) of low-sodium cheese are substituted for the $1^1/_2$ cups of meat. In addition, up to two servings (total) from any of the dessert, fat, fruit, vegetable, and calorie-supplement lists may be provided to enhance palatability and intake of the diet.

Gastrostomy Tubes

FEEDING A PET THROUGH A STOMACH TUBE

Successful feeding of and caring for an animal with a stomach tube in place is not difficult if instructions are closely followed.

- It is very important that careful observations are made when a pet is fed through a feeding tube. If any of the problems described later in this appendix occur, if difficulty arises when the client uses the feeding tube, or if questions arise at any time, owners should not hesitate to contact the veterinarian.
- Gastrostomy tubes must be tightly capped (usually with a catheter adapter) when not in use. A three-way valve can be used when the valve of the stopcock is in the off position so that food or liquid cannot flow toward the patient or into the patient's stomach (see Figure 5-5).
- If a liquid diet is fed, only the plug is removed, and the syringe fits into the catheter adapter.
- If a blenderized diet is used, both the plug and the adapter are removed and the syringe fits directly into the tube.
- The animal should be offered a small amount of fresh food before being fed through the tube. If appetite returns, the veterinarian is consulted for guidance on reduction of tube feedings.
- To ensure that the tube is clear, 3 to 6 ml of water is injected through the tube before feeding. If the water cannot be injected, or if the animal begins to cough or vomit or shows signs of pain, feeding is stopped immediately.
- If the pet can be fed, it should sit up or lie on its right side and be fed slowly over 5 to 10 minutes, no more than 20 ml per minute.
- Gruels or solutions should be warmed to room temperature before feeding.
- If pushing the syringe becomes difficult, feeding is stopped and the tube checked to ensure that it has not kinked. If the tube is not kinked and the food still does not flow properly, or if the pet vomits at any time, the veterinarian should be called.
- After feeding, the tube is thoroughly flushed to prevent clogging with dried food. Approximately 3 to 6 ml of water is used to flush the tube. The pet is watched closely for any signs of discomfort.

Problems

The veterinarian should be called if any of the following signs are present.
- Abdominal swelling
- Drainage where tube exits the body
- Vomiting

Nothing but the feeding solution should be administered through the tube without permission of the veterinarian.

TUBE SITE MAINTENANCE

The tube site is checked before each feeding. If a wrap or covering is present over the feeding tube site, it is removed before each feeding and examined for the following.
- Redness
- Tenderness
- Swelling
- Irritation
- Pus
- Leakage of stomach contents

Inspection of the position of the mark that was made during placement of the tube reveals inward or outward movement. If the tube appears to have migrated, feeding is stopped and the veterinarian contacted.

CLEANING THE TUBE SITE

- Most dogs and cats keep the skin around the feeding tube site clean.
- Skin is cleaned with antibacterial soap and water only when necessary. A spiral pattern is used, starting close to the tube site and moving outward. The cleaned area is dried thoroughly.
- If the tube has a rubber bumper on the outside, the bumper is cleaned if necessary.
- If a crust is present, it is removed by use of hydrogen peroxide diluted to half strength with water.
- After removal of the crust, the area is rinsed with water and dried well. If a dressing or bandage is used and becomes wet, it is changed immediately.

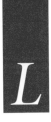

Exchange Lists

MEAT GROUP

Each serving contains approximately the following.
- 7 to 10 g of protein
- 25 to 30 mg of sodium
- 70 to 150 mg of phosphorus
- 50 to 150 kcal (values vary widely)

Food	Amount per Serving
Cheese, low sodium	$\frac{1}{4}$ cup
Cottage cheese, 2% fat	$\frac{1}{3}$ cup
Egg, large	1
Fish	
Fresh	$\frac{1}{2}$ cup
Low-sodium salmon or tuna	$\frac{1}{4}$ cup
Shellfish	
Fresh clams, oysters, or shrimp	5 small or $\frac{1}{4}$ cup
Scallops	$\frac{1}{4}$ cup
Meat or poultry	$\frac{1}{4}$ cup
Peanut butter	2 tbsp
Soybean curd (tofu)	$\frac{1}{2}$ cup

FAT GROUP

Each serving contains approximately the following.
- 0 g of protein
- 45 kcal

The following food items may be regular or low sodium.

Food	Amount per Serving
Butter	1 tsp
Margarine	1 tsp
Mayonnaise	2 tsp
Salad dressing	
French	1 tsp

Roquefort or blue cheese	1 tsp
Thousand Island	1 tsp
Italian, low sodium	2 tsp
Lard	1 tsp
Oil, cooking	1 tsp
Oil, salad	1 tsp
Vegetable shortening	1 tsp

STARCH GROUP

Each serving contains approximately the following.
- 2 g of protein
- 70 kcal (values vary)

Food	Amount per Serving
Barley, uncooked	$1\frac{1}{2}$ tbsp
Biscuit or muffin	1 small
Bread, any	1 slice
Bun, hamburger or hot dog	1 small or $\frac{1}{2}$ large
Cereal, dry, any	$\frac{3}{4}$ cup
Cereal, hot, cooked without salt	
(do not use "quick" or "instant")	$\frac{1}{2}$ cup
Cornbread	2-inch square
Creamer, nondairy	1 cup
Flour, cornmeal, tapioca	$2\frac{1}{2}$ tbsp
Graham crackers	2 squares
Macaroni, noodles, spaghetti,	
rice cooked without salt	$\frac{1}{2}$ cup
Melba toast	5 slices
Pancake or waffle, homemade	1
Tortilla	1 (6 inch)
Holland rusk, regular	1
Roll, any	1 small or $\frac{1}{2}$ large

DESSERT GROUP

Food	Amount per Serving
Brownies	1 ($2 \times 2 \times \frac{3}{4}$ inches)
Cake—angel food cake, sponge cake, layer cake,	
pound cake, any kind	1 small slice
Cookies, any	2 medium
Cupcake, any	1 medium
Danish pastry, doughnut, sweet roll	1 small or $\frac{1}{2}$ large
Popcorn, popped, unsalted	$1\frac{1}{2}$ cups
Sherbet	$\frac{3}{4}$ cup

FRUIT GROUP

Fruit listed is fresh or frozen unless otherwise specified. Each serving contains approximately the following.

- 0.5 g of protein
- 80 kcal

Food	Amount per Serving
Apple	1 small
Apple juice	$\frac{1}{2}$ cup
Applesauce, canned, sweetened	$\frac{1}{2}$ cup
Apricots	3 medium
Apricots, canned, in heavy syrup	4 halves
Apricots, dried	5
Avocado	$\frac{1}{4}$
Banana	$\frac{1}{2}$
Blackberries	$\frac{1}{2}$ cup
Blueberries	$\frac{1}{2}$ cup
Boysenberries, raw	$\frac{1}{2}$ cup
Cantaloupe	$\frac{1}{2}$ cup
Casaba	$\frac{3}{4}$ cup, cubed
Cherries	10
Cherries, canned, with syrup	$\frac{1}{2}$ cup
Cranberries	1 cup
Cranberry juice cocktail, bottled	$\frac{1}{2}$ cup
Cranberry sauce, jellied, canned	$\frac{1}{2}$ cup
Dates, dried	5
Figs, canned, in heavy syrup	3 (with liquid)
Figs, dried	2
Figs, raw	1 medium
Fruit cocktail, canned, in heavy syrup	$\frac{1}{2}$ cup
Fruit salad, tropical, in heavy syrup	$\frac{1}{4}$ cup
Gooseberries, raw	$\frac{1}{4}$ cup
Grapes	10
Grape juice, canned, bottled, or from frozen concentrate	$\frac{1}{2}$ cup
Grapefruit, canned, with syrup	$\frac{1}{2}$ cup
Grapefruit, pink, red, white	$\frac{1}{2}$ medium
Grapefruit juice, canned or from frozen concentrate	$\frac{1}{2}$ cup
Guava	1
Honeydew	$\frac{1}{2}$ cup
Kiwi fruit	1 medium
Lemon, fresh	1
Lime, fresh	1
Mandarin oranges, canned, with syrup	$\frac{1}{2}$ cup
Mango	1
Nectar—apricot, pear, peach	$\frac{1}{2}$ cup
Nectarine	1 medium
Orange juice, fresh, canned, or from frozen concentrate	$\frac{1}{2}$ cup

Orange, navel	1 medium
Papaya	$\frac{1}{3}$ medium
Peach	1 small
Peach, canned, with syrup	2 halves
Pear, canned, with syrup	$\frac{1}{2}$ cup
Pineapple, raw	$\frac{1}{2}$ cup
Pineapple, canned, with syrup	$\frac{1}{3}$ cup
Pineapple juice, canned	$\frac{1}{2}$ cup
Plums	1
Plums, canned, with syrup	2
Pomegranate	$\frac{1}{2}$ medium
Prunes, canned	5
Prune juice, canned or bottled	$\frac{1}{3}$ cup
Prunes, dried	5
Raisins, seedless	$\frac{1}{4}$ cup
Raspberries	$\frac{1}{2}$ cup
Rhubarb, frozen, cooked	$\frac{1}{2}$ cup
Strawberries	$\frac{1}{3}$ cup
Tangelo	1 medium
Tangerine	1
Watermelon	1 cup, diced

VEGETABLE GROUP

Vegetables listed are fresh or are frozen and cooked unless otherwise specified. Pickles, pickle relish, olives, sauerkraut, and other pickled vegetables should be avoided if sodium is restricted.

Each serving contains approximately the following.

- 2 g of protein
- 35 kcal

Food	Amount per Serving
Artichoke, cooked	1 medium
Artichoke hearts, frozen, cooked	$\frac{1}{3}$ cup
Asparagus, canned, cooked	$\frac{1}{2}$ cup
Asparagus, frozen	$\frac{1}{4}$ cup
Bamboo shoots, canned	$\frac{1}{2}$ cup
Bean sprouts, mung	$1\frac{3}{4}$ oz
Bean sprouts, soybean	$\frac{1}{2}$ cup
Beans, green (snap)—canned or cooked, frozen	$\frac{1}{2}$ cup
Beans, green, fresh, cooked	$\frac{1}{2}$ cup
Beans, wax, cooked	$\frac{1}{2}$ cup
Beet greens	$1\frac{3}{4}$ oz
Beets, cooked	$\frac{1}{2}$ cup
Broccoli	$\frac{2}{3}$ cup
Brussels sprouts, cooked	3 or 4 medium
Cabbage, all varieties	$\frac{1}{2}$ cup
Carrots	$\frac{2}{3}$ cup

Cauliflower, raw	$\frac{1}{2}$ cup
Celery, cooked, diced	$\frac{1}{3}$ cup
Celery, raw	$\frac{1}{2}$ stalk
Corn on cob, sweet	$\frac{1}{2}$ ear
Corn, sweet, cooked	$\frac{1}{2}$ cup
Cucumber	$\frac{1}{2}$ cup sliced
Eggplant, cooked, 1-inch cubes	$\frac{1}{2}$ cup
Greens—collard, dandelion, mustard turnip, kale	$\frac{1}{2}$ cup
Hominy, grits, cooked	$\frac{1}{2}$ cup
Lettuce, iceberg	$1\frac{3}{4}$ oz
Lettuce, romaine, raw, shredded	1 oz
Mixed vegetables	$\frac{1}{2}$ cup
Mushroom, raw	3 small
Okra, frozen, cooked, sliced	$\frac{1}{2}$ cup
Onion, all varieties	$\frac{1}{2}$ cup
Parsnips, cooked	$\frac{1}{2}$ cup
Peas	$\frac{1}{2}$ cup
Pepper, jalapeño, canned, solid	$\frac{1}{2}$ cup
Pepper, sweet, raw	$\frac{1}{2}$ cup
Potato, cooked without skin	$\frac{1}{2}$ cup
Potato, frozen, French fried	10 strips
Pumpkin, cooked or canned	$\frac{1}{2}$ cup
Rutabaga	$\frac{1}{2}$ cup
Spinach	$\frac{1}{2}$ cup
Squash, summer, all varieties, cooked	$\frac{1}{2}$ cup
Squash, winter, all varieties, baked	$\frac{1}{2}$ cup cubed
Sweet potato	$\frac{1}{2}$ cup
Tomato, canned whole	$\frac{1}{2}$ cup
Tomato, raw	1 small
Tomato juice, unsalted	$\frac{1}{2}$ cup
Vegetable juice cocktail, unsalted	$\frac{1}{2}$ cup
Watercress, chopped	$1\frac{3}{4}$ oz
Yam, cooked or baked	$\frac{1}{3}$ cup

CALORIC SUPPLEMENTS

Each serving contains approximately 60 kcal.

Ingredient	Amount per Serving
Arrowroot flour	2 tbsp
Supplements	
Polycose	1 tbsp
Controlyte	2 tbsp
Butterballs	1 medium
Butterscotch drops	3 pieces
Cornstarch	2 tbsp
Cotton candy	2 cups
Cranberries, raw	$\frac{1}{4}$ cup
Gumdrops	2 large

Gumdrops	15 small
Hard candy	2 pieces
Honey	1 tbsp
Jam	1 tbsp
Jelly	1 tbsp
Jelly beans	10
Lollipop	1 small
Marmalade	1 tbsp
Marshmallows	3 large
Mints	2 medium
Sugar, confectioners'	1 tbsp
Sugar, granulated	4 tsp
Syrup, corn, light	1 tbsp
Syrup, flavored (not chocolate)	2 tbsp

BEVERAGES

Beverage	Amount per Serving
Artificially flavored fruit drinks; carbonated cola, lemon-lime, root beer	6 oz
Ginger ale	1 cup
Lemonade	$\frac{1}{2}$ cup
Popsicle	1 average
Tang orange drink	$\frac{1}{3}$ cup

INDEX

A

AAFCO. *See* Association of American Feed Control Officials
Abdomen, tucked up, 29
Abdominal bandage, usage, 66
Abdominal distention, 83
Abdominal pain, 81
Abdominal walls, exit, 66
Absorptive hypercalciuria, 130
Accidental contaminants, presence, 145
Accutane. *See* Retinoid 13-*cis*-retinoic acid
ACE. *See* Angiotensin-converting enzyme
Acid-base abnormalities, 101
Acid-base balance, 104
Acid-base imbalance, 128
Acid-base status, normalization, 59
Acromegaly, 78
Action stage, 157
  plan, creation, 160
Active diversion, 160
Activity
  impact. *See* Obesity
  level. *See* Pets
Acute gastroenteritis, 82-83
Acute-onset diarrhea, 82
Acute-phase protein synthesis, 58. *See also* Enhanced acute-phase protein synthesis
Ad libitum. *See* Free-choice
Adult cats, 30-31, 37
  client communication tips, 31
  commercial diets, 176t-177t, 184t-185t
  tech tips, 31
Adult dogs, 15-18, 25
  client communication tips, 16-17
  nutrition/behavior, 16-18
Age-related diseases, presence, 21
Aggression. *See* Dominance aggression; Fear-related territorial aggression
  pathophysiology/therapy. *See* Dogs
Aging, physical signs, 21, 25
Alanine, 36
Alaskan malamutes, syndrome I, 117
Albumin. *See* Serum albumin
  evaluation, 7t
Aldosterone, impact, 94, 136
Alkali, sources, 102
Alkaline phosphatase
  increase, 129
  levels, 140
Allergens, presence, 145
Allergies. *See* Foods
Allopurinol, 132
Alpha-linolenic acid, 120
Altered urine pH, 125
Alternative veterinary medicine, 143-147
Aluminum hydroxide, usage, 102

American Botanical Council, 145
American College of Veterinary Dermatology, 121
American Veterinary Medical Association (AVMA), Executive Board recommendation, 197
Amino acids
  catabolism, 35
  metabolism strategies, 34
  providing, 117
  release, 58
Ammonia
  concentrations, 93
  production. *See* Renal tubular ammonia production
  toxicity, 35
Ammonium urate, flocculation, 132
Anabolic steroids, usage, 61
Anemia. *See* Iron-deficiency anemia
  laboratory findings, 60
Angiotensin-converting enzyme (ACE) inhibitors, 94
Angiotensin II, impact, 95
Animal milk, composition, 11t
Ankylosis, occurrence, 139
Anorectum, obstruction, 89
Anorexia, 56, 92-93, 104, 135-136. *See also* Anxiety-induced anorexia; Fear-induced anorexia; Psychogenic anorexia
Antitension suture, usage, 66
Anxiety, anticipation, 160
Anxiety-induced anorexia, 60
Appetite
  loss. *See* Chronic disease
  stimulation, drugs (usage), 60, 61t
Aquasol A, recommendation, 124
Arachidonic acid
  biosynthesis, 120f
  formation, 119
  presence, 29
  requirement. *See* Cats
  synthesis, 36. *See also* Endogenous arachidonic acid
  usage, 117
Arginine
  increase, 136
  presence, 35
  requirement. *See* Cats
  usage, 67
Arteries, blockage, 110
Ascorbic acid. *See* Vitamin C
Association of American Feed Control Officials (AAFCO)
  feeding trials, 23, 31-32, 37
    protocols, 14, 193
  foods, oversight, 163
  ingredients, listing, 44
  labeling rules, 43t
  labels, guarantees (problem/limitation), 45, 48
  pet food labeling rules, 43
  regulations, changes, 43
Atherosclerosis, development, 21
Atopic dermatitis, 118-121
AVMA. *See* American Veterinary Medical Association
Azotemia, 107t. *See also* Postrenal azotemia
  onset, 101

Page numbers followed by b indicate boxes; f, figures; t, tables.

B

Bacterial infections, 78
Balanced
  definition, 43
  usage, 44
Basal energy needs, 56
β-amino acid. *See* Taurine
BCS. *See* Body condition score
Beagles
  idiopathic hyperlipidemia, 80
  studies, 18
Behavioral change, transtheoretical model, 156-162, 156t
Behavioral measures, 17
Beta carotene (β-carotene), 13, 152
Beta-cell dysfunction, combination, 76
Beverages, exchange list, 240
Bicarbonate (potassium citrate), 104
  usage, 102
Bile acid, production, 35
Bilirubin, concentrations, 93
Biotin, dietary deficiencies, 124
Birds, nutrition Web site, 167
Biscuits, usage. *See* Treats/biscuits
Blood glucose
  concentrations. *See* Postprandial blood glucose concentrations
  control, 78
    improvement, 76
  postprandial fluctuations, minimization, 137
Bloodletting, 143
Blood lipids, elevation, 110
Blood pressure, increase, 110
Blood urea nitrogen (BUN), 153
  evaluation, 7t
Body care, characteristic. *See* Cats
Body condition
  achievement, feeding (impact), 14
  maintenance, 21
  scoring, 2, 4f
Body condition score (BCS), 4f-5f
  assignation, 16, 193
  decrease, 109
  determination, 76
  evaluation, 13, 28
  importance, review, 15, 16, 20, 31, 33
  level, 14-15, 19, 25
  maintenance, 135
  sheet, 31
Body weight, 57
  desired level, 57f
  rule of thumb calculation, 114
  time, comparison, 10f
Bone pain, 6t
Book values. *See* Pet foods
Borborygmus, 63, 82, 84
Bovine milk protein, allergies, 119
Bovine protein allergy, 119
Bowels
  diarrhea. *See* Chronic small bowel diarrhea; Large bowel diarrhea; Small bowel diarrhea
  disease. *See* Inflammatory bowel disease
Brachycephalic breeds, oral health problems, 73
Breast cancer, development risk, 110
Breeding, effect, 9
Briard dogs, hypercholesterolemia, 80
Bulking-fermenting fibers, usage, 88
BUN. *See* Blood urea nitrogen
Burn wounds, presence, 56

C

C. *See* Contemplation
Cachexia, 6t, 21, 49. *See also* Digitalis cachexia
  signs, 53
Calcitrol
  effectiveness, 104
  treatment. *See* Low-dose oral calcitrol treatment
Calcium
  imbalance, 140
  ionization, increase, 104
  levels. *See* Extracellular fluid calcium levels
Calcium oxalate
  dihydrate (weddelite), 130
  monohydrate (whewellite), 130
  stones, 130-131
    dissolve, attempts, 131
  urolithiasis, 130
Calcium phosphate, presence, 129
Calculolytic diets, 128-129
Calculus, control, 74
Caloric density, decrease, 111
Caloric intake, 56
  calculation. *See* Obesity
Caloric needs
  determination, 114
  estimation, 58
  review. *See* Total daily caloric needs
Caloric supplements, exchange list, 239-240
Calories, determination. *See* Obesity
Cancer, 50-54, 136
  client communication tips, 55
  obesity, relationship, 110
  prevalence. *See* Cats; Dogs; Humans
  risk
    nutrition, effects. *See* Humans
    reduction. *See* Mammary cancer risk
  tech tips, 55
  types, distribution, 51
Canine CliniCare, 67
Canine discoid lupus erythematosus, 124
Canned diets, mixing. *See* Medications
Canned foods, 42
  palatability/digestibility, 41
Cannula, fitting, 65
Carafate. *See* Sucralfate
Carbohydrates. *See* Soluble carbohydrates
  impact. *See* Sled dogs
Carbonate, usage, 103
Carbonate apatite, presence, 128
Cardiovascular problems, obesity (relationship), 109-111
Carmalt forceps, usage, 64
Carotene, increase, 136
Carpus, hyperflexion/extension, 13
Casein-based liquid diets, 35
Catabolic factor, 53
Cat bite abscess, 134
Catecholamines, impact, 18
Cats. *See* Adult cats
  arachidonic acid, requirement, 36
  arginine, requirement, 35
  behavior, 198-199
  body care, characteristic, 200
  cancer, prevalence, 52t
  DCM, 97-99
  dental diets, 220t
  dental treats, 72t
  diagnoses, 50t
  energy needs, 57f

Cats—(*continued*)
  enrichment recommendation. *See* Indoor cats
  feeding. *See* Geriatric cats
  foods
    characteristic, 199
    nutrient comparison tables. *See* Commercial cat
      foods
    palatability, 36
  gestation, 27-28, 36-37
    tech tips, 28
  hairballs, incidence, 84
  high-fiber diet, high-protein diet (contrast), 77t
  housing, ideal, 199
  hyperchylomicronemia, 79
  IC, 133-134
  IHL, 93-94
  interaction, 198
  lactation, 26-27, 36-37
    tech tips, 28
  linoleic acid, requirement, 36
  lipoproteins, characteristics, 80t
  litter type preferences, 198
  megacolon, 89-90
  metabolism, differences, 52
  modified fiber diets, 221t-222t
  movement, characteristic, 199
  neonate milk replacers, 182t
  neutering, dietary recommendations, 29
  niacin, requirement, 36
  novel protein diets, 216t-217t
  nutrient
    needs, 34-36
    needs specificity, 34f
    supplementation, value, 29
  nutrient-dense diets, 218t-219t
  phosphorus diets, reduction, 108t
  preformed vitamin A, requirement, 139
  protein diets, reduction, 109t
  reduced-energy diets, 225t
  reduced-fats diets, 223t
  reduced-phosphorus reduced protein diets, 228t-229t
  reduced-sodium diets, 224t
  rest, characteristic, 199
  serum lipid concentration increase, causes, 79t
  social contact, characteristic, 199
  stone types, prevalence, 127t
  summary, 36-38
  thiamin
    deficiency, 139-140
    requirement, 36
  urinary citrate, increase, 131
  urolithiasis diets, 226t-227t
  veterinary diets, 216-229
  vitamin E deficiency, 139-140
  water intake, characteristic, 199
Cats, growth, 28-30, 37
  client communication tips, 30
  diet, 183t
  tech tips, 30
Cats, homemade diets, 231-232
  ingredients, 231
  nutritional information, 231
  preparation, 231-232
CAVM. *See* Complementary and alternative veterinary
  medicine
Cervical cancer, development risk, 110
Change
  costs, 161

processes, relationship. *See* Transtheoretical model
  sustaining, 161
Charisma, 144, 147
CHF. *See* Congestive heart failure
Chinchillas, nutrition Web site, 167-168
Cholesterol
  concentrations, 93
  serum concentrations, 81
Chronic diarrhea, 82
Chronic disease
  appetite loss, 56
  protein depletion, 59
Chronic inflammatory diseases, 121
Chronic kidney disease, nutrient recommendations, 107t
Chronic large bowel diarrhea, 85
Chronic liver disease, 92
Chronic pancreatitis, 78
Chronic primary renal failure, 101
Chronic renal failure (CRF), 100-107, 135-136
  accelerated progression, 104
Chronic small bowel diarrhea, 84
Chylomicrons
  production, 79
  serum concentrations, 80
Cimetidine, 101
Circulatory problems, 110
Cisapride, usage. *See* Propulsid
Clients. *See* Owners
Clinical dietetics, 49
  recommended readings, 141
Clinical expertise, definition, 152
Clinical nutrition, issues, 143
Clofibrate, usage, 81
Coax-feeding, 71
Colectomy, recommendation. *See* Subtotal colectomy
Collagen, loss. *See* Skin
Colon
  cancer, risk, 111
  obstruction, 89
Colonic bacteria, fermenting process, 90
Coma, occurrence, 139
Comfort foods, consumption, 144
Commercial cat foods, nutrient comparison tables,
  182-186
Commercial diets, 39-46. *See also* Adult cats; Adult dogs
  quality, 9
Commercial dog foods
  digestibility, 18-19
  nutrient comparison tables, 172-179
Complementary and alternative veterinary medicine
  (CAVM), 144-145
Complementary veterinary medicine, 143-147
Complete
  definition, 43
  usage, 44
Condition scoring. *See* Body; Muscle
Confidence-based alternatives, 155
Congestive heart failure (CHF), 94-96, 137
Consciousness-raising, 157
Consolidated Standards of Reporting Trials
  (CONSORT), 154
Constipation, 87-88. *See also* Drug-related constipation
ConsumerLab, 146
Contemplation (C) stage, 157, 159
Copper deficiency, 121
Coprophagia. *See* Feces
Coronoid processes, fracture, 13
Cranial abdomen, 63

Creatinine. *See* Serum creatinine
    evaluation, 7t
CRF. *See* Chronic renal failure
Critical care, 54-71
    diet, selection, 67-68
    feeding, impact, 68-69
    nutritional assessment, 59-60
Crystal
    formation
        impact, 127
        pH impact, 128t
    growth. *See* Urine
Crystallization, inhibitors (absence), 126
Current best evidence, definition, 152
Cyproheptadine, usage, 60
Cystein, synthesis, 97
Cystine, increase, 136
Cytokines, responsibility, 53

D

Dalmatians, protein intake, 97
Dams
    drying off, 11
    health, 9
Database maintenance. *See* Obesity
DCM. *See* Dilated cardiomyopathy
Decision results. *See* Owners
Dehydration, 89
Delayed food allergies, 118
Dental aids. *See* Nonnutritional dental aids
Dental diets. *See* Cats; Dogs
Dental disease, 72-75
    client communication tips, 75
    feeding, impact, 74
    grades, 75t 75f
Dental Ring (Omega Paw Inc.), 74
Dental treats, 72t. *See also* Cats; Dogs
Dermatitis. *See* Atopic dermatitis; Flea allergy dermatitis
Desaturation enzymes, 120
Dessert group, exchange list, 236
Developmental orthopedic disease (DOD), 49
    avoidance. *See* Puppies
    occurrence, 14
    pathogenesis, 15
DHA. *See* Docosahexaenoic acid
Diabetes
    impact, 112
    obesity, relationship, 110
    onset, 21
Diabetes mellitus, 75-79, 133, 137. *See also* Insulin-
    dependent diabetes mellitus; Non-insulin-
    dependent diabetes mellitus
Diarrhea, 124. *See also* Acute-onset diarrhea; Chronic
    diarrhea; Chronic large bowel diarrhea; Chronic
    small bowel diarrhea; Small bowel diarrhea
    definition, 82
    impact, 60
    occurrence, 68
Diazepam, usage, 60
Diet. *See* Cats; Commercial diets; Dogs; Novel protein diets;
    Puppies; Raw food diets; Reduced energy diets
    change, 47-48
    characteristics, 39, 48
    consumption. *See* Protein-restricted diet
    factors, 39
    feeding. *See* Hypoallergenic diet
    information, 188
    label information. *See* Dogs

palatability, fat impact, 23, 26
plan, completion. *See* Obesity
problems, history/clinical signs, 3t
selection. *See* Critical care
summary, 48
usage. *See* Natural diets
Dietary fiber, impact. *See* Physiologic function
Dietary Supplement Health and Education Act of 1994
    (U.S. Food and Drug Administration), 144
Dietetics. *See* Clinical dietetics
Diet history, 76. *See also* Dogs
    evaluation form, 187-189
    obtaining. *See* Obesity
    sheet, 187-189
Diet-induced disease, 49
Diet-induced food intolerance, 118
Diet-induced primary/secondary deficiencies, 121
Diet-induced problems, 138-140
Diet-related orthopedic problems, 13
Diffidence-based alternatives, 155
Digitalis, impact, 136
Digitalis cachexia, 138
Dilated cardiomyopathy (DCM), 94. *See also* Cats; Dogs
Dioxygenase (digestive enzyme), 36
Dirt/rocks, eating (pica), 90
Diseases
    grades. *See* Dental disease
    lipid abnormalities, 81t
    relationship. *See* Obesity
Diuretics, impact, 136
DL-Alpha-tocopherol acetate. *See* Vitamin E
DMB. *See* Dry matter basis
DNA binding site, 104
Doberman pinscher, GDV, 83
Docosahexaenoic acid (DHA), 97
DOD. *See* Developmental orthopedic disease
Dogs. *See* Performance dogs
    aggression, pathophysiology/therapy, 16
    aging, weight/age (factors), 21t
    cancers, prevalence, 51t, 52t
    care/feeding. *See* Puppies
    DCM, 96-97
    dental diets, 205t
    dental treats, 72t
    diagnoses, 50t
    diets
        history, 19
        label information, 46t
    doggie push ups, 115
    feeding. *See* Giant-breed dogs; Large-breed dogs
        management. *See* Geriatric dogs
    foods
        nutrient comparison tables. *See* Commercial dog foods
        selection. *See* Geriatric dogs
    gestation, feeding, 9-11
    growth
        diet, 174t-175t
        tech tips, 16
    lactation, 23-24
        feeding, 9-11
    lipoproteins, characteristics, 80t
    metabolism, differences, 52
    modified fiber diets, 206t
    neonate milk replacers, 173t
    novel protein diets, 202t-203t
    nutrient-dense diets, 204t
    nutrient needs. *See* Geriatric dogs
    nutrition/behavior. *See* Adult dogs

Dogs—(*continued*)
  pancreatitis, clinical scoring system, 91t
  phosphorus diets, reduction, 109t
  pregnancy, 23-24
  protein
    diets, reduction, 108t
    feeding, amount, 21
    requirement, 121
  reduced-energy diets, 209t
  reduced-fat diets, 207t
  reduced-protein reduced-phosphorus diets, 212t-213t
  reduced-sodium diets, 208t
  serum lipid concentration increase, causes, 79t
  stone types, prevalence, 127t
  summary, 23-26
  urinary citrate, increase, 130
  urolithiasis diets, 210t-211t
  veterinary diets, 202-213
Dogs, homemade diets, 231-232
  ingredients, 231
  nutritional information, 231
  preparation, 231-232
Dominance aggression, 17
Double bond, 119
  addition, desaturation, 36
Drug-related constipation, 89
Drugs, usage. *See* Appetite
Dry foods, 41-42
  advantages, 40
  consumption, impact, 133
  volume, usage, 88
Dry matter basis (DMB)
  calculation, 41b
  level, 16-17
Dynamic steady state, 58
Dysphagia, 65

E
Early kidney failure, 102
EBS. *See* Epidermolysis bullosa simplex
Edema (hypoproteinemia), 21
EFAs
  deficiency, 121, 124
  providing, 117
Effect
  biologic plausibility, 155
  consistency, 155
  dose-response relationship, 155
  specificity, 155
  strength, 155
Eicosapentaenoic acid (EPA), 97
Electrolyte
  correction, 128
  replacement, 59
Elizabethan collar, usage, 63
Elongation enzymes, 121
Eloquence-based alternatives, 155
Eminence-based alternatives, 154
Endocrine disease, 75-81
  client communication tips, 81
  tech tips, 83
Endogenous arachidonic acid, synthesis, 121
Endothelial cell surfaces, 79
Energy
  densities, 96
  diets. *See* Cats; Dogs
  increase, lipid amounts (usage). *See* Foods
  intake level, 109

needs. *See* Basal energy needs; Cats; Parenteral nutrition
  requirements, life stage (impact), 40f
Energy-dense food, 161
English bulldog, urate urolithiasis development, 131
Enhanced acute-phase protein synthesis, 58
Enostosis, 13
Enteral (oral) nutrition, 92
Enteral (oral) tube feeding, 93-94
Environmental information, 189
Enzymatic coating, 74
Enzymes. *See* Desaturation enzymes; Elongation enzymes;
      Liver-specific enzymes
  concentrations, 35
  destruction, cooking (impact), 139
EPA. *See* Eicosapentaenoic acid
EPI. *See* Exocrine pancreatic insufficiency
Epidermolysis bullosa simplex (EBS), 124
Epiglottic entrapment, 64
Equal-energy basis, 193
Esophageal dysfunction, occurrence, 64-65
Esophagostomy feeding tubes, complications, 65
Esophagostomy tubes, usage, 64-65
Esophagus
  passage, 63
  scarring, 65
Etretinate, usage, 124
Evidence-based medicine, 147, 151-156
  results, 153-156
Exchange lists, 235-240
Exercise, 160
  categories, 20t
  metabolic effects, 23
Exocrine pancreatic insufficiency (EPI), 78, 90-91
Exotic pets, nutrition, 163
  World Wide Web sites, reviews, 165t-169t
Extensor rigidity, development, 139
Extracellular fluid calcium levels, 140
Extrusion, process, 39-40
Eye lesions, 98

F
Famotidine, 101
Fasting hyperinsulinemia, 80
Fat
  consumption, 91
  density. *See* Pet foods
  diets. *See* Dogs
  disease. *See* Yellow fat disease
  group, exchange list, 235-236
  impact. *See* Diet; Sled dogs
  intake, reduction, 85
  metabolism strategies, 34
  overcoat, 60
  reserves, 105
Fat-soluble vitamins, 123-124
Fatty acids
  consumption, 121
  content. *See* Lipid sources
  family. *See* Polyunsaturated fatty acids
  formation, 119-120
  levels. *See* Polyunsaturated fatty acids
  release, 79
  usage, 36. *See also* Omega-3 fatty acids
Fear-induced anorexia, 60
Fear-related territorial aggression, 17
Fecal consistency, 88, 90
Feces
  application, 143

eating, coprophagia, 91
Feeding. *See* Coax-feeding; Dogs; Force-feeding;
    Gastrostomy tubes; Puppies; Self-feeding
amount. *See* Puppies
complication. *See* Overfeeding
considerations. *See* Geriatric cats
directions. *See* Nutrition-related developmental
    orthopedic disease prevention; Puppies
factors, 39, 47-48
    summary, 48
frequency, 15, 193
impact. *See* Critical care; Dental disease
regimens, 159
stomach tube entrance. *See* Pets
success. *See* Oral feeding
syringe, 66f
tubes, distal end, 64
Feeding-related diseases, treatment, 49
Feline CliniCare, 67
Ferrets, nutrition Web site, 168
Fever, presence, 56
Fiber
    amounts. *See* Foods; Pet foods
    content, 85
        increase, 88
    diets. *See* Cats; Dogs
    impact. *See* Physiologic function
    increase, 115, 137
Fiber-containing diets, 86
Fiber-supplemented diets, 84, 90
Fiber-supplemented food, 87
Fibric acide derivatives, usage, 81
Filler, increase, 115
Finches, nutrition Web site, 168
Fish, nutrition Web site, 167
Flatulence, 82, 84, 124
Flavorings, usage, 106
Flea allergy dermatitis, 118
Fluid therapy, goals, 59
Flushing, 68
Food intake, 109-112, 123
    characteristic. *See* Cats
    maintenance, 106
    normal levels, 72
    problems, history/clinical signs, 3t
Foods
    additives, 118
    adverse reactions, 118-121
    allergies, 118-121. *See also* Delayed food allergies;
        Immediate food allergies
    aspiration, 64
    challenge, 119
    contrast. *See* Soft foods
    deprivation, 35, 59
    diets. *See* Raw food diets
    excessive restriction, 93
    fiber, amounts, 77t, 86t. *See also* Pet foods
    intolerance, 118. *See also* Diet-induced food tolerance
    labeling. *See* Pet foods
    net weight, 43-44
    non-immune-mediated reaction, 118
    nutrient content, comparison, 41-43
    palatability/digestibility. *See* Canned foods
    prolonged deprivation, 93
    transition sheet, 191-192
    type, definition, 43
    usage. *See* Textured food
Force-feeding, 61

Forceps, usage. *See* Carmalt forceps; Kelly forceps
Free-choice basis, 9, 16, 30-31, 36-37
    diets, 47
    importance, discussion, 55
Fruit group, exchange list, 237-238

G
Gluconeogenesis, 58
Gastric acid secretion, 102
Gastric dilatation-volvulus (GDV), 83-84. *See also*
    Doberman pinscher; German shepherd; Great
    Dane; Irish setter; Saint Bernard
Gastric emptying, slowing, 89
Gastric walls, exit, 65
Gastroenteritis. *See* Acute gastroenteritis
Gastroesophageal reflux, 64-65
Gastrointestinal (GI) bandage, 102
Gastrointestinal (GI) disease, 77, 82-94
    client communication tips, 93
    mechanisms, 82
    signs, 82-83
Gastrointestinal (GI) disturbances, 88
Gastrointestinal (GI) enzymes, usage, 85
Gastrointestinal (GI) microbes, 85
Gastrointestinal (GI) tract, 58, 118
Gastrointestinal (GI) ulcers, 101
Gastrostomy feeding tubes, maintenance, 67
Gastrostomy tubes
    feeding, 66f
    usage, 65-67
Gastrotomy tubes
    site
        cleaning, 234
        maintenance, 234
    usage, 233-234
GDV. *See* Gastric dilatation-volvulus
Gemfibrozil, usage, 81
Genetic juvenile periodontitis, development.
    See Greyhounds
Genetic life expectancy, 138
Geriatric cats, 31-34, 37-38. *See also* Sick geriatric cats
    client communication tips, 33
    diet, 186t
    feeding, considerations, 33-35
    health, 31-33
    nutritional recommendations, 33
    protein requirements, 32, 37
    tech tips, 34
Geriatric diets, necessity, 32
Geriatric dogs, 20-23, 25-26. *See also* Sick geriatric cats
    client communication tips, 24
    diet, 179t
    feeding management, 23
    foods, selection, 23
    nutrient needs, 22-23
    tech tips, 24
Geriatric survey, results, 21t
German Federal Health Agency, Commission E, 145
German shepherd, GDV, 84
Gestation. *See* Cats
    client communication tips, 13
    diet, 172t
    feeding. *See* Dogs
    tech tips, 13
GFR. *See* Glomerular filtration rate
GI. *See* Gastrointestinal
Giant-breed dogs, feeding, 13-14
Gingival health, assessment, 72

Gingivitis, control, 74
Glomerular filtration rate (GFR), 100
Glucocorticoids, usage, 61
Glucose
    abnormalities, 71
    advantages, 70
    dose, adjustment, 78
    intolerance, 80
Glucose-based formula. *See* The Ohio State University
    (OSU)
Glucose-based solution, 70
Glutamate, conversion, 35
Glutamine, increase, 137
Glycine, usage, 130
Glycogen, 105
Glycolytic tissues, 58
Google, usage, 148
Gourment products, formulation, 41
Government-sponsored site, 149
Great Dane, GDV, 83
Greyhounds, genetic juvenile periodontitis (development),
    73
Growth failure, 49
Guaranteed analysis, 44
Gumabone toys (Nylabone Products), 74

H
Hagedorn, usage, 79
Hair
    keratinization, 123
    resynthesis, 117
Hairballs, incidence. *See* Cats
Haircoat, 21, 121
Hard foods, contrast. *See* Soft foods
HDL. *See* High-density lipoprotein
Heart
    abnormalities, 139
    damage, echocardiographic signs, 98
    failure. *See* Congestive heart failure
        functional classification, 95t
    murmur, 134-135
    valves, diseases, 94
Heart disease, 94-98
    client communication tips, 100
    dietary therapy, 98
    tech tips, 99
Hedgehogs, nutrition Web site, 168-169
Heme synthesis, 121
Heparin, usage, 79
Hepatic isoenzyme, 129
Hepatocytes, reduction, 93
Herbal preparations, contradictory pharmacologic effects,
    146
High-density lipoprotein (HDL), serum concentrations, 80
High-fiber diet, high-protein diet (contrast). *See* Cats
High-priority protein synthesis, 58
High-protein diet, contrast. *See* Cats
Hip dysplasia, 13
Histamine-2 receptor-mediated gastric acid secretion,
    inhibition, 101
Histidine, 36
Homemade diets, 125b. *See also* Cats; Dogs
    feeding, 15
Homemade treats, 125b
Home-prepared diet, formulation, 92
Humans
    foods, increase. *See* Low-fat human foods
    metabolism, differences, 52

pets, bond (maintenance), 54
Humans, cancer
    prevalence, 52t
    risk, nutrition (effects), 52t
Hydration. *See* Dehydration
    maintenance, 88
Hydrochloric acid, addition, 40
Hydronephrosis, 129
Hydropulsion, 128
Hydroxyapatite, 129
Hyperadrenocorticism, 75, 78
    onset, 21
Hypercalciuria, 130-131. *See also* Absorptive hypercalciuria;
        Renal leak hypercalciuria; Resorptive hypercalciuria
Hypercholesterolemia, 80. *See also* Briard dogs
Hyperchylomicronemia, 80. *See also* Cats
Hyperglycemia, 70
Hyperkeratinization, 124
Hyperkeratosis, 6t, 123
Hyperlipidemia, 75, 79-81. *See also* Idiopathic
        hyperlipidemia
    development. *See* Primary hyperlipidemia
    nutritional management, 81
Hyperparathyroidism. *See* Nutritional secondary
        hyperparathyroidism; Renal secondary
        hyperparathyroidism
Hyperpigmentation. *See* Lesions
Hypertension, 81
    increase, 110
Hyperthyroidism, 78, 134, 136
Hyperventilation
    presence, 56
    syndrome, 127
Hypoalbuminemia, 58
    laboratory findings, 60
Hypoallergenic diet, feeding, 85
Hypokalemia, 89, 104
    control, 135
Hypoproteinemia. *See* Edema
Hypothermia, impact, 11
Hypothyroidism, 75, 78
    impact, 112
Hypoxanthine, conversion, 132

I
IBD. *See* Inflammatory bowel disease
IC. *See* Idiopathic cystitis
IDDM. *See* Insulin-dependent diabetes mellitus
Idiopathic cystitis (IC). *See* Cats
    therapy, diet (impact), 133
Idiopathic hepatic lipidosis (IHL). *See* Cats
    nutritional therapy, 93
Idiopathic hyperlipidemia, 80-81. *See also* Beagles;
        Miniature schnauzers
Idiosyncratic sensitivities, 118
IHL. *See* Idiopathic hepatic lipidosis
Immediate food allergies, 118
Immunogenicity. *See* Protein
Impacted feces, evacuation, 90
Incubator
    construction, instructions, 12f
    usage instructions, 12f
Indoor cats, enrichment recommendation, 197-200
Infection rates, 72
Inflammatory bowel disease (IBD), 82, 88-89
Information, 148-151
    basis, 149
    evaluation. *See* World Wide Web

providing, 159
source, 149
Insensible losses, 56
Insulin
    effects, 76
    formulations, 79
    injection, usage, 78
    resistance, 81
Insulin-binding antibodies, 79
Insulin-dependent diabetes mellitus (IDDM), 76, 110-111
Intake, functional classification. *See* Sodium
Intercostal space, holding, 64
Interferon (IFN), responsibility, 53
Interleukin (IL)
    mediation, 58
    responsibility, 53
Intervention, risk-benefit ratio, 53
Intestinal lymphangiectasia, presence, 90
Intestinal microflora, 98
Intestinal transit time, decrease, 89
Intestinal vitamin K transport, antagonism, 124
Intracolonic pressure, reduction, 89
Intradermal tests, 119
Irish setter, GDV, 83
Iron-deficiency anemia, 121
Isotretinoin. *See* Retinoid 13-*cis*-retinoic acid

J
Jejunostomy
    feeding tubes, placement, 66
    tubes, 66
Joints, pressure, 110

K
Kelly forceps, usage, 64
Keratinization. *See* Hair
Keratosis. *See* Hyperkeratosis; Parakeratosis
Kidney disease, 100-106
    client communication tips, 107
    nutrient recommendations. *See* Chronic kidney disease
    severity, 100f
    tech tips, 108
Kidney failure. *See* Early kidney failure
Kidney-friendly veterinary foods, 102
Kittens, 37. *See also* Orphaned kittens; Queen-raised kittens
    weaning, 27-28

L
Labeling, descriptive terms, 45
Laboratory evauulation, 6, 115
    results, 7t
Lactation. *See* Cats
    client communication tips, 13
    diet, 172t
    failure, 11
    feeding. *See* Dogs
    tech tips, 13
Lactose
    content, 85
    usage, 89
Lactulose, usage, 89
Lameness, 140
Large-breed dogs, feeding, 13-14
    directions, 16
Laryngeal obstruction, 65
Laxatives. *See* Osmotic laxatives
L-Carnitine deficiency, 96
Learned aversion, inducing (risk), 33

Least-cost formulation, 41
Lente, usage, 79
Lesions. *See* Thorax; Ventral abdomen
    hyperpigmentation, 123
Lethargy, 135
Lidocaine hydrochloride, usage, 62
Life stage, impact. *See* Energy
Life-style, questions, 159
Linoleic acid
    requirement, 120. *See* Cats
    usage, 117
Linolenic acid. *See* Alpha-linolenic acid
Lipid abnormalities. *See* Diseases
    impact. *See* Secondary hyperlipidemia
Lipid amounts, usage. *See* Pet foods
Lipid-based formula. *See* Michigan State University
Lipid-based PN, 70
Lipid sources, fatty acid content, 122t
Lipoproteins
    characteristics. *See* Cats; Dogs
    lipase, activation, 79
    metabolism, disorders, 80
Liquid diets. *See* Casein-based liquid diets
    usage, 67
Liver disease, 82. *See also* Chronic liver disease
Liver-specific enzymes, 93
Long bones, bowing/folding, 140
Long-term intake, anticipation, 93
Long-term patient management, dietary therapy, 61
Low-dose oral calcitriol treatment, 104
Low-fat cottage cheese, usage, 85
Low-fat diets, 89
    recommendation, 85
Low-fat human foods, increase, 46
Luminal nutrients, 83
Lymphadenopathy, 123
Lymphangiectasia, 90-91
Lymphopenia, laboratory findings, 60
Lysine, 36

M
Magnesium
    loss, 96
    wasting, 136
Magnesium-restricted diets, 136
Maintenance stage, 157
Malassezia sp. *See* Yeast
Malic acid, addition, 40
Malnutrition. *See* Protein-energy malnutrition
    form, 21
    physical signs, 6t
    risk factors, 60
Mammary cancer risk, reduction, 51-52
MCS. *See* Muscle condition score
ME. *See* Metabolized energy
Meat group, exchange list, 235
Medications, canned diets (mixing), 91
Medicine. *See* Alternative veterinary medicine;
        Complementary veterinary medicine;
        Evidence-based medicine
Medline, 155
Megacolon. *See* Cats
Metabolic acidosis
    commonness, 136
    control, 104
Metabolic rate, increase, 56
Metabolic water, usage, 56
Metabolized energy (ME), estimates, 42

Methionine, synthesis, 97
Metoclopramide, usage, 101
Michigan State University (MSU)
  lipid-based formula, 70
  PN solution, 69
Milk
  composition. *See* Animal milk
  protein, allergies. *See* Bovine milk protein
  replacers. *See* Cats; Dogs
    supply, 12
Minerals
  deficiencies, 121-123
  needs, 59
  oversupplementation, 138
Miniature schnauzers
  idiopathic hyperlipidemia, 80
  urinary calcium excretion, 130
Modified fiber diets, 88. *See also* Cats; Dogs
Molds, presence, 145
Morris Animal Foundation, recommendations, 83-84
Motivational interviewing, 158
Movement, characteristic. *See* Cats
MSU. *See* Michigan State University
Mucosal cells, absorption, 79
Multicat houses, 198
Muscle
  condition scoring, 2, 5f
  mass, 5f
    acceptability, 2
    replacement, 53
  wasting, 5f
Muscle condition score (MCS), 5f
  determination, 76
  discussion, 60
  evaluation, 13, 28

N

Nandrolone decanoate, usage, 61
Nasoesophageal tubes, usage, 62-63
Nasogastric tubes
  characteristics, 63t
  placement, 63f
  removal, 68
  usage, 62-64
Nasopharynx, passage, 62-63
National Cancer Institute, 148-149
National Center for Complementary and Alternative
    Medicine (NCCAM), 144
National Institutes of Health, 144, 148-149
National Research Council, zinc intake recommendations,
    123
Natriuresis, 131
Natural diets
  denotation, 72-73
  usage, 73
Nausea. *See* Transient nausea
NCCAM. *See* National Center for Complementary and
    Alternative Medicine
Necrosis, 139
Neonate milk replacers. *See* Cats; Dogs
Neonates (dogs), 24
Neoplasia, 65
Nervousness-based alternatives, 155
Neuromuscular diseases, 89
Neurotransmitters, balance, 18
Neutral protamine, usage, 79
Newborn animals, physiological immaturity, 11
Niacin

dietary deficiencies, 124
  requirement. *See* Cats
Nicotinic acid, usage, 81
NIDDM. *See* Non-insulin-dependent diabetes mellitus
Nitrogenous wastes, production (decrease), 135
Nonacidifying diets, 136
Non-immune-mediated reaction. *See* Foods
Non-insulin-dependent diabetes mellitus (NIDDM),
    76, 110
Nonnutritional dental aids, 74
Novel protein diets, 125. *See also* Cats; Dogs
NSHP. *See* Nutritional secondary hyperparathyroidism
Nutriceutical intakes, 53
Nutrient-dense diets, 136. *See also* Cats; Dogs
Nutrient-restricted diets, 105
Nutrients
  assimilation, 56
  comparison tables. *See* Commercial cat foods;
    Commercial dog foods
  deficiencies, 1
    possibility, 21
  delivery, routes, 60-67
  digestibility, 67
  intake, 54
  needs. *See* Cats; Geriatric dogs
  recommendations. *See* Chronic kidney disease
Nutrient-sensitive diseases, 49
Nutrient-sensitive skin problems, 117-125
Nutrition. *See* Exotic pets; Parenteral nutrition
  effects. *See* Humans
  impact. *See* Sick/injured animals
  issues. *See* Clinical nutrition
Nutritional orthopedic disease, 14
Nutritional secondary hyperparathyroidism (NSHP), 140
Nutritional support, 101-102
  guidelines, 69
Nutrition assessment, 1. *See also* Critical care
  depth, determination, 2t
  history, 1-2
  questions, 2
  summary, 6-7
Nutrition-related developmental orthopedic disease
    prevention, feeding directions, 193
Nutrition-related diseases, 137
Nylafloss (Nylabone Products), 74

O

Obesity, 49, 109-117
  activity, impact, 115
  caloric intake, calculation, 113
  calories, determination, 113
  client communication tips, 116
  database maintenance, 115
  diet
    history, obtaining, 112-114
    plan, completion, 114
  disease, relationship, 109-111
  excuses, 159t
  photographs, 115
  physical examination, 112
  prevention, 111
  relationship. *See* Cancer; Cardiovascular problems;
    Diabetes; Osteoarthritis; Skin; Surgical risk
  screening, 112
  technician, tasks, 112-115
  therapy, transtheoretical model (role), 156-162
  therapy program, 112-116
    follow-up, 114-115

veterinarian, tasks, 112
weight, determination, 113-114
Obesity-related diseases, 114
The Ohio State University (OSU)
    glucose-based formula, 70t
    PN solution, 69
    program, 111
    study, 104-105
Oleic acid, 120-121
Omega EFAs, requirement, 120
Omega-3 fatty acids
    increase, 137
    usage, 81
Omeprazole, 102
Oral disease, 134, 135
Oral feeding, success, 60
Oral health
    care, 72
    problems. *See* Brachycephalic breeds; Shetland
        sheepdogs; Toy poodles
Oral nutrition. *See* Enteral nutrition
Organic bone matrix, production, 140
Ornithine, synthesis, 35
Orogastric tube, usage, 61-62
Orphaned kittens, 28
Orphaned puppies, 12
Orthopedic disease. *See* Nutritional orthopedic disease
    avoidance. *See* Puppies
    prevention, feeding directions. *See* Nutrition-related
        developmental orthopedic disease prevention
Orthopedic problems, 13, 25. *See also* Diet-related
        orthopedic problems
    prevention, 14
OS. *See* Overcoat syndrome
Osmotic laxatives, 89
Osteitis fibrosa, 140
Osteoarthritis, obesity (relationship), 110
Osteochondrosis, 13
Ostriches, nutrition Web site, 169
OSU. *See* The Ohio State University
Overcoat. *See* Fat
Overcoat syndrome (OS), 5f
Overfeeding, complication, 58
Owners (clients)
    change, TTM stages, 159t
    commitment, confirmation, 160
    decision results, 160t
    information, 189
    satisfaction. *See* Pets
    self-assessment questionnaire, 161b
    work schedules, 115
Oxalate urolithiasis, development, 130
Oxazepam, usage, 60
Oxypurinol, 132

P

Pancreatic disease, 82
Pancreatic enzymes, usage, 68
Pancreatitis, 91-92. *See also* Chronic pancreatitis
    clinical scoring system. *See* Dogs
Parakeratosis, 123
Parathyroid hormone (PTH)
    action, 102
    concentration, 102
        achievement, 103
    secretion, 140
    synthesis, 104
Parenteral nutrition (PN), 69-71. *See also* Lipid-based PN

formulas, 69t
patients, energy needs, 70
solution. *See* Michigan State University; The Ohio State
        University
    macromineral portion, 70
    water-soluble vitamins, addition, 70
Parenteral solution ingredients, 71f
PC. *See* Precontemplation
Pelvic canal, narrowing, 140
Pelvic fracture malunion, 90
Pelvic reconstructive surgery, 90
PEM. *See* Protein-energy malnutrition
People foods, 99
Peptides, usage, 36
Performance dogs, 18-20, 25
    client communication tips, 20
    diet, 178t
    tech tips, 20
Periosteal bone production, 139
Peroxidized polyunsaturated fats, accumulation, 139
Pet foods, 39-43
    book values, 44
    energy increase, lipid amounts (usage), 123t
    fat density, 42
    fiber, amounts, 86t
    ingredients/functions, 45t
    labeling, 43-46, 48
        rules. *See* Association of American Feed Control
            Officials
    labels
        descriptive terms, usage, 46t
        ingredients, list, 44
Pet Nutrition (Hill's), 53
Pets
    activity level, 20
    care, owner satisfaction, 147t
    diet, change, 191-192
    feeding, stomach tube entrance, 233-234
    information, 187
    nutrition. *See* Exotic pets
Pharyngostomy tubes, usage, 64-65
pH impact. *See* Crystal formation
Phosphoric acid, addition, 40
Phosphorus
    concentrations. *See* Serum phosphorus concentrations
    diet, reduction. *See* Cats; Dogs
    impact, 135
    intake, 131
        restriction, 102, 106
    restriction, 101-103, 136
    variation, 140
Physical activity, increase, 114
Physical examination, 2-6. *See also* Obesity
Physiologic function, dietary fiber (impact), 86t
Pica. *See* Dirt/rocks
Pig-nose technique, 62
Plaque
    control, 74
    level, assessment, 72
    removal, 73
Plaque Attacker (Nylabone Products), 74
Plasma calcium, variation, 140
Plasma concentrations, increase, 58
Plasma taurine concentrations, 97-98
PN. *See* Parenteral nutrition
Pollens, presence, 145
Polyunsaturated acids, accumulation. *See* Peroxidized
        polyunsaturated fats

Polyunsaturated fatty acids
    levels, 140
Polyunsaturated fatty acids, family, 120f
Polyuria, 107t
    induction, 132
Postprandial blood glucose concentrations, 76
Postrenal azotemia, 128
Potassium
    depletion, 135
    impact, 135
    loss, 96
Potassium citrate. *See* Bicarbonate
    administration, 131
Precontemplation (PC) stage, 157
    clients, 158
Preformed vitamin A, requirements. *See* Cats
Preparation stage, 157
Prescription Diet (Hill's), 73
Pressure sores, 21
Primary-care setting, 152
Primary hyperlipidemia
    development, 22
    type, 80
Prochaska, James, 156
Proline, 36
Proparacaine hydrochloride, usage, 62
Propulsid (cisapride), usage, 89
Propylene glycol, safety, 40
Prostate cancer, risk, 111
Protein
    allergy. *See* Bovine milk protein; Bovine protein allergy
    breakdown, 56
    calculation sheet, 195
    depletion. *See* Chronic disease
    diets. *See* Novel protein diets; Veterinary hydrolyzed
        protein diets
        level, 16-17
        reduction. *See* Cats; Dogs
    evaluation, 195
    fermenting. *See* Undigested protein
    hydrolysates, 36
    immunogenicity, 118
    impact, 135
    intake, 135. *See also* Dalmatians
        calculation, 195
    metabolism strategies, 34
    needs, 92
        calculation, 59
    requirements, 114. *See also* Geriatric cats
    reserves, maintenance, 21
    restriction, 101
    synthesis. *See* Enhanced acute-phase protein synthesis;
        High-priority protein synthesis
    turnover, 58
Protein-energy malnutrition (PEM), 117, 121
Protein-restricted diet, consumption, 47
Proteus spp., presence, 129
Prothrombin time
    evaluation, 7t
    increase, 124
Protocol testing, 44
Pruritis, causes, 118
Psychogenic anorexia, 61
Psyllium, usage, 88
PTH. *See* Parathyroid hormone
Puberty, growth rate, 51
Puppies. *See* Orphaned puppies
    care/feeding, 11-15

developmental orthopedic disease (avoidance), feeding
    directions (usage), 14-15
    eating, time, 10
    feeding amount, 13
Puppies, growth, 13-15, 25
    client communication tips, 15
    diet, 13-14
    feeding, 14
Purine metabolism, 132
Pyrroline-5-carboxylate synthase, 35

Q
Quackery, definition, 145
Queen-raised kittens, 28

R
Rabbits, nutrition Web site, 169
Radius curvus, 13
Ranitidine, 101
Raw food diets
    benefits, 146
    client communication tips, 148
Rectal cancer, risk, 110
Red blood cells
    indices, 19f
    parameters, evaluation, 7t
Reduced-energy diets, 116. *See also* Cats; Dogs
Reduced-fat diets. *See* Cats; Dogs
Reduced-phosphorus reduced-protein diets. *See* Cats; Dogs
Reduced-sodium diets. *See* Cats; Dogs
Regression to the mean, definition, 152
Regurgitation, signs, 82
Rehydration, 59
Relaxation, 160
Remnant kidney model, 102
Renagel. *See* Sevelamer hydrochloride
Renal failure. *See* Chronic renal failure
Renal function, preservation, 21
Renal insufficiency, 106
Renal leak hypercalciuria, 130
Renal secondary hyperparathyroidism, 103
Renal tubular acidosis, 127
Renal tubular ammonia production, 132
Reproductive failure, 49
RER. *See* Resting energy requirement
Research studies, evidence (grading), 154t
Resorptive hypercalciuria, 130
Respiratory stridor, 64
Rest, characteristic. *See* Cats
Resting energy needs, 53
Resting energy requirement (RER), 20
Reticulocyte numbers, 40
Retinal degeneration, 6t
Retinoid 13-*cis*-retinoic acid (isotretinoin [Accutane]), 124
Retinol, oxidation, 124
Riboflavin, dietary deficiencies, 124
Risk-benefit ratio. *See* Intervention
Rubber jaw, 6t

S
Saint Bernard, GDV, 83
Salt restriction, 101
Scaling, characterization, 124
SCr. *See* Serum creatinine
Secondary hyperlipidemia, lipid abnormalities (impact),
    80t
Secondary zinc deficiency, syndrome II, 123
Self-evaluation, 160

Self-feeding, 30-31
Self-reevaluation, 157
   continuation, encouragement, 160
Semimoist foods, advantage, 40
Sepsis prevention protocols, 71
Serologic tests, 119
Serotonin, impact, 18
Serum albumin, 21
   concentrations, 129
Serum biochemistry, 140
Serum creatinine (SCr), 100-101
Serum lipid concentration increase, causes. See Cats; Dogs
Serum phosphorus
   concentrations, 100
      achievements, 103
   decrease, 129
Serum urea nitrogen (SUN), 100-101
Sevelamer hydrochloride (Renagel), 103
Shetland sheepdogs, oral health problems, 73
Siberian huskies, syndrome I, 123
Sick geriatric cats, 134-137
Sick geriatric dogs, 137-138
Sick/injured animals, nutritional impact, 54-59
Skeletal radiodensity, decrease, 140
Skin
   collagen, loss, 60
   problems. See Nutrient-sensitive skin problems
      obesity, relationship, 111
   resynthesis, 117
   scaling, 124
Skin disease, 117-125
   client communication tips, 126
   diagnosis, 116-125
   tech tips, 126
Sled dogs
   stamina, fat/carbohydrates impact, 19
   studies, 18
Small bowel diarrhea, 82-83. See also Chronic small bowel
      diarrhea
Smooth-coated dogs, 14
Social contact, characteristic. See Cats
Social liberation, 157
Sodium
   amounts, 95
   diets. See Reduced-sodium diets
   excretion, 94
   intake, 95-96
      functional classification, 95t
   restriction, 106
Soft foods, hard foods (contrast), 73
Soluble, definition, 85
Soluble carbohydrates, 77
Soluble-insoluble ratio, 85
Somogyi phenomenon, occurrence, 79
Spores, presence, 145
Stages-of-change perspectives, 157
Stanozolol, usage, 61
Staphylococcus, presence, 128
Starch
   gelatinization, 40
   group, exchange list, 236
Steatitis, 139
Stomach, peritoneum adhesions, 65
Stomach tube entrance. See Pets
Stone-forming pets, urine, 128
Stones. See Calcium oxalate; Struvite stones; Urate stones;
      Urinary tract
   formation, 127

types, 125-128
   prevalence. See Cats; Dogs
Stresses, questions, 159
Struvite stones, 128-129
Struvite urolithiasis, risk reduction, 46
Substrate accumulation, assessment, 73
Subtotal colectomy, recommendation, 90
Sucralfate (Carafate), 101
Sugar gliders, nutrition Web site, 169
SUN. See Serum urea nitrogen
Supplemental oral taurine, 97
Surgical risk, obesity (relationship), 111
Surgical trauma, 59
Surrogate physiologic measurement, 153
Systemic hypertension, 105

T
Table scraps, 21, 139
Taurine (β-amino acid). See Supplemental oral taurine;
      Whole blood taurine
   concentrations. See Plasma taurine concentrations
   inadequacy, problem, 99
   increase, 136
   presence, 29, 35
   supplementation, 97
   taurine-deficiency-induced dilated cardiomyopathy,
      35
   usage, 67
Taurine (β-amino sulfonic acid), synthesis, 97
Termination stage, 157
Teryptophan, impact, 18
Textured food, usage, 73
Thiamin deficiency. See Cats
Thoracic duct, circulation, 79
Thorax, lesions, 124
Tissue uptake, 79
TNF. See Tumor necrosis factor
Topical anesthetic, usage, 62
Total daily caloric needs, review, 55
Total iron-binding capacity, evaluation, 7t
Total lymphocyte count, evaluation, 7t
Toxicities, 1. See also Ammonia
Toy poodles, oral health problems, 73
Transcription factor, 104
Transient nausea, 124
Transtheoretical model (TTM), 156. See also Behavioral
      change
   role. See Obesity
   stages, change. See Owners
      processes (relationship), 158f
Treats/biscuits, usage, 73-74, 113
Triglycerides, 79
   concentrations, 93
   resynthesis, 79
   secretion, 93
   serum concentrations, 81
Triple phosphate, detection, 128
TTM. See Transtheoretical model
Tumor necrosis factor (TNF), 53
Tumors, 134
Turtles, nutrition Web site, 169
Two-carbon fragment (elongation), 36
Type 1 diabetes, occurrence, 76, 109
Type 2 diabetes, 110
   development, risk, 78
   occurrence, 76
Type II error, definition, 153
Tyrosine, impact, 18

U
Ulcers. *See* Gastrointestinal ulcers; Uremic ulcers
  formation, 102
Ultralente, usage, 79
Undigested protein, fermenting, 92
University of California at Berkeley, 148
Urate stones, 131-133
Urate urolithiasis, development. *See* English bulldog
Urea cycle
  control, 34-35
  intermediaries, control, 35
Urea generation, 56
Urease-positive urinary tract infection, 128
Uremia, 107t
Uremic ulcers, 135
Ureteral obstruction, 129
Uric acid
  derivation, 132
Uric acid metabolism, defect, 132
Urinary calcium excretion. *See* Miniature schnauzers
Urinary citrate, increase. *See* Cats; Dogs
Urinary disease
  client communication tips, 134
  tech tips, 134
Urinary tract
  disease, 125-134
  health, 46
  infection. *See* Urease-positive UTI
  obstruction, 128
  stones, 125-133
Urination, frequency, 127
Urine
  alkalization, usefulness, 132
  crystals, growth, 127f
  flow, reestablishment, 128
  pH, 127. *See also* Altered urine pH
Urine specific gravity (USG), 100, 128
Urolithiasis diets. *See* Cats; Dogs
U.S. Food and Drug Administration, 147. *See also* Dietary
    Supplement Health and Education Act of 1994
USG. *See* Urine specific gravity
Uterine cancer, development risk, 110

V
Vegetable group, exchange list, 238-239
Vehemence-based alternatives, 155
Ventral abdomen, lesions, 124
Ventriflexion, 136
Vertebral foramina, 139
Very-low-density lipoprotein (VLDL), 79
  serum concentrations, 80
Veterinary diets. *See* Cats; Dogs
Veterinary hydrolyzed protein diets, 119
Veterinary medicine. *See* Alternative veterinary medicine;
    Complementary veterinary medicine
Vitamin A
  amount, excess, 139
  intoxication, 124
  oversupplementation, 124
  presence, 29
  problems, 117
  requirements. *See* Cats
  storage, increase, 124
Vitamin B_6 deficiency, 130
Vitamin B injections, 60
Vitamin C (ascorbic acid), metabolism, 130
Vitamin D activation, increase, 131

Vitamin E
  deficiency. *See* Cats
  DL-Alpha-tocopherol acetate, 124
  problems, 117
Vitamin K transport, antagonism. *See* Intestinal vitamin K
    transport
Vitamins. *See* Fat-soluble vitamins; Water-soluble vitamins
  deficiencies, 123-125
  metabolism strategies, 34
  needs, 59
  oversupplementation, 138
VLDL. *See* Very-low-density lipoprotein
Vomiting, 64, 80-82
  impact, 60
  signs, 82, 135

W
Water
  intake
    characteristic. *See* Cats
    decrease, 126
  loss, 56
Water-soluble contrast medium, usage, 63
Water-soluble vitamins, 125
  addition. *See* Parenteral nutrition
Web sites, favorites, 150-151
Weddelite. *See* Calcium oxalate
Weekend athletes, 18, 25
Weight
  acceptability, 2
  determination. *See* Obesity
  gains, 53
  loss, 96, 104, 134
    efforts, 76
    impact, 110
Whewellite. *See* Calcium oxalate
Whole blood taurine, 98
Wobbler syndrome, 13
World Wide Web
  information, evaluation, 147-151
  links, 150-151
  sites
    recommendation, 150t-151t
    reviews. *See* Exotic pets
Wounds
  healing, delay, 21
  presence. *See* Burn wounds
  regeneration, 58

X
Xanthine
  conversion, 132
  crystals, formation, 133
  oxidase, inhibitor, 132
Xerophthalmia, 6t

Y
Yeast (*Malassezia* sp.), treatment, 119
Yellow fat disease, 139

Z
Zinc
  deficiency, 123
    syndrome II. *See* Secondary zinc deficiency
  intake recommendations. *See* National Research Council
  problems, 117
  sulfate, supplementation, 124